Promotion of Mental Health
Volume 2, 1992

Edited by

DENNIS R. TRENT
COLIN REED

Avebury

Aldershot · Brookfield USA · Hong Kong · Singapore · Sydney

Published by
Avebury
Ashgate Publishing Limited
Gower House
Croft Road
Aldershot
Hants GU11 3HR
England

Ashgate Publishing Company
Old Post Road
Brookfield
Vermont 05036
USA

British Library Cataloging in Publication Data

Promotion of Mental Health - Vol 2: 1992
   I. Trent, Dennis R. II. Reed, Colin
   362.2

ISBN 1 85628 430 1

Printed and Bound in Great Britain by
Athenaeum Press Ltd, Newcastle upon Tyne.

Contents

Section Two: The Presentations

Section Three: Plenary and Workshop

List of contributors

Afzalnia, Mohammed Reza, B.A., M.A., M.Sc., E.Ds., Ph.D. University of Keele, Staffordshire

Albee, George, W., M.S., Ph.D. University of Vermont, USA

Armstrong, Elizabeth, R.G.N., R.H.V. Kensington, Chelsea and Westminster FHSA

Barry, Margaret, M.A., Ph.D. Health Research Unit, University College of North Wales

Barry, Robina. B.A.Hons., M.Clin.Psychol., C. Psychol., Mental Health Foundation of Mid Staffs

Benn, Sally. Cert.Ed., B.Ed. Mid Staffordshire Health District

Bostock, Janet, B.A., M.Phil., M.Sc., Nottingham Psychology Service

Brockington, Professor I. A.

Buglass, Dorothy, B.A., M.Phil. Lothian Region Social Work Department

Collins, Louize, B.A.(Hons), Dip.A.S.S., C.Q.S.W. Chapel Orchard Health Project, Merton Social Services

Coutts, Margret. Lothian Regional Council

Cox, John, L., B.M., B.Ch., D.M.(Oxon), F.R.C.P(Edin.), F.R.C.Psychol. School of Postgraduate Medicine, University of Keele, Staffordshire

Coyle, Adrian, Ph.D. University of Surrey and Frances Harrison College of Healthcare

Daniels, Michelle, M.Sc. Enfield Health Authority's Health Promotion Service

Goodbody, Louise. South Devon Healthcare

Graham, Helen, B.A., M.Phil. University of Keele, Staffordshire

Hall, Peter, M.B., B.S., Ph.D., F.R.C.Psych. The Woodbourne Clinic, Birmingham

Harrison, Margaret, O.B.E. HOME-START Consultancy, Leicester

Hartley, James. University of Keele, Staffordshire

Hazell, J., R.M.N., B.Sc., M.Phil. Bromsgrove and Redditch Health Authority

Holden, Robert, W. Laughter Medicine Clinic, Birmingham

Hopkins, Jeffrey, M.Phil. Dept. of Applies Social Studies, University of Keele, Staffordshire

Horridge, Paul, B.Sc., D.Phil., M.Sc., C.Q.S.W. Principal Social Services Officer, South Glamorgan

Hughes, Jane, B.A.,(Econ), D.S.W., C.Q.S.W. Cheshire Social Services, Macclesfield District

Humphris, Gerry, Ph.D., M.ClinPsychol., Cpsychol., Dip.Soc.Econ. Department of Clinical Psychology, Liverpool University

Hunter, Sarah. Tyneside Women's Health Project

Jebali, Christine, R.M.N., CPN.Cert., B.A.(Hons). Shropshire and Staffordshire College of Nursing and Midwifery

Jenkins, Rachael, M.A., M.B., B.Chir.(Cantab), F.R.C.Psych., M.D.(Cantab), F.R.I.P.H.H. Principal Medical Officer, Department of Health

Keddie, Kenneth. Sunnyside Royal Hospital, Montrose

Kenyon, Zoe, M.B., C.H.B., F.R.C.G.P. Independent Medical Adviser, Kirklees Family Health Service Authority

Ledwith, Frank, B.A., M.A., Ph.D. Preston Community Health Services

Lorenc, Louise, B.A., M.Sc., Ph.D. Bromsgrove and Redditch Health Authority

MacDonald, Glenn, B.Ed., M.Ed. First Community Health NHS Trust of Mid Staffordshire

Manktelow, Roger, B.A., M.Sc., Ph.D. Northern Health and Social Services Board, Northern Ireland

McDougall, Liz, M.A., B.A.(Honours). Equality Services, Coventry City Council

McGuire, Alex, M.A., M.S.L.S., M.R.S.H., B.A.C.(Acc). Leeds Crisis Centre

McKenzie, Patricia, B.A.Hons., Cert. Counselling. Family and Child Health, First Community Health, Stafford

Miller, Edgar. President, British Psychological Society

Money, Mike. Liverpool John Moores University

Moore, Lilley, R.M.N. Dip in Nursing (London University). St. George's Hospital, Stafford

Murphy, Dr. C.

Murray, Chris, B.A., C.Q.S.W., Dip. Community Development, B.A.C. Accredited. Community Support Team Macclesfield

Murray, Michael Charles, M.S.(Econ), B.A., D.M.A., M.M.S., M.I.P.M., M.Inst. A.M.(Dip). The Mental Health Foundation of Mid Staffordshire NHS Trust, Stafford

Nadirshaw, Zenobia, M.A., Dip.Psychol., C.Psychol., A.F.B.Ps.S. Dacorum and St. Albans Community (NHS) Trust

Najarian, Bahman, B.Sc., M.A., Ph.D. Shahid Chamran University, Iran

Norman, Annemarie, B.A., Tyneside Women's Health Project

Ormston, Cathy, Dip.C.O.T. Northern Regional Drug and Alcohol Problem Service, Newcastle Mental Health NHS Trust

Phillips C.W. Derek, F.R.C.G.P. General Practitioner, Slaithwaite

Poppleton, Wendy. 'Ease Your Mind' user group

Powell, Jackie. Social Work Studies, University of Southampton

Pritlove, Jeremy, M.A., M.Phil., C.Q.S.W. Social Services Department, City of Leeds

Rayner, Claire, R.G.N. Writer and Broadcaster

Richards, Doris. London Borough of Richmond upon Thames

Rowe, Dorothy. Psychologist

Smith, Jo, B.Sc., M.S.C., Ph.D. Bromsgrove and Redditch Health Authority

Sullivan, Kevin, B.A.(Hons), M.Sc., Dip.Clin.Psychol, C.Psychol. The Mental Health Foundation of Mid Staffordshire NHS Trust

Tate, Jenny. Lothian Regional Social Work Department

Thornton, Jacqui, Dip.C.O.T. Northern Regional Drug and Alcohol Problem Service, Newcastle Mental Health NHS Trust

Trent, Dennis, B.A., M.A., Ph.D., A.F.B.Ps.S. Chartered Clinical Psychologist, c/o The Mental Health Foundation of Mid Staffordshire NHS Trust

Tumim, His Honour Judge S. Her Majesty's Chief Inspector of Prisons

White, Ian. Northumbria Probation Service

Wills, Steve, B.A., C.Q.S.W., Dip.S.W. Community Support Team, Macclesfield

Wonham, Margaret, M.A. The Mental Health Foundation of Mid Staffordshire NHS Trust

Woodward, Raie. B.Sc., M.Sc., M.Psychol, Dip.Psychotherapy. Psychology Dept, Victoria Cental Hospital, Wallasey.

Wylie, Ann, M.A. Health Promotion & Education Centre, Prospect Park Hospital, Reading

Yeo, Tim, M.A. Parliamentary Under Secretary, Department of Health

Introduction

The Second Annual Conference on the Promotion of Mental Health took place in September, 1992. Following on from the success of the first year, we anticipated an exciting and provocative second conference. We were overwhelmed by the response we got. The quality and the quantity of papers for the second conference were wide ranging while clearly focused on the issues inherent to the conference.

Heading into our third year, the Mental Health Promotion Unit (MHPU) was growing and the direction was changing to meet the needs of The Mental Health Foundation of Mid-Staffordshire NHS Trust, its co-sponsor along with the University of Keele. As a first wave trust we were acutely conscious of the need to look at ways in which we could best meet the needs of the local, regional and national communities and the changing role of the NHS. The conference became one of the major focal points for that effort. By continuing to support the idea of research and discussion within mental health promotion, the conference brought to light the efforts of many like minded people who said that they had heretofore often felt as though they were functioning in an intellectual vacuum.

We were fortunate to have an outstanding list of internationally known guest speakers and presenters from around the world. Their wit and wisdom made the conference both enjoyable and stimulating. None of it, however, could have been done without the support and guidance of those few people who often hide behind the scenes to let others gain the centre stage. The people at St. George's Hospital again carried the brunt of the effort. Special mention must be made of the MHPU Team, Michael

Tiernan who read through so many papers, Sue Johnson who typed them all and Peter Davies, the individual who organised and managed the day to day running of the conference. Professors John Sloboda and James Hartley in the Department of Psychology at the University provided stability and moral support through trying times.

The next year offers even greater challenges. The focus of mental health promotion activities always needs re-definition as needs change within the Foundation and the communities it serves. Each year brings us a new conference and a new direction for mental health promotion. While the plans are well under way for Conference '93, I am sure that it will be different from this year's while remaining true to the goals of the conference; to promote mental health, de-stigmatise mental illness and de-mystify psychology for the increased understanding of all. I have been proud to be a part of the last two conferences and I look forward to the future with a sense of excitement and anticipation.

D.R.T.

Section One
GUEST SPEAKERS

1 Guest speaker presentation

G.W. Albee

It is a great pleasure for me to come to a conference such as this; it is encouraging to know that an interest in prevention spans the Atlantic. I have listened to a number of British speakers, over the last three days. It took me a day or so to begin to understand them, but I think now my ear is tuned to proper English. There are certain things that I still haven't learned; last evening I sat next to Lord Stafford at dinner, so I knew which of the 17 utensils I was to use, at the proper time. I still can not figure out how you can get peas on the back of a fork, but I'm going to go home and practice that. I am always afraid of making a gaff when I am speaking in a different culture or different society. A friend of mine who is a woman who is a Professor of Political Science at my University, married a Russian intellectual. He was telling us the other night about the first gaff he made. He had gone to a health club and he was in the shower and he asked the man next to him if he would mind washing his back. I don't know if that's done here; it certainly is not done commonly in America.

I was heartened to learn that Government Ministers here share the US officials' problems in arithmetic. Let me try to explain what I mean. If I listened correctly to the Minister's talk on the first morning, there are 6 million cases a year of mental disorder in the United Kingdom. Now I sat around last evening doing some arithmetic. If each case requires just 10 hours of therapy a year, which I reckon is a fairly modest estimate, that means 60 million hours of therapy. Now if each therapist who works 50 weeks a year, I assume has a vacation of at least 2 weeks, and if they see 30 clients a week, then each therapist can really only do 1,500 hours of therapy a year; so if you do the arithmetic this means that we in Britain would require 40 thousand full time therapists, but perhaps 20 hours a year is a better estimate, which means that 80 thousand therapists would be required. Many clients or patients as I think they have been referred to this week would require as much as 50 hours a year which would mean 200 thousand therapists. If we hit a happy average of these estimates it may be safe to say that in order to provide for the 6 million cases a year you would require a 100 thousand therapists. The only conclusion that I can draw from this is the same conclusion that I draw back home in the States, that one to one intervention is hopeless. I mean it's humane, it's kind, but it's hopeless, because we simply don't have anywhere near the number of therapists. Every year no matter how great an effort we make to try to train more therapists we never have them. I picked up from a number of talks that there are 40 spaces open for Psychiatrists in this District. The possibility of training enough Psychiatrists is absolutely slim. In the United States each year more Psychiatrists die than enter the field. When I said this recently in the States someone said 'Well what's the bad news?' but I won't say that here.

Now we have also had a recent epidemiological survey by a major Government agency which chose 6 different regions of the country, rural and urban, and carefully selected random families. Then they randomly selected an adult in each family, I won't go through all the detailed design, but it is an adequate research design, and they went with well trained interviewers and spent a 2 hour interview with each of the preselected adults, and then they came back and punched their data into a big computer, and then headlines all over the country reported that 20% of the US population has a psychiatric, that is DSM3, diagnosis; 1 person in 5. Now in Britain it is apparently 1 in 10, but it may not surprise you that there are twice as many crazy people in the United States as there are in Britain. But the end is not yet; if 20% of US adults have a diagnosis of mental disorder, you have to remember that they didn't interview children and adolescents, and homeless people, because you had to be part of a household. A very large number of homeless are mentally disordered. Also they didn't interview people in institutions, and according to my calculations if you add all the children, adolescents, institutionalised people and homeless people you add another 20%, which means that 40% of the US population is mentally disordered. But there is one more fact we know from our own research and clinical experience; for every disturbed person two other people are also reflectively emotionally disturbed, so if you have a schizophrenic mother you have got two other people who are emotionally distressed, if you get an alcoholic father you have got two more, or a mentally retarded sibling. Which means that if you double the

2

40%, that's 80%, add the original 40%, and so 120% of the US population...... Actually it turns out there are only 17 normal people in all of the United States, I know I'm one of them.

The point is, and I can't say this enough times, that the thought that we can do anything significant about the vast numbers of people who are troubled, by one to one therapy, is just absolute nonsense. But no one, in or out of our fields, seems to understand this.

Jane Brady is one of the most distinguished Science writers in America, she writes for the New York times and she usually get things right. She also has a very good health cook book which I recommend to you, but she wrote an article 2 years ago in which she said 'in a survey of all different forms of psychotherapy' and she said 'today in the United States 34 million people are in psychotherapy' and then she went on to a long description of each kind, from analysis to cognitive to primal scream. She had a very good review, but something kept bothering me. 34 million people in psychotherapy, and if you assume that each therapist can see 34 people a week which is a heavy load according to my friends who are psychotherapists, that would mean there would have to be 1 million therapists and I didn't think there were that many. So I went to the library and I found a book and a series of articles by Charles Kiesler who had actually counted the number of therapists, full time equivalent, adding together the part timers, and he said 'at least there are 50,000 therapists full time equivalent in the United States' so I wrote Jane Brady a friendly letter and double spaced it in case she wanted to print it. I had back a very friendly hand written note that she was aware after my letter that she had made a mistake and she thought there would have to have been 20 times as many therapists than there actually were, 'but people don't remember what they read in yesterday's newspaper so I am not going to call any attention to this, and the next time I write about therapy I will get it right.'

There is this example of a view of a well informed writer who thinks that there are therapists available when as a matter of fact there aren't. Most of our therapists, psychologists, Psychiatrists, Social Workers etc are to be found in five states; there are 50 states in the US so five of the States have like 90% of the therapists. Well one of the States is the District of Columbia which really isn't a State, but that's where our Government is. Actually there are more Psychologists per head in Washington DC than any place else in the Country, again not necessarily surprising!

So I want to make a few points while I have your attention. I want to tell you a little bit of my personal history, not out of narcissism, but to explain to the young people in the audience that life is a series of accidents, if you want to write that down I will wait a minute. Back in 1954 when I was a young assistant Professor I had an argument with the Chair of our Psychiatry Department in Cleveland Ohio, we were arguing over lunch over why he couldn't get enough residents, that is people to train in psychiatry, to put into all the hospitals and clinics he was responsible for. I said because there weren't enough to go around, and he said no it was because they didn't want to come to Cleveland, which is sometimes referred to locally as 'the mistake on the lake'. I went back to my office all charged up and I wrote a letter to Karl Meninger, now that name may not quiver you up but Karl Meninger was the number one Psychiatrist in the nation, head of all Psychiatry during World War 2, head of the Meninger Clinic in Topeka Kansas, and I thought that if anyone knows how many people are in training, he will. So I wrote him a letter with some trepidation, I didn't really know whether I would get anything back, but about a week later I got back a six page single spaced letter from Karl Meninger telling me an awful lot of things including the fact that even some psychiatrists are obsessive compulsive, because he told me in endless detail that no-one knew how many people were in training in psychiatry, and this is way back before computers, because there had been IBM punch card errors, and at the end of the six pages he said 'if you want to do a service to the field you will find out how many people are available and in training in psychiatry, psychology and Social work, psychiatric nursing etc.' So I took this letter to my Dean, he was a hard bitten old mister, and I said 'Dean, look, I need some money because I need to hire a doctoral student to work with me this summer, because see, look, Karl Meninger says I have got to do this study'. The Dean said 'how much do you want?' I said 'I need 75 dollars because I have to hire a woman for the whole summer to work with me', that's about £40. He said 'Will you take 60' (£30) that's how long it was ago, when you could hire a doctoral student for the whole summer. So Margaret Dicky and I spent the summer collecting data (and I apologise for the word Manpower, that was what it was called back then; we have had our consciousness raised since, about sexist language) we wrote an article about 'Manpower trends in the mental health professions', and it was about 8 pages long. We sent it to the 'American Psychologist' which is the flagship journal of the APA. I got a call right back from the editor saying 'we have just received your article and we would like to publish it in the next issue', and I said 'I am delighted that you think it's that important'. He said 'no, we just don't have enough articles to fill up'.

But this is another tip for young people. If you write an article about something which everyone is interested in and if you were the first, you then become the 'national authority'. On the basis of that one article

4

Margaret Dicky and I became authorities on mental health manpower. About a year later I got a call from the Eisenhower Commission Director, a Psychiatrist named Jack Ewall at Harvard, saying 'would you come up to Cambridge Massachusetts and write a book about mental health manpower?' I said, 'I have said everything I know in this seven page article,' he said, 'you know, stretch it.' All of this is absolutely true. I went to Cambridge and I wrote a 300 page book on mental health manpower and I learned so many important things during that year in Cambridge.

I was sitting one evening with a Social Psychologist named Marie Hoder. Has anyone ever heard of Marie Hoder? She was an American Social Psychologist who married a member of Parliament and moved to England and I'm glad she had some visibility here. She told me that 'all mental disorders are interpersonal disorders or intrapersonal', and she went on to explain that 'you don't become neurotic or psychotic about sheep or horses or automobiles, only about your relationship with other human beings.' That it is all interpersonal problems, and I was so delighted to hear Dorothy Rowe talk about our learning to use people as objects and about the importance of parenting. But then Marie Hoder explained to me that all mental disorders, with a few small exceptions, are learned disorders, and she went on to explain that if they are learned they can be unlearned; now this is in the early 1950's before psychologists and Social Workers were doing psychotherapy. And so as she was saying, 'before long everyone in the treatment field will be doing psychotherapy and helping people unlearn their learned problems', this was very heady stuff in those days. She also said 'if these problems are learned they can be prevented. We can change the learning environment in which infants and children are reared!' I became at that moment a 'born again' preventionist. It was possible to prevent mental disorders by controlling the social environment in which people grew up. On another evening I learned the second thing. There are only two, so I won't regale you with more. John Gordon who is Professor of Epidemiology at Harvard, explained to me that the way to prevent disorders is to use a method of public health, and he spent the whole evening in telling me about the triumphs in the field of public health. One of these triumphs was the action of John Snow who as you probably know removed the handle from the Broad Street pump in London. In fact the American Public Health Association each year gives the 'pump handle award' for the person who has done the most for the prevention of illness in the United States. In fact there is a John Snow pub on that corner and the city has recently installed a replica of the original pump which John Snow chained so people couldn't use it, so they had to go to other wells and he stopped a cholera epidemic around Broad Street in London. So this weekend while I was in London I paid a nostalgic visit to the John Snow Pub to toast his memory. They have a guest book that public health people can sign and I have a number of friends at home who respect John Snow, and in their memory I will also toast his honour. Anyway, John broadly explained to me that many great plagues which have afflicted human kind have been eliminated through successful efforts at primary prevention, he explained how the observation was made in England that milkmaids who milked cows never caught small-pox. I'm sure most of you know this story, but that led to the discovery that they contracted 'cowpox', a modest cousin of smallpox, and somehow that protected them. As a consequence British Physicians began experimenting with giving people cow pox, and this was the vaccination, and smallpox has now disappeared from the face of the earth. Now I have to point out that treating individual smallpox sufferers didn't eliminate the disease. It was finding a way to strengthen the potential host in order to keep them from succumbing to the noxious agent which causes smallpox.

Now I am going to try and make a case for translating this model into the field of mental disorders. John Snow taught me this; no mass disorder afflicting human kind has ever been eliminated or controlled by attempts at treating the affected individual, or by training large numbers of individual practitioners. I make my students memorise this, if they feel they have to carve it in marble and carry it around for a week, and I hope you will ponder this because I offer it in all seriousness 'no mass disorder afflicting human kind has ever been eliminated or brought under control by attempts at treating the individual'. We will never reduce the incidence, which means the number of new cases of mental disorders, by individual treatment. Now as I have said before, individual treatment is humane, it's appealing, a very large number of young people coming into Psychology today envisage themselves as Psychotherapists. This has become a big growth industry in the mental health field in the United States and there is something very satisfying about being a therapist because when it's all over the client wrings your hand and says 'thank you, I don't know how you did it but I feel better, I'm cured' and you say 'just part of my job' but you feel warm fuzzy success, whereas I have to warn you if you work in the field of Primary Prevention you never know who has been saved. You don't know and they won't thank you because they don't know. I have another friend, that's two, who works for the Vermont Department of Health and she spends all of her time keeping people healthy and she says to me one day 'you know that no one ever calls to thank me that they haven't caught Typhoid Fever'. I remind people that they should at the proper holiday season send a card to their Department of Health thanking them for keeping them healthy for another year.

The point is that if you work in Primary Prevention your satisfaction has to come from seeing the incidence curve decline. Fewer people are anxious, fewer people have phobias, there is a reduced rate of child sexual abuse, so you have got to get your kicks from seeing that declining curve. Primary prevention is what it's all about, Primary prevention is proactive, and as it's instituted before the problem appears it's aimed at groups, generally groups at high risk. We identify those groups who are at high risk for some future pathology, mental or physical, and then we take steps to reduce the future incidence. Incidence is the key word, incidence means new cases of the disorder. The purpose of Primary Prevention is to reduce incidence, a rate change.

Now Emily Collins, who has written extensively about Primary Prevention, divides efforts into those that are person centred or those that are centred on institutional change. Sometimes we work with high risk groups of individuals, we know that the children of schizophrenics or the children of alcoholics are at high risk for becoming later casualties. There is a danger here (and I won't take time to digress down that road) but there is a danger that this will become a self fulfilling prophesy if you tell them they are at risk. But there are effective programmes of teaching interpersonal skills, interpersonal problem solving. Again Emily Collins, of the University of Rochester, has a national programme for helping children in the first grade at school by bringing in volunteer adult, usually women, tutors who not only tutor them in their school work but also form a relationship with them. Anyway, it's possible to demonstrate that these children have far fewer difficulties later in school. At the High Scope Educational Foundation in Ypsilanti Michigan there have been programmes of working with pre-school kids who are at high risk, for a year or two before they start kindergarten. That's all they do; this very intensive two year intervention programme which involves teaching them not only academic skills but interpersonal relation skills, and then following these kids until they are 18 or 20. The result is very clear, children who have had that early experience commit fewer than half as many acts of delinquency. They are significantly more likely to graduate from high school and to go on to college. They are significantly less likely to become premature parents. You can write to them at Ypsilanti Michigan and they will send you a basket full of their reports of their effective early intervention with measured results in terms of the reduction of later psychopathology. The important thing for prevention efforts is that there be measurable results, because our opponents, and there are many, will constantly say 'well you really don't have any evidence that

7

prevention works.' I have heard this so many times I simply ask them to read the books that we have published from our Vermont Conference on prevention. I have put a batch of them on a table out near the registration area for you to look at and I'll take a commercial break 'They are on sale at half price if you will send your order to me at the University of Vermont, and we will pay the postage'.

Alright, let me go on with some specific points about primary prevention. I mentioned that in the field of public health there basically are three approaches. You identify the noxious agent and you neutralise or get rid of it. John Snow in London suspected that there was a noxious agent in the water, he wasn't sure, but by removing the handle of the Broad Street pump and keeping people from using that water he stopped the cholera epidemic in that neighbourhood. A second strategy in public health is to strengthen the resistance of the host. Now each of us is a potential host for whatever the noxious agent is, so we have found various ways of strengthening the resistance of the host. The third and final method in the field of public health is to prevent transmission of the noxious agent to the host. Interrupt that transmission. When there was an attempt to build the Panama Canal the French were the first to try. They finally had to give up because so many of the workers digging the canal died of a disease called Yellow Fever which was endemic in the isthmus of Panama. Finally, Walter Reed and some other American army physicians said 'If we got rid of the mosquitos (they had just discovered that mosquitos transmitted malaria) perhaps we could get rid of Yellow Fever.' So they went to Panama, drained the swamps and poured oil on the breeding grounds so that they couldn't breed and they got rid of the specific mosquito that carries the yellow fever agent. They ended yellow fever and the Panama Canal was built, largely as a result of the successful efforts at preventing transmission.

Now if we look at the present scourge of AIDS, the acquired immunal deficiency, the HIV virus that causes the disease, what we want to do is prevent the transmission of the noxious agent to the host and I don't know what the present status is in AIDS education in the United Kingdom. We have a book out there on education as a way of preventing AIDS, we do not have any treatment for AIDS that is effective, and I don't think that we will ever have a vaccine to strengthen the resistance of the host. There are a lot of very technical reasons why it seems impossible, because the AIDS virus keeps changing its characteristics. So we finally have to talk openly about sex and sexuality and how the AIDS virus is transmitted, and so we frequently advertise the importance of condoms. Now 10 years ago in the United States I couldn't have used the word condom from the vicar's

8

platform. Now in Vermont where I come from the buses all have signs on the billboards outside the bus saying 'Don't forget your rubbers' and people are now comfortable talking about safe sex and the use of condoms. I heard a story last week about a man who came into an American drug store and said out loud 'I want a dozen condoms' and then very quietly 'and a pack of cigarettes'.

If we look at the historic public health methodology and then we contrast this with a strategy for the prevention of mental and emotional disorders, the noxious agent in a great many mental disorders is stress. It's interpersonal stress, I'm becoming high tech here, the noxious agent is often stress. The most important stress currently in the United States, and I suspect here, is involuntary unemployment. We have endless research data to indicate that people who are involuntarily unemployed are very high risk for all kinds of mental and emotional disorders. When a steel mill closes in Gary, Indiana and moves to Japan or Taiwan or Singapore we have a lot of very macho type steel workers who are now out of work. There is no new industry coming in to Gary, Indiana and so there is a high rate of social withdrawal, schizoid withdrawal, with a very high rate of alcoholism among these unemployed steel workers. There is a dramatic increase in physical and sexual abuse of spouse and children. There is an increase in depression and the point here is that each of these different so called mental illnesses, depression, schizoid withdrawal, alcoholism, spouse abuse, do not each have a separate cause. One of the arguments you hear from the enemies of primary prevention is 'you really can't prevent something until you know what's the cause, and since we have not yet discovered the separate cause of each mental illness we can't do anything about preventing that'. Now this is nonsense! Stress and exploitation is a major cause of a variety of different forms of mental disorders.

Who or what is the group in the United States at the greatest risk of developing both physical illness and mental disorder? The answer is the five million migrant farm workers who pick our crops, starting from southern California and moving north up the Pacific coast and the same way through the Mid West. Our crops are picked by migrant farm workers, a great many of them are minority members, their children don't go to school, their children work in the fields along with their parents because they can help add modestly to the family income. Their life expectancy is 48 years, compared to the life expectancy of the middle class American, which is somewhere up in the late 70's. Migrant farm workers have more tuberculosis, more cancer, (they work with the pesticides in the fields). They also have a significantly high rate of schizophrenia. So it is poverty and hopelessness that are major factors, that's the cause, not a separate specific cause for each form of mental disorder.

One of my favourite examples is the successive waves of immigrants that have arrived in the United States, and their rates of what we used to call idiocy and lunacy. I just reviewed a book called 'Idiocy and Lunacy in Massachusetts in 1855,' that's the title. Now I don't know if it's taken that long to get a book reviewed. It was recently reprinted by Harvard University Press and the author is Edward Jarvis, and I commend it to you to read. It's a reproduction of a book that Jarvis published in 1855 or 56. He was asked by the Massachusetts state legislator to study the distribution of idiots and lunatics in Massachusetts, and so he wrote from his study in Cambridge to each Town Clerk and he said 'Please send me a list of the names of each idiot and each lunatic in your town'. That's how you did epidemiological research in the 1850's. So he collected all of these data and he made a dramatic discovery, he discovered that people with Irish names contributed far, far more than their proportional share of idiots and lunatics, and he made the perhaps unwarranted conclusion that the Irish were constitutionally defective, that they were an inferior race and he recommended to the Massachusetts Legislator that separate a Mental Hospital, separate but equal, be built for the Irish because they were incurable. The native yankees could be cured. Now I hope this sounds ridiculous to your ears, because we know now that as the Irish got educated and their children moved up into respectability and responsibility their rate of idiocy declined, but then came a huge wave of Swedish peasants and they arrived, and their rates of idiocy and lunacy were the highest in the land, and the vaudeville joke of the day was 'What's dumber than a dumb Irish man?' and the answer was 'a smart Swede'. Now that simply illustrates the low regard with which the Scandinavians were held in the 1860's and 70's but then they moved up, they moved to Minnesota and became prosperous farmers and their rates declined, but then there were a couple of million of Russian Jews who arrived on the Eastern shores of the United States, and terrible things were said about their high rates of idiocy and lunacy. Then they moved out of the slums and into the middle class and they were followed by millions of Southern Italians and it embarrasses me to read what the psychological text books of the 1910-1925 period had to say about the Southern Italians 'Why are they subject to higher rates of Dementia Praecox, why are they or their children slow learners in school? It's because they are inferior, they are one standard deviation below the mean in terms of measured intelligence.' My late first wife was the eldest daughter of an immigrant Sicilian couple and she went from living in a fifth floor walk up on the lower side of Manhattan, which was the melting pot, to become a Professor of Social Work. She moved a considerable distance because she had opportunities to do so and free College education at Brooklyn College in New York. I have four half Sicilian children, two of whom got part of their Graduate Education here in England. I don't think they are one standard deviation significantly below the average of the population. Now the people who are at the bottom of the economical ladder in the United States are the Chicanos, the Hispanic Americans on the West Coast, blacks who have migrated from Southern small farms to the North looking for industrial jobs and Puerto Ricans from the island of Puerto Rico which is a Commonwealth of the United States. These are the so called slow learners and the people who produce the highest number of schizophrenics. Well perhaps this is a too likely illustration of what I do regard as a very important point; it is poverty, it is discrimination, it is a feeling of powerlessness, that puts people at risk of psychopathology and school learning problems. What happened, and I keep looking at bookshelves here and elsewhere, is that the people who hold the microphone (at least in the United States) currently are claiming that all mental disorders are genetic in origin; those bad genes are what's responsible for schizophrenia, for anxiety, for alcoholism, for even juvenile delinquency and crime. This is contradicted completely by the experience in America of seeing each poverty stricken group move up and their rates of idiocy and lunacy decline, we have had this 140 year history of whole successions of immigrant groups from outside and inside the country who in turn have been at high risk of school learning problems and mental and emotional disorders.

Well what does this suggest about primary prevention? It is this, and I have got a lot of data to support what I am going to say. Political conservatives favour explanations for mental disorders that stress internal defects. Political conservatives are very supportive of the argument that this group of people is inferior, they have bad genes, and so now we have a whole succession of spokes-persons in the United States supporting a bio-chemical genetic explanation for, not only schizophrenia, but for alcoholism, for obsessive compulsive disorders, for anxiety, and these people hold the microphone and they constantly produce articles in the popular medical journals like Time and News Week, and The Reader's Digest. They support the argument that people who have mental and emotional disorders are somehow twisted and disturbed inside their skin. On the other hand, people who support a social, environmental explanation of mental and emotional disorders are those that say it is unemployment, it is powerlessness, it is discrimination, it is prejudice, it is sexism, it is racism, it is ageism, it's all of the negative social pressures that we put

11

on groups of people that make them at risk. Now, when I spent a year working for the Carter Commission we reviewed all of the studies from the field of prevention and we found that every study in the field of Primary Prevention could be fitted into this formula. Now it's not as awesome as it appears, if our goal is to reduce the incidence of disorder then what we have to do is to reduce the noxious agents, which are these agents in the numerator right back to the public health model. Or increase these factors that strengthen the host by improving these factors in the denominator.

Now I could spend the rest of the morning giving you examples, now let me just pick one for each, we know that a major source of organic difficulty is premature birth. Women who are heavy smokers or heavy drinkers are at risk for giving birth either to premature and or low birth weight infants or at much higher risk for survival and also for forming close bonds and relationships with the mother or parents. We also know now that heavy metals are extremely dangerous to the central nervous system and therefore we should avoid eating fish that are heavily contaminated with mercury and we should avoid drinking water that comes through lead pipes where the water has stood. We find that while we have outlawed lead paint which is a major prevention effort, in the inner city slums where the buildings and the rooms and the window sills have not been repainted in years, children still chew on the window sill and still ingest lead paint, so lead poisoning is more common in the inner city poor children than in the suburban children. We now use titanium or latex paint. I mentioned the stress of involuntary unemployment which is a major form of stress. Another major form of stress is sexism and racism, people who are the targets of sexist beliefs, of macho television programmes, of male dominated work places, are at risk. Why are (at least in the United States) three times as many women subject to depression as men? I don't believe that there is anything on the Y chromosome that protects men. I think that women tend to have more of a conscience and that the more conscience a group has the more likely they are to be subject to fits of depression. But women, I think, are also more sensitive to the injustice that exists around them, so that's another major source of stress. Exploitation; people who are exploited and can't escape exploitation, a good example here are American Indians, so called native Americans, but the same thing is true of minority adolescents, they form a giant pool of potential low paid person power and so they are at significant risk. Whatever we can do to neutralise or change these noxious agents will result in reducing the incidence of disorder. Now we can do more to the denominator, which is more the focus of this Conference. What can we do

12

about the competency feelings, the social coping skills of people? Well, again, in our book display out there we have several books about improving the competence of children, improving the competence of adults and elderly people. Several times in the course of listening to papers at this Conference I have heard about ways that are being used to improve the self esteem of groups with whom you work. Clearly people with good self esteem are much more resistant to stress than people with lower self esteem. One of the characteristics of people with mental and emotional disorders is that they tend to be social isolates. One of my public health heroes worked in South Africa, worked with the Zulu tribe and then moved to the University of North Carolina where he spent the rest of his life, name of John Seely. He said 'People with social isolation feelings are at greater risk for suicide, a greater risk for alcoholism, a greater risk for schizophrenia; do something to reduce their feelings of social isolation and that's a primary prevention set of programmes'. Raising their self esteem can have the effect of reducing their susceptibility to mental and emotional disorders. Well I've got to find a way to finish. Social support I have left till last because I think it's the most important form of primary prevention, there are dozens and dozens of different strategies for providing social support, one of the most frequently referred to is Phyllis Severman's Widow to Widow programme. She developed in Boston a technique which involved taking experienced widows and having them offer help and support to new widows so the new widows got a call from the widow group who volunteered to go over and spend time helping them sort their lives out and decide what was going to be different. They provided a built in support group of experienced widows and this has worked dramatically well, but there are lots and lots of others. Just before I left a friend of mine, who is very much concerned with child abuse, handed me this little story which I thought I might share with you because it illustrates a support system. This is an essay written by a third grade little girl in Oakland, California, third grade means that she was about nine years old.

What is a Grandmother?

A Grandmother is a lady who has no children of her own. She likes other people's little girls. A Grandfather is a man Grandmother, he goes for walks with little boys and they talk about fishing and tractors and things like that. Grandmothers don't have anything to do except be there. They are so old they shouldn't run. It's enough if they drive us to the Supermarket, where they pretend horses and have lots of dimes (little coins), or if they take us for a walk and slow down past things like pretty leaves, or caterpillars. They never say 'hurry up.' Usually they are fat, but

13

not too fat to tie your shoes. They wear glasses and funny underwear, they can take their teeth and their gums off. It's better if they don't typewrite or play cards, except with us. They don't have to be smart, only have to answer questions like,Why do dogs hate cats? or how come God isn't married? They do not talk baby talk like visitors do because it's so hard to understand. When they read to us they don't skip over anything or mind if it's the same story again. Everybody should try to have one. Especially if you don't have a television, because Grandmas are the only grown ups who have got time.

A beautiful illustration of a support network, 'Everyone should have a Grandmother or Grandfather'. If I may take one more minute I have a poem that I didn't write but it was shared with me by a colleague and I will close with this.

It was a dangerous cliff as they freely confessed, though to walk near its crest was so pleasant that over its terrible edge there had slipped a Duke and for many, a peasant. The people said 'something will have to be done,' but their projects did not at all tally. Some said 'Put a fence along the edge of the cliff,' some 'an ambulance down in the valley.' The lament of the crowd was profound and was loud as their hearts over flowed with their pity but the cry for the ambulance carried the day as it spread through the neighbouring city. A collection was made to accumulate aid and the dwellers of highway and alley gave dollars and cents not to furnish a fence, but the ambulance down in the valley. For the cliff is alright if you are careful they said and if folks ever slip and are dropping it isn't the slipping that hurts them so much as the shock down below when they are stopping. For years we have heard as these mishaps occurred, quick forth with the rescuers sally, to pick up the victims who fell from the cliff with the ambulance down in the valley. Said one in her plea 'it's a marvel to me that you give so much greater attention to repairing results than to curing the cause, you much better aim at prevention. For the mischief of course should be stopped at its source, come neighbours and friends let us rally, it makes far better sense to rely on a fence than an ambulance down in the valley.' 'She's wrong in her head', the majority said 'she would end all our earnest endeavour, she is the one who would shirk this responsible work, but we will support it for ever. Aren't we picking up all just as fast as they fall, and giving them care liberally? A superfluous fence is of no consequence if the ambulance works in the valley.' Now the story looks queer as we have written it here but things oft occur that are stranger. More humane, we assert, than to suffer the hurt, is the plan of removing the danger. The best possible course is to safeguard the source, and attend to things rationally. Yes let's build the fence and let us dispense with the ambulance down in the valley.'

2 Guest speaker presentation

J.L. Cox

Introduction

I suppose I am entitled to give a welcome on behalf of the Post-Graduate Medical School and of the University to you. It is really absolutely splendid that Dennis Trent and Mid Staffordshire Trust and others have put on this national conference on promoting mental health here at Keele. We have worked very closely in North Staffordshire with the other psychiatrists in Mid Staffordshire and in South East Staffordshire over the last year and it has, as Chris Cooper implied, been very gratifying to see the development of psychiatric services in this part of England. For example, our trainee psychiatrists rotate through to Stafford and down to Wolverhampton as well and of course we are moving into a new era in the Health Service - we shall be a Trust in eighteen months time and consultants are getting more involved with management, going on management courses etc. It has been very interesting and very impressive in its way to see what work the Mid Staffordshire Mental Health Foundation Trust has been able to do and incidentally, we are about to make another bit of history. I expect the National Health Service executives will pick out that the South East Staffordshire is a Trust as well and they are about to advertise an academic post within our Department, a senior lecturer post which they are funding entirely which has four sessions actually on site in North Staffs so they have sussed out that somehow it is something good for them to make formal academic links with us.

The background

The background to my talk, I suppose, is the link up with the developments I have just been talking about, and that is that the developments here both at this University in terms of the School of Postgraduate Medicine, which has eight or nine professors and supporting staff in different specialties, is funded entirely by the National Health Service and so that people who work in this Medical School certainly can't go back on clinical work. We are much closer to NHS structures and managers them we would be in a more traditional development funded by the UIC. So I think that probably underpins a little bit of my feeling for the subject and certainly any knowledge or knowhow one has had or picked up over the last few years in terms of thinking about the development of services as they relate to purchaser/provider splits and trusts etc.

With that sort of introduction and perhaps just to amplify a little bit more - I am a general adult psychiatrist, as Chris Cooper says. I have those particular interests as well as an interest in psychotherapy, and that is really my background. What I want to do in this talk is to discuss some of the broader issues relating to mental health promotion and its relationship to the provision of services for mental illness. I thought, and I know Dennis and others wouldn't disagree in that sense, that of course if one is talking about promoting mental health, I fully recognise that that is and must be independent to a large measure of health professionals and mental health professionals it is working on a very broad political plain and is to do with the sort of subjects that I wouldn't have any particular close acquaintance with. Nevertheless of course, I don't really see how we can talk about the promotion of mental health without recognising that the prevention and treatment of mental illness must be a component of that in some place, and that though health care professionals and lay workers and user groups who have particular interests and concerns about mental illness of course must indeed, and as this conference has shown, do have a key contribution to the much more global issues of promoting mental health. Incidentally, I was somewhat apprehensive about the sort of tone to communicate in my talk, particularly at such a late stage of the day and I was reassured I must say by the content of the Minister of Health's talk this morning and by the follow on talk from the Director of MIND, which really placed mental health promotion within the field, to an extent, of the services necessary to treat mental illness. I think that is an important point that one should not forget despite, of course, the WHO definition here, with its wonderful Utopian ideals of this wonderful state of Nirvana of a complete physical, mental and social wellbeing and not merely the absence of disease or infirmity. Of course that is important for doctors, particularly for those with rather a restrictive bio-medical reductionist approach, who may well by training, through no fault of their own, forget that there is more to physical, personal wellbeing than the treatment of physical and mental disorder or disease. There was a conference held in Manchester about two years ago when Aston Jeblenski, who is one of the senior workers in the Mental Health Unit in the WHO, was talking about the role of a social psychiatrist, it was a conference on social psychiatry, and he is a social psychiatrist and so am I really by background and orientation. He made the point that of course, social psychiatrists, people who are involved in this particular field, and social psychologists too, endorse explicitly or implicitly, the promotion of mental health, so hopefully the psychiatrists that you relate to, especially if they are social psychiatrists, will have an awareness of the promotion of mental health. Nevertheless, I know as well as you that the realities of the job and the pressures under which we operate, and I am sure many of you operate as well, means that that interest may well get squeezed out by the sheer pressure of work of dealing with disturbed individuals with mental health problems and psychiatric disorders of varying degrees. Nevertheless, it is important to make the point that in social psychiatry, and I would argue within good general psychiatry, the prevention of mental illness and thinking about the promoting of mental health is a part of our job. Although I suppose by training we all can't do everything, and maybe your psychiatrist is best spending his job doing those things that perhaps he or she is trained to do, which will indeed relate more to the mental illness field.

I was interested in the Conference aims as they were put out on the information about the Conference - very thought provoking and stimulating. 'A Published Forum for pro-active activities which encourage the wellbeing of an individual'. 'Seeks to de-stigmatize and de-mythologise mental health'. Now, I sort of stuck on that, and I will tell you why I stuck on it - because I fully agree with the sentiment but it just so happened that that afternoon there had been a local discussion about what our community mental health centre should be called, and I expect you may have gone around this particular circle yourselves. There was a debate going on between the mental health professionals, and we have had two new mental health resource centres, about whether it should be called a mental health resource centre or whether word mental or mental health should be taken out of it - whether this was in some way giving not a good image to the people who wanted to use it - it wasn't 'user friendly' enough. I don't know whether you have come across that particular debate but it was a debate that went on and of course makes the point that in some people's thinking, the term 'mental health' or 'mental' is in some way stigmatising itself which seems to me personally a very extraordinary things as though we could actually go round without having a mental life at all - for if we haven't got a mental life what have we got? So then it just sharpens up and reminds ourselves of the views of users and we have to listen to what users say, but heaven knows what you call a mental health resource centre if you don't call it something like that. I was doing out-patient clinics this afternoon, actually within a medical out-patient department, there is a big 1000 bedded hospital here, and I am bound to say that I think that was probably one of the least stigmatising environments in which one could see patients, clients, users, whatever, with mental health problems. It was close to cardiology, the actual receptionist was sometimes manning other clinics etc. and if you wandered in it wasn't clear you were going to a psychiatric clinic. So I think the arguments about where is the least stigmatised place in which to seek your help is still an unresolved one, but of course a very very important one. I had to look up what a euphemism was - I expect you clever people knew exactly what the definition of a euphemism was but in the dictionary it is defined as 'an inoffensive word or phrase', and as I have just made the point there seemingly is a view, which seems a bit far-fetched to me, that the phrase 'mental health', in some people's way of looking at it, carries some offence. I think we have to educate the public basically, and the users, and I think it will just add to stigma if we yield to these sorts of pressures. That is my personal view.

'Mental health' said James Mathers, who is a lecturer in counselling in Birmingham, 'could be seen from various perspectives'. The assumption of absence of mental ill health may be, yes, and it seems to me if you've got mental illness you can't be at one level mentally healthy, although I suppose you could have a healthy adjustment to a mental illness as you could have a healthy adjustment to a stroke or to diabetes. He then links up this idea with preventing mental ill health and looking at interpersonal factors, considering making contact with people who often don't regard themselves as ill - that is very important and I think that is where team work within the mental health field is so fundamentally important that we who see mostly people who have got mental health problems and mental illness do need to be reminded that it must be others who are aware that in terms of mental health promotion there are others who aren't suffering in the way that we see people suffer. That was some of my background thinking about the subject of mental health promotion and its relationship to mental illness.

What I want to do in my main talk is to just review a little bit more the

Health of the Nation document, and I am sure in other workshops and other sessions, we have all been thinking about this extraordinarily encouraging statement from the Department of Health about putting mental illness and mental health problems way up on the priority list. I think if they can put the resources there and stick at it then I think this could well be a good time to be working in this field, at least better than it has been in the past. I want to look a little bit at the Health of the Nation. I then want to outline to you some of the response to Health of the Nation that the Royal College of Psychiatrists has made - a document called 'Mental Health of the Nation' which I am afraid costs £5.00 - I thought it could at least be sent round to all members and fellows of the College (9000 of them). I am afraid that in this commercial age that we are in, that hasn't happened. It is a 20 page document produced by a working party of different specialities. I want to tell you a little bit about that and then more or less in conclusion, perhaps the last ten minutes of my talk, I want to describe the way in which the post-natal mental illness services, both nationally and locally, illustrate some of the themes that I am touching on, which is the relationship of the mental illness service to mental health promotion within a field in which I have specific interest, from a clinical and research perspective and from publication.

To take the 'Health of the Nation' document. I have a shrewd idea where these objectives came from and I have a shrewd idea who wrote Mr Yeo's speech this morning, and it was very much containing information and ideas that have been around within the Department of Health and discussed within the College and with other mental health user groups as well, I am sure that Dr Rachel Jenkins will have been very influential in that - I am sorry I couldn't hear her talk this afternoon and John Read as well. Of course these objectives, from the point of view of mental health professional work and psychiatrists and from the users with mental illness are very very searching are they not! I mean to take the mortality of suicide and to say that by eight years time we can have a 15% reduction in the overall suicide rate and a one third reduction in those with severe mental illness, that is giving a target that is a bit utopian but nevertheless, in order to fulfil, to begin to meet those targets one has to look very globally at the type of psychiatric services and mental health services that we have. Above all I would say we must look at the coordination between the various health professionals providing a mental health service, and also the links with user and voluntary groups. I say that without glossing over it, I say it because I mean it. I personally believe that a mental health service that becomes fragmented becomes an inefficient and an unsafe mental health service, and I say that out of experience because I have seen

19

what happens when clinical psychologists don't talk to psychiatrists and vice versa. I have seen what happens when the CPN service gets entirely lost to the secondary psychiatric services and are restricted solely to general practice based work, however important that may be, and I have seen what happens when there is no communication, when there are no social workers on the team and so on. I firmly believe that, and I would want to champion the idea that the days when we sort of threw mud at each other really should belong to the past in the mental health field, and I and most psychiatrists, I should have thought, would have been on the receiving end of a fair bit of flak, some of it quite deserved, but cumulatively, most of it not, and some of the arguments of clinical psychologists for example, have been quite heavy. I think with increasing training and improved training, and I will say a bit more about this in a moment, of psychiatrists - I can only speak for the training of psychiatrists, may be those times should be restricted to the past. I think it is not just the Keele tradition, but it is the Keele tradition of inter-disciplinary communication that makes me underline that particular point, and if we are to come anywhere near to reducing the suicide rate by 15% in the mentally ill and 30% of severely mentally ill, then we have to work very closely with each other and acknowledge each other's skills, look for appropriate leadership wherever that may be and operate closely with Social Services to see that the patients and the clients/users - those patients with chronic schizophrenia, don't slip through the net and that their co-existing depressive illness is not unrecognised. Of course it is in that way that one would begin to cut back the suicide rate because those are the high risk groups, the severe depressions and those patients with chronic mental illness such as schizophrenia with a co-existing depression. Of course the way in which the Government sets this out and tries to achieve these aims are briefly summarised - `improving information and understanding; more extensive national and local data collection'. Marvellous, I mean no one in Staffordshire knows what the epidemiology of mental illness is in this part of the world, at least there is no published literature in Staffordshire. There will be hopefully over the next five years. So of course one is lacking the scientific epidemiological base in a very distinctive area such as the Potteries, which is working class but cohesive, geographically very stable. I remember when I first came here that I didn't quite know where a meeting was in Birmingham and I thought I would ring up the Switchboard at the City General Hospital, which is three miles from here, a 1000 bedded District General Hospital, and I spoke to the telephone operator and said `Can you tell me where the Woodburn Clinic is?' and he said `Where's that?' and I said `Oh, that's actually in Birmingham' to which he said `Oh, in Birmingham - I've never been there' and I thought he was pulling my leg but in fact the local population, allowing for generalisations, is really very geographically stable. I don't know about Stafford, I can't speak for Stafford but the point that there is a need to look at local epidemiological needs and look at unmet needs goes without saying.

Then they talk about further development of good practice, to education, training, protocols and standards of good practice. Now in discussion after my talk, I would be very interested to know what you think about the feasibility of preparing protocols on the optimum management of let us say a severe depressive psychosis - is that or is it not feasible? I gather in America there are some consensus statements about what is good practice about the management of severe depression, let us say with severe retardation or stupor or the management of anxiety state or what is the optimum management of an acute schizophrenic psychosis. We are being asked by the Minister and the Department of Health to produce those sorts of protocols on a sort of consensus - what is the consensus of the professionals working in that field about optimum managements, and I don't know whether you think that is feasible. I think it actually is a rather good idea; it would probably pull into line a few people who are rather way out of line on their management and that is a good thing. Some of my colleagues would say 'well you can't regiment your colleagues, they are qualified doctors, they are consultant psychiatrists or consultant clinical psychologists, they are working within their own professional knowledge and who is to say that your view about the optimum management of, let us say Anorexia Nervosa, is the right one?' I think myself, that that is a task which is not insurmountable, although I would be very interested to know what other mental health professionals think about that; but those are the sort of directions in which we are being asked to move.

So as the Minister said this morning, the objectives, if they are to be achieved, clearly link up with mental illness services and the prevention of mental illness and of course that, I would say, is a good thing, and to bring before the public the recognition that psychiatric disorders have a certain mortality is important and necessary. Although as they say in the document, of course, it is very difficult to develop targets for the equally disabling but perhaps not quite so life threatening and apparently less severe psychological disorders, whether you call them neuroses or those more chronic, lower grade problems. So that was the challenge, and of course it is a challenge to all the different health professional groups here and to managers I am quite sure, and it is a challenge to the Royal College of Psychiatrists and to that body. The College has produced its own

21

'Mental Health of the Nation' report which was I suppose a sort of consensus statement, but it was a bit 'Heath Robinson' to an extent. It was a group of about ten people who were representing different specialist sections, whether that be forensic psychiatry or child and adolescent psychotherapy, general adult, learning disabilities and so on, to see what we could say corporately to the Department of Health about in what way mental health services could be improved.

There were some broad statements which I think broadly speaking I went along with, about the need for a more person orientated service and above all of course there was a recognition that the work, if we are thinking of psychiatrists and our contribution to the mental health field, it is very clear to anyone working as a consultant psychiatrist that the demands, the work load, has increased very very substantially for all sorts of reasons. Now you can probably think of various ways in which the role of a psychiatrist is different now from what it was ten years ago or twenty years ago when I trained. For example, management issues would be one; who would have thought that I would be going to a course on management and one of my colleagues would be a clinical director spending two thirds of his time on management issues. As we were discussing over tea, I am sure the future is going to be that our medical students and people doing postgraduate training will be doing management courses and they will come up through the system and there may be courses on health economics and so there will be a different type of doctor being produced. Those are new demands and they are time consuming demands. If you are spending four sessions per week on management issues clearly you are not spending four sessions per week on face to face meetings with client sufferers and families. The other major factor that has made us look at the manpower constraints for psychiatry is doing what we were doing anyhow but we are doing much more explicitly now; looking at what users want, and what users want, seemingly and understandably, is more time with a single mental health team, with a designated consultant, and they are wanting more psychological treatments, whether it be cognitive therapy, Rogerian counselling, dynamically orientated psychotherapies, and they are much more suspicious, sometimes too suspicious in a way, of the role of biological treatments in mental illness, not least the anti-depressants. Of course the training needed and the time taken for the psychological treatments are really very time consuming, and so that is another way in which the role of the psychiatrist has increased the demands made and there are other demands, for audit and for training of trainee psychiatrists. If you have to give an hour to an hour and a half to supervising a registrar and you are lucky enough to have a senior registrar

22

and he has an hour's supervision as well, that is a half day on supervision. So those were some of the background factors, and I think each of the other health professionals could draw up a similar list, which made us go very strongly for hoping that the Government would release more monies for personnel. Now, just to sharpen up this argument in case you think or expect me to say that because I am a psychiatrist I just want more of us or something. In the West Midlands where we are now, which has a population the size of Scotland, and I worked in Scotland so I can imagine the population of Scotland and I can imagine the population of the West Midlands, and if I tell you that the West Midlands Regional Health Authority, assuming we still have regional health authorities, and I gather Virginia Bottomley has reassured regional health authorities that they are going to be there, it extends from where we are now, Stoke-on-Trent, the Potteries, right down to Hereford in the South West, Birmingham obviously, Stratford, Rugby, Coventry, Burton. That is the West Midlands Regional Health Authority with the population of Scotland, and it has only one medical school, in Birmingham. Keele has its bid all ready if the Tomlinson Report should suggest relocation of a medical school and it would be a rather good place to have a medical school here in some respects. In terms of manpower in the mental health field, if you accept the argument that it is difficult to run an optimum psychiatric service without psychiatrists - I know there may possibly be some here who may want to dispute that but if you would accept for one moment that it would be difficult to have a comprehensive psychiatric service without psychiatrists, if I then tell you that there are 40 unfilled consultant psychiatrist posts in the West Midlands Regional Health Authority (they are unfilled by substantive posts, that is not to say there are not locums in post) you realise what the situation is in the West Midlands and it is not that much different in other parts of the country. So there is a real manpower - sorry, forgive the word, I know some people are very jumpy about manpower as being a sort of gender type issue but we now have a lady president elect of our College who is a manpower expert and Fiona Caldicott doesn't mind the use of 'manpower' - issue of some proportions, and of course it has the disadvantage that not only are trusts competing against each other, which our beloved Government wishes us to do and I just hope the competition doesn't get so destructive, but it makes us compete even more for attracting people into posts so that one of the recommendations is that there should be an increase in the number of senior registrars, which are the training posts for consultants, and a big increase in consultant establishment, and that is important. The other two issues which are highlighted in the report relate to the numbers of consultants per unit of the population and that is linked up with what I was just saying basically, that probably in Stafford and in North Staffordshire you would have one consultant maybe for 60,000 of the population if you are sectorised and zoned. Clinical experience, and I have my ear close enough to the ground to be pretty confident about what I am saying, I think if we are to have a high quality mental health service and to cut back the suicide rate by 15% over eight years then we have to begin to approach the ratio of consultants per population that is the situation in New Zealand and Australia at the present time which is one consultant for about 20,000 or less, 15,000 of the population. So the recommendation landing on the Minister's desk is for an increase in manpower and of course it starts at the training registrar grade. Now I dare say that other health professionals will be making exactly the same case and I would support them personally in exactly the same way, but it has resource issues for government and is certainly directly related to whether care in the community is going to be operational and feasible in April next year.

I noticed in the speech this morning, I don't know whether you did, talking about who was going to be the key worker and the case manager and talking about CPNs or social workers and then actually slipped in, and this is how and I think rightly, was the consultant psychiatrist for whom he is treating somebody who is currently attending an out-patient clinic and that actually makes sense to me for that small group. That is not to say there isn't a much larger group who won't need consultant psychiatrists at all but it just makes the point of the demands made at this particular time. The other issue, which I wouldn't expect you to be so sympathetic with, assuming you are sympathetic with that broad manpower issue, would be the question of in-patient beds and the number of those, and I know it's old hat, particularly when I'm treading on difficult ground talking to managers about beds, but still. There is a national crisis to an extent that because of the reduction of acute beds, which is policy as you get more into the community and better CPN service and crisis intervention and so on, the reduction in beds has had an effect certainly in areas which are demoralised or inner city areas and particularly in areas where the mental health services are poor with problems of recruitment as I have described, of making those acute units almost intolerable places to work in or to be in as a patient because they are much more disturbed. There are many more disturbed patients/clients/users in that unit and of course there are then morale issues for health professionals working there, not least consultants and psychologists, and psychiatric nurses. I work on an acute unit just down the road so I know the efforts that have to go in to maintain morale and demonstrate to managers and to others that of course mental illness doesn't go away. A lot of it can be treated in the community, can be looked after in the community but there is still a need for residential accommodation and there is still a need for acute beds, not as many as we needed. The estimate in the Royal College Report was of 20 to 50 per 1000 of the population. Now that is a very big range, 20 to 50, which is right because if you are working in North Staffordshire which is almost as high up the Jarman indices as Mid Staffordshire, a little bit below, you don't need as many beds as you would do in the middle of Birmingham or Manchester or Tower Hamlets where I did my medical training at the London Hospital. If you are working in an area with a higher or a lower Jarman index, you may well need the 50 beds per 1000 to provide any credible safe service. By safe service I am talking of safety in the sense that the Health of the Nation talks about it in terms of preventing mortality, and of course it lays us open to criticism from others saying 'Good Lord if I was admitted to that hospital I would feel even more suicidal - what a horrible place to be'. So it does give fuel to those sorts of arguments, but basically the problems are to do with resources and will.

Those were some of the points of 'Mental Health of the Nation' that were put out from a working party from the College, and we hope that the Department of Health will listen and we hope (you have to be optimistic in the mental health field) that it will indeed lead to greater resources and I think lead to much better team work between all health professionals and in that way we might begin to meet those targets in the eight years that we are given. I commend that report to you - it can be obtained from the Royal College of Psychiatrists and it is a public document, a bit wordy in places but it makes points that I think many mental health professionals would agree with and go along with and it gives one ammunition when one is debating about resources within a service, and of course it goes along with the philosophy that we need a local accessible community orientated service, of course that is right. My only concern about that, taken to extreme, would be that if you are rigidly sectorised or zoned, it can diminish the need for and the resources allocated to District specialities who are not geographically zoned, such I feel in a big District like we are here in North Staffordshire, 400,000, we need our substance abuse, psychotherapy, post-natal illness, neuro-psychiatry - it is not just because we are teaching, but because we believe that provides a better service for the population.

Now for the last ten minutes, to illustrate a bit of what I am saying, I would like to take you through, if you need that, some of the background aspects of post-natal mental illness and its services. I think you will see

25

that it really illustrates many of the points I have made so far in my talk in terms of resources, in terms of users and in terms of what is the particular role of the doctors and the psychiatrists.

I do have an interest in Psychotherapy and I am very ashamed that my generation of psychiatrist were not trained in counselling or cognitive therapy, the next generation is/will be. I have made it up, mostly, and this is a good book but I just make the point that if you have a psychiatric disorder which happens to be affecting in this instance, the mother at that stage, it has a knock on effect on the family clearly and can produce which is in ICD-10, the new child and adolescent psychiatry category of sibling rivalry disorder - it seems to be stretching classifications a little bit more than they can really go, but sibling rivalry I am sure we are all familiar with in various settings, and of course it reminds us that the partner, the husband, may well be depressed himself, he certainly looks pretty uptight, and the evidence is that 50% of partners at that time, more specially if the mother is psychiatrically disturbed, are themselves unhappy, with minor depression but also suffering from major depression bordering on mental illness. Then of course there are the previous generations, shadows from the past who are very relevant in that setting. And so that gives you a sort of taste of what is special and unusual about psychiatric disorder when it occurs at that time and it perhaps gives some of its distinctive features, both resource issues as it relates to what do you do if the mother is grossly psychotic, fortunately only two per 1000 have a florid psychosis, but it is a most pathetic and difficult emergency, more specially if you haven't got a mother and baby unit, which alas, until our new building goes up we don't have a mother and baby unit here, it stopped three years ago and I know what it is like to try to muddle through these managements on an acute admission wards - it is not good news and the management is much less satisfactory.

This is the sort of terminology in case there is a semantic problem; I am sure you here would not get muddled between the 'blues', the fifth day emotionalism and the neurotic depressions which are the 10-13%, and the psychoses, which are two per thousand and have remained about two per thousand over the last twenty years.

I am very interested in this subject so I must make quite sure I don't say more than is appropriate at the end of a long, hot day. This is the bit of history; Escurol noted that the incidence of psychiatric illness following childbirth was greater than the statistics from psychiatric hospitals would indicate, and large numbers of mild to moderate cases were cared for at home and never recorded. That is just what it is like in Stoke-on-Trent now, and Stafford and Dundee and Kent or wherever. These are the grumbling, the hidden, I call them illnesses, you may have another name for them, but it is a disability, and I think it strains credibility to regard it as a sort of gross experience that people are better going through than not going through - that is not how most of the women that we see express themselves. This is just to remind you with the complexity of the subject, and there is a substantial reading material on this subject. I was interested to see the book called 'Depression' edited by Katie Hurbst outside there and there is a chapter on post-natal mental illness that I wrote which covers some of these issues. You have got psychodynamic factors impinging, socio-cultural role change - that is the sort of trans-cultural bit for me where one is interested in these factors but of course there are enormous biological considerations which one can't ignore, massive hormonal changes which can certainly affect mood. Genetic determinants of puerperal psychosis certainly, so that is the fascination and that is why I think any mental health professional worth their salt, needs to be as conversant as possible with the varieties of different, sometimes conflicting, but mostly complementary, aetiological models. This really just makes a point very quickly, that something happens in the few months after childbirth to give this increase of admissions to psychiatric units compared with the months either after two years post-partum or two years before, and really any studies that are carried out show that to be so, and you can imagine the debate about whether that is biological or psychological stress or both. I think it is important in the mental health field that when one talks, one talks from facts and scientific facts I suppose is what I mean, published reports that you can chew through, and the interesting thing about this whole field is that the figure 10-13% sort of sticks out throughout all the prospective studies, so one can confidently say, not with a smile on one's face, that at six to eight weeks post-partum, one in ten of women and a slightly smaller proportion of their partners will indeed be suffering from a depressive disorder. I shall hasten on a little. I shall be tempted to pause there longer than I should. I said earlier on that there are no epidemiological studies of affective disorder in Staffordshire. I think broadly speaking that is true. In six months time there will be this study published in the British Journal of Psychiatry, which was a controlled study - we had 232 matched pairs of puerperal women and matched women who had not had a baby in the previous year and were not currently pregnant and we screened using the Edinburgh Screening Scale. We interviewed high scorers etc. and we found that the prevalence, the total amount of depression in the two groups, and this was a surprise, was absolutely identical. You could not distinguish the post-natal group from the non post-natal group on prevalence, on the total

27

amount, and that is an interesting finding. However, we did find that within the five weeks following delivery, if you looked at onsets of incidence, there was a three fold increased onset rate of these depressions, neurotic depressions, general practice type depressions or CPN type depressions occurring which suggests that again whether this is physiological or psychological, nevertheless this is a stressful event which initiates depression.

A few points on prevention. I think one of the interests of this field is that in post-natal illness, we do know from research quite a bit about what is effective in terms of prevention and we can go through the list, as I imagine, other speakers will have gone through at the Conference, about primary, secondary and tertiary. Primary prevention, we can detect high risk mothers in ante-natal clinics, if it wasn't such a lovely day I would go on for more than that - you can pick out those with a family history of previous puerperal psychoses, those with disturbed family relationships etc. You could consider prophylactic medication, you could give ante-natal education with a CPN or a health care worker, you could educate primary care workers, and we have taken a lot of initiatives locally in that field. You can educate psychiatrists, believe you me, that is a big job in itself. There is a college report that I was chairman of, which had a very stormy ride through some of my closest colleagues - 'now what is this about post-natal illness, post-natal psychoses, it is no different from psychoses occurring at any other time,' and they were mostly males by the way, I think, on the whole it tended to be males who held the most extreme views on that. You need your adequate co-ordinated post-natal illness service for the reasons outlined earlier on.

Secondary prevention. Early detection - here, to fly my own flag, humbly a little bit high, we have developed a very good screening scale called the Edinburgh Post-Natal Depression Scale, which is being very widely used. It is absurdly simple. It has ten items, it has excellent psychometrics bearing in mind the distinguished psychologists we have here, and it is user friendly etc., and it picks out depression. To give you an idea of how acceptable it is, on that study I described, and elsewhere, you can get a 90% response rate from a postal questionnaire so it has got user friendly aspects and I won't get stuck on it because that is another too long time but, those are some of the items on the EPDS - it is derived from Snaith's Hospital Anxiety Depression Scale but it has modified items that have good face validity for the puerperium and omits silly items like 'I have read a good book or watched television - as much as usual/not so much as usual' - now obviously that sort of item as a measure of lack of interest is not so sensible in the puerperium, and we can go on like that.

28

It has been translated a lot into different languages, which is incorrect actually, because you can't translate self-report scales from one culture into another, well if you do you should re-validate them, certainly not if there are big differences between cultures. Secondary prevention, early treatment, yes I did a study with Jennifer Holden, Ruth Sikorsky, which showed that non-directive counselling, listening visits by health visitors, are effective and in a third of depressed women, they were effective alone. This was the study published in the BMJ about four years ago. There were 26 women who had counselling, which really consisted of eight sessions of non-directive counselling, listening visits. I mean, if there are any Rogerian counsellors here you would regard this as not 'the real McCoy' Rogerian counselling, but it was on that sort of continuum. We saw from the control group that a third got well with just routine treatment from their GP and, very important to mental health services - this is the group I see at Charles Street, a third did not get well with counselling, and it is that group who require more specialist mental health services such as those we have had available at the day hospital that Dr Cooper kindly made mention of.

Tertiary prevention - well here we are into couple therapy, family therapy, self-help groups. That is where the self-help groups and the associations for post-natal illness, manic depressive illness and other associations, interlocking with health professional work, makes such a powerful lobby and it is enormously encouraging to researchers and clinicians and others working in the field. It is also surprising that some of the things that worry some people about labelling, about using the term illness, don't actually bother so much the people in these self-help groups. I mean that is always I find, rather interesting, the association for post-natal illness is the National Association - they like the term post-natal illness, it is not 'good lord this is medical model illness stuff' - in that sense.

That is a reminder that our Unit at Charles Street is called a Parent and Baby Day Unit and is deliberately called a Parent and Baby Day Unit because we set out to try and take on board the partners, the husbands, and to do something about the 30% of them who are distressed and who require explanation and some of them requiring psychiatric support and direct treatment. I think on that note, I will summarise my talk. I haven't shown you a slide of Charles Street. It is in Hanley, which those of you who don't know Stoke-on-Trent, is the centre of Stoke-on-Trent, one of Arnold Bennett's towns, and is opposite the Bus Station. It is a Victorian building, believe you me it is falling down but morale within it is very high because it is an extremely good team but there are resource issues there. There are other issues about, is this going to be a sub-directorate of post-natal mental illness, am I going to spend three sessions doing that, holding a budget with a nurse manager? If I do that I can't run an acute admission ward or help with a mental health resource centre. So these are the issues that confront us. I think they are issues, Chairman, that we have been reminded of already today, by the minister and I was very very encouraged by the lead given by MIND on this particular subject and that actually made me say more about the post-natal illness service here, because this is to do with women's issues and men's issues and I was very encouraged the tone of the talk and I think that sort of degree of collaboration amongst mental health workers and with users and with clients is basically what it is all about, and I think if we can increase resources, if we can get our act together with general practitioners, with CPNs, if we can acknowledge some of the key leadership roles of consultant psychiatrists, then I think we might approach, if not a 15% reduction, perhaps a 5-10% reduction by the year 2000. So on that note I would like to close and thank you very much for your attention on this very very hot and pleasant evening.

3 Promoting better mental health in the elderly: The problem of Alzheimer's disease

E. Miller

As a neuropsychologist, my interests tend to be rather different from those of most of the other contributors to this conference. Neuropsychologists do not usually consider their work in terms of concepts like the 'promotion of mental health' or 'prevention'. Nevertheless, being asked to provide a presentation in a context like the present sharpens the mind and acts as a catalyst to thought. Having worked extensively with people suffering from neurodegenerative disorders, it became apparent on reflection that certain aspects of work with these conditions do have health promotional or preventative aspects.

One of the most prevalent of the neurodegenerative disorders is Alzheimer type dementia. This form of dementia is a major source of mental ill-health in older people. Estimates suggest that 5-15% of those above retirement age will be clearly suffering from some form of dementing illness of which the largest proportion will be those with Alzheimer's disease (Kay & Bergmann, 1980). Given that the elderly now constitute almost 20% of the whole population of the UK, it can be seen that Alzheimer's disease is responsible for a considerable amount of mental ill-health and constitutes a major social and economic problem.

Two questions then arise from a health promotion perspective. Firstly, can anything be done to prevent the occurrence of Alzheimer type dementia and, secondly, what can be done to ameliorate the impact of this disorder in those who are afflicted. The first question relates to primary prevention and this paper will discuss one line of work in relation to the primary prevention of Alzheimer's disease.

Primary prevention

Understanding of the underlying causes of Alzheimer's disease is limited. It is well established that the brain shrinks or atrophies and that certain neuropathological features, such as plaques and neurofibrillary tangles, can be found in the brain (e.g. Tomlinson et al, 1970). A range of different neurotransmitter systems have been also implicated (Rossor, 1987). There are considerable problems in this work in determining exactly what is cause and effect but a least some basic neuropathological changes have been identified.

One hypothesis that has received considerable attention, not only in scientific circles but at a more popular level as well, is that aluminium may be implicated in the causation of Alzheimer type dementia. If this is so, then it might be possible to base preventative measures on a reduction in exposure to aluminium. There was in the UK a short period in the 1980s when some people disposed of their old aluminium based cooking utensils and replaced them with pots and pans made from other substances. This was because of the alleged association between aluminium and Alzheimer's disease. The potential problem here is that aluminium is a ubiquitous element that is found in small traces in a wide range of substances, including foodstuffs, and so a complete reduction in exposure to aluminium would not be feasible. Nevertheless some reduction in exposure might be beneficial.

All this presupposes that aluminium does have a causal role in the production of Alzheimer's disease. There are a number of lines evidence that suggest that aluminium might play a role in the production of this disorder. This is summarised in Table 1.

Table 1
Sources of evidence linking aluminium to Alzheimer's disease

1. Aluminium identified in the neuropathological features of Alzheimer's disease (plaques and tangles)

2. Dementia occurring in renal dialysis linked to absorption of aluminium

3. Inhalation of 'McIntyre powder' by miners

4. Link between incidence of dementia and levels of aluminium in local water supplies

Whilst this evidence is consistent with the notion that aluminium might produce Alzheimer's disease it stops far short of proving this hypothesis to be true. In the case of the neuropathological evidence, whilst it is true that the plaques found in such profusion in the brains of those with Alzheimer's disease do contain aluminium (e.g. MacLachlan, 1986), this does not demonstrate that aluminium produces plaques. It could be that once formed, plaques have a propensity to attract the small traces of aluminium that would be present in the brain anyway.

The available evidence does suggest that dementia can occur in those subject to renal dialysis (e.g. Alfrey et al, 1976) and it also appears that this relates to aluminium getting into the body through the dialysate. However, patients on renal dialysis have compromised renal function and aluminium entering the body normally tends to be excreted through the kidneys. Possibly the crucial factor here is the failure of kidneys to excrete aluminium satisfactorily rather than such dialysis patients being subject to levels of aluminium outside the range that the body can sustain. Furthermore, dialysis dementia appears to be clinically different from Alzheimer type dementia (Hughes, 1989).

There is a report that Canadian miners subject to having 'McIntyre powder' (a finely ground mixture of elemental aluminium and aluminium hydroxide) pumped into the atmosphere as a prophylactic against silicotic lung disease, may have suffered some intellectual deterioration (Rifat et al, 1990). Whilst this report does suggest that inhaled aluminium may have a deleterious effect on cognitive functioning there are problems with the design of the investigation and it is not clear whether the relatively mild effects resemble Alzheimer type dementia. It should also be noted that in this study the aluminium was inhaled rather than ingested through the gut.

Finally there have been reports that the prevalence of Alzheimer type dementia varies with the level of aluminium in the local drinking water (e.g. Martyn et al, 1989). Again this is a finding which tends to raise more problems than it solves. Only a very small proportion of the typical daily intake of aluminium comes through water, the vast majority is contained in foodstuffs. When considered in this light the effective variation in total aluminium intake that could be related to water supplied is very small. It is surprising that, given all the other sources of 'noise' in the data as well, significant correlations between the incidence of dementia and water levels of aluminium have emerged. One suggestion (Birchall & Chappell, 1989) has been that possibly aluminium levels in the water are not the crucial factor. In water supplies, there is a marked trend for aluminium levels to be inversely correlated with the levels of silicic acid. There are levels to be inversely correlated with the levels of silicic acid. There are reasons to relate silicic acid to the handling of aluminium by the body and so it could be that it is the level of silicic acid that was the crucial factor.

To summarise the evidence relating aluminium to Alzheimer's disease, there do appear to be very good grounds for linking the two. What is less clear is whether aluminium truly plays a causal role, as would be necessary if preventive measures based on reducing exposure to aluminium were to be effective, or whether its role is less central. Those situations where aluminium is associated with intellectual deterioration also suggest that it is long-term exposure that is critical and the link is especially likely where aluminium enters the body other than through the gut. The possible exception to this last statement is the work linking aluminium levels in the water supply to the incidence of dementia.

The oral ingestion of aluminium as a possible cause of cognitive decline

In view of this evidence, the possible influence of ingested aluminium in producing cognitive decline merits some further exploration. A colleague, Lindsey Williams, and I have recently completed a study looking at the effects of considerably increased aluminium intake on cognitive functioning. Many antacids contain aluminium hydroxide and people who need to take antacids typically do so over long periods of time. We therefore studied a group of 20 subjects with gastroenterological problems who had been taking antacids for a least two years. Because antacids are taken on an irregular basis as symptoms fluctuate, it is impossible to estimate actual aluminium intake with any accuracy. What does appear to be the case is that the average aluminium intake for this group over the period that they were taking antacids would have been very considerably greater (e.g. 3 to 5 times greater) than the usual population levels.

Two comparison groups were also used. The first consisted of a similar number of normal controls and the second a small group of 10 patients with Alzheimer type dementia. The second comparison group was included in order to show that, should no difference emerge between antacid and control groups, then the measures employed were actually sensitive to the changes produced by Alzheimer type dementia.

A number of measures were used which included memory tests, the Trail Making Test (Reitan, 1958), the FAS test of verbal fluency (see: Lezak, 1976), a test requiring the judgment of spatial relationships adapted from Benton et al (1978) and the Paced Auditory Serial Addition Test (PASAT) which involves information processing and requires considerable attention and concentration (Gronwall & Wrightson, 1974). Memory testing was based on the free recall of lists of words (10 lists, each of 12 words) based on the material used by Miller (1971). Immediate recall was determined by the total number of words produced from the immediate recall of words in each list. Delayed recall without previous warning with the subject being required to produce as many words as possible from any all of the lists was required after a delay of 5 minutes. This was followed by recognition testing in which subjects were presented with 20 cards, each containing three words, and had to indicate which of the three had appeared in the original lists.

As Table 2 demonstrates the antacid and control groups produced very similar results and none of the relevant comparisons emerged as being even remotely close to the usual levels of statistical significance (by t test). In contrast there is a clear difference in performance between the group with Alzheimer type dementia and the other two. This latter finding

Table 2
Comparison of subjects exposed to aluminium containing antacid medication with controls and a reference group with Alzheimer type dementia

	Antacid takers (Means)	Control (Means)	Alzheimer type dementia (Means)
Immediate recall	46.5	47.3	11.5
Delayed recall	5.6	5.6	0
Delayed recognition	11.6	12.4	6.7
Verbal fluency	51	47.7	17.1
Trails `A'	8.4	8.6	1
Trails `B'	4.7	4.2	*
PASAT	31.4	31.4	*

* no data recorded because an appreciable number of subjects unable to meet requirements of this test

indicates that the measures used are unlikely to have failed to discriminate between the antacid and control groups simply because they lacked any sensitivity at all to the predicted effects.

This single investigation does not of course finally prove that aluminium ingested through the gut can have no deleterious effect on cognitive functioning. Such an effect may have been manifest if different kinds of measures had been employed or if the antacid group had been taking this medication for very much longer lengths of time than was typically the case in this study (median length of use 3 years).

Whatever the limitations of the work that has just been described, it does not support the notion that the oral ingestion of aluminium is a significant factor in the production of Alzheimer's disease. The consequence of this is that measures that might be taken to reduce the oral intake of aluminium, such as the use of non-aluminium cooking utensils or the reduction of aluminium in the water supply, are unlikely to have any effect on the incidence of Alzheimer's disease.

Viewed from this standpoint, findings of the kind that have just been described are disappointing since they do not lead to any action that can be taken to prevent Alzheimer's disease. On the other hand, the fact that traces of aluminium are found so extensively in so many things, including foodstuffs, means that reduction of exposure to aluminium beyond certain limits would be extremely difficult. That the oral ingestion of aluminium does not appear to be a significant factor can therefore be seen as a relief from one potential source of concern.

All this is also not to deny that other putative causal mechanisms for Alzheimer's disease could be postulated and that some of these, if confirmed, could lead to preventive measures. Given the limitations of space it is necessary to leave possible causal mechanisms and prevention to look at the possibilities for ameliorating the effects of Alzheimer type dementia once it has occurred.

The amelioration of dementia

Once a dementing illness has developed the crucial issue then becomes whether it is possible to halt or even reverse the disease process. Where continuing impairment exists, as it inevitably does in the case of Alzheimer type dementia, the key question is whether the impairments can be ameliorated in any way. In other words, can anything be done to assist afflicted individuals to function as well and independently as possible despite their impairments.

One potential approach here is pharmacological. Increasing knowledge about such things as the neurotransmitter systems (e.g. Rossor, 1988) involved in dementia give some hope that drugs can be identified that will in some way counter the neurochemical processes underlying the disease process. So far pharmacological research in this field has certainly not been accompanied by spectacular success but the possibility remains that successes may one day accrue. It is not the purpose of this paper to pursue the pharmacological aspects. For present concerns it is sufficient to note that pharmacology may have something worthwhile to offer in the future.

The other approach to amelioration is psychological or psychosocial. This approach aims to manipulate environmental features in order to help the individual maintain functional capacities or to relearn skills that have been lost. As will be seen some small gains have been made in endeavours of this kind.

If there is a real possibility that pharmacological interventions may one day be able to counteract the pathological processes it might be argued that psychological interventions, no matter how successful, are destined to be made redundant. This is only so if pharmacological interventions can completely reverse the disease process. It seems inherently unlikely that this will be the case. It is more probable that such interventions will act merely to slow down the rate of progression of the dementing process (as in the case with L Dopa and Parkinson's disease). In which case pharmacological success could mean that sufferers from Alzheimer's disease will remain mildly impaired for much longer. In this case the potential role of psychological interventions to enhance functioning could be seen as even more rather than less important.

A preliminary point that arises is whether people with dementia really are sensitive to environmental manipulations and can respond with appropriate behavioural change. This might be doubted and it is well established that subjects with Alzheimer type dementia perform very poorly on many memory tests (e.g. Morris & Kopelman, 1986). In fact the data from the antacid study briefly described in the previous section (see: Table 2) illustrates this quite well.

Despite this there is some encouraging evidence that even subjects with quite moderate degrees of dementia can learn and change their behaviour. Various studies have shown such people to be capable of classical eye-blink conditioning (Solyom & Barik, 1965), operant conditioning (Ankus & Quarrington, 1972), pursuit motor learning (Eslinger & Damasikon, 1986), and so on. the acquisition and retention may not always be quite up to normal levels in these experiments but the degree of impairment is slight. There is thus evidence that some forms of learning and retention are possible to at least useful levels even though others, especially verbal learning and memory, may be markedly impaired.

So the evidence of at least adequate response relates only to experimental tasks. However, similar findings have emerged from studies of 'real life' situations. One example of this is a series of reports which have shown that elderly psychogeriatric patients with dementing illnesses and living in residential units are susceptible to environmental changes. A good early example of this is provided by Sommer & Ross (1958). They noted that the chairs in a day room were all in straight lines with their backs against the walls of the room. Moving the chairs so that their were placed in small groups around coffee tables increased the amount of social interaction between residents. Admittedly this was not to a high level but it was a clear improvement on what had been the case before. There have been a number of similar demonstrations since the sommer & Ross (1958) early report.

In more recent times a growing literature has attested to a variety of attempts to enhance functioning in those with dementia. These are best discussed in terms of the various approaches adopted.

Reality orientation

Reality orientation (RO) was the first psychological approach specifically designed for use with the intellectually impaired elderly. RO was initially devised by Folsom (e.g. Folsom, 1968) to enhance orientation because he had noted that such patients were disoriented in space, time and person. RO was rapidly applied and extended in a number of centres and there became a tradition of describing a range of different interventions with psychogeriatric patients as RO (see: Holden & Woods, 1987). This trend of slowly expanding what is regarded as being part of RO has two disadvantages. Firstly, to the degree that the RO becomes all things to all people it can then become difficult to know what sort of things are involved when an intervention is described as RO. The term loses its precision and meaning. Secondly, to describe most psychological interventions with this client group as RO tends to reinforce the view that older people are different and need different kinds of intervention from those used with younger populations. It can lead to an undesirable form of 'ageism'.

This account will therefore stick with a fairly narrow definition of RO. As originally devised, RO has two elements. These are, firstly, ' 24 hour RO' and, secondly, 'classroom RO'. (In the UK the term 'classroom' carries rather more negative connotations for adult groups than it does in America and so alternative terms, such as 'group RO' have been used.)

The first form of RO, 24 hour RO, is implemented through all people who come into contact with intellectually impaired patients. It involves using all interactions to emphasise information relating to orientation. In consequence, the nurse handing out tablets instead of saying 'here are your pills' will say something like 'it is 12 o'clock Mrs Jones and time to take your pill'., This emphasises for Mrs Jones the time of day, what happens at that time of day, and what her name is.

In contrast classroom RO involves getting patients together in small groups in which the therapist introduces activities that relate to enhancing orientation. For example the session may start by having the group determine where they are, what day it is, the date, the time of year, etc. It may then go on to a discussion of what happens at that time of year, for example the flowers to be seen in Springtime if the current season happens to be Spring, and so on.

Undoubtedly RO has a number of advantages. It has a simple and easily understood rationale, it is easy to implement and has proved popular with direct care staff, occupational therapists, and so on. It appears to have played a useful role in combating the therapeutic nihilism that has all too often been endemic in psychogeriatric units.

On the other hand, any proper evaluation of RO has to go beyond this. Evidence relating to the effectiveness of RO has been summarised in a number of sources (e.g. Powell Proctor & Miller, 1982; Miller, 1987). It is classroom RO that has been most extensively investigated and this seems to produce definite, if small improvements in subjects' ability to provide information relating to orientation (e.g. by answering questions like 'what day of the week is it', 'where are we now', and so on. These gains are at the expense of considerable effort and appear to be lost if the intervention is terminated. There is also no real benefit to other aspects of functioning not targeted by the intervention.

RO procedures can be extended. For example, Hanley et al (1981) found that adding a special training procedure whereby residents were given additional 'ward orientation training' in order to learn to orient themselves within the residential unit. In this residents would be escorted round the building and have signposts pointed out to them. This last component was found to be necessary in order to enhance the actual ability to find their way around the building.

A final point that can be made about RO is whether it is directed at the right aspects of functioning. Is it more important for a people with moderate dementia to be able to say that today is Wednesday, or whatever it is, than to dress or feed themselves? Where these particular self-care skills are being lost it could be argued that they should take precedence over knowing what day of the week it is.

For all its limitations RO has been important in introducing a more positive approach to the care of those suffering from dementia. The fact that it is relatively easy to implement and catches the enthusiasm of direct care staff means that it can be used as a base from which to build a more extensive range of interventions.

Behavioural approaches

Behaviour modification, as based on the principles of operant conditioning, has been applied to the problems presented by elderly populations. Since the basic principles and typical applications of behaviour modification are well known it would be redundant to set them out yet again here.

As far as elderly populations, and particularly those suffering from dementing illnesses, are concerned there have been a number of reports of the successful application of behaviour modification techniques to the resolution of specific problems (e.g. Burgio et al, 1988; Downs et al, 1988; Rinke et al, 1978; Schnelle et al, 1983). These largely refer to such things as the re-establishment and maintenance of fairly basic skills such as dressing, feeding and toileting.

Behaviour modification does appear to be able to create beneficial changes, at least under some circumstances, but the established value of this technique lies mainly in the realm of basic self-care skills. Nevertheless, in this population the maintenance of such skills can be important in ensuring maximum independence.

Memory rehabilitation

There is now a set of techniques developed to ameliorate the consequences of memory loss in people who have suffered brain damage or injury (often such things as closed head injury). These are based on such things as mnemonics, the use of imagery and memory aids like lists or diaries). A basic description of many such procedures has been given by Wilson (1987) and there is a more recent review by Miller (1992).

An example of the application of such methods with a patient suffering from Alzheimer's disease has been reported by Hill et al (1987). This patient was taught to identify the names of people depicted in photographs by linking the name with a prominent facial feature as a linking image or mnemonic. In this way a feature that reminded the patient of a turtle was used to identify the individual's real name which was 'Tuttle'.

It is worth noting that these techniques can be based on the use of what Harris (1980) has described as 'internal' or 'external' strategies. Internal strategies are such things as the use of imagery or mnemonics which require the individual to make some form of internal mental manipulation to link things to be remembered (e.g. a face with a name). Harris (1980) has shown that normal people use internal strategies very little in helping to supplement memory. Normal people tend to rely very heavily on external strategies like noting appointments in a diary, making a list of things to buy at the supermarket, and so on. There are reasons to suspect that external strategies of this kind may also be more helpful with those who have impaired memories (Miller, 1992).

Those whose dementia is more advanced will have considerable difficulty in employing strategies of the kind mentioned to improve memory related performance. If these techniques have a useful role in dementia it is likely to be with very early cases.

Reminiscence

This is an approach that has been increasingly used as an alternative to RO. It was initially developed for elderly people in general (Butler, 1963) but has been extensively employed with those who suffer from dementia. It is conducted in a group setting and starts by eliciting memories from the past. This has an intuitive appeal since it is recollections of the distant past that remain most intact in Dementia. Memories from the past are often elicited by using special materials such as pictures of the local town as it used to be several decades ago. These can then be used as a focal point for discussion and to link with the present. For example, this is a picture of the Market Square in the late 1930s, how has this part of town changed between then and now?

Reminiscence has not been as extensively evaluated as RO although it has considerable popularity with those who work with elderly people suffering from dementia. There is evidence that both reminiscence and reality orientation lead to greater staff-patient interaction as well as increasing staff knowledge about the people they look after (Bains et al, 1987; Head et al, 1990). The trial by Baines et al (1987) compared reminiscence with RO using a cross-over design. the group receiving RO followed by reminiscence showed statistically significant gains on a range of both cognitive and behavioural measures. The group receiving the two interventions in the reverse order showed much more transient improvements.

Validation therapy

This arose out of what was perceived to the insensitive use of reality orientation. Like RO and reminiscence it has been used as a group procedure. Accounts of this approach are provided by Bleathman & Morton (1988) and by its originator (Feil, 1982).

Validation therapy is more concerned with the client's feelings and involves trying to listen with empathy to what the sufferer is trying to communicate about their feelings and to respond accordingly. Thus, if an elderly sufferer talks about her husband as if he is still alive despite having been widowed for some considerable time, then the factual error would be ignored. The response would be to empathise with the person's sense of loss and insecurity.

Although Feil (1982) has made strong claims about the effectiveness of validation therapy so far there appears to be no more concrete evidence as to its effectiveness. Unlike the other approaches described above it also makes alternative interpretations of what, at first sight at least, appear to be manifestations of memory impairment. In the example briefly outlined above the elderly widow's reference to her husband as if he were still alive is assumed to reflect a sense of continuing loss as well as, or instead of, a marked memory impairment. It would be useful to explore the validity of assumptions of this kind.

Conclusions

The ideal way of responding to the problem of Alzheimer type dementia would be by primary prevention if effective preventative methods could be developed. This paper has not explored all possible approaches to primary prevention but has concentrated on one suggested means, that of reducing aluminium intake. The balance of evidence, including the new data reported above on the use of aluminium hydroxide based antacids, indicates that reducing the oral ingestion of aluminium is not likely to have any beneficial effect on incidence. At one level this conclusion is disappointing but, as already indicated, there would be marked practical difficulties in reducing aluminium intake even if this was considered desirable.

In the present state of knowledge, promoting better mental health in those suffering from a dementing illnesses has to concentrate on ameliorating the consequences of the disorder. The increasing understanding of impairments in the underlying neurotransmitter systems may well eventually lead to useful pharmacological interventions. Such possibilities have not been explored in this paper but it is worth noting that the development of drugs which may produce some beneficial effect is unlikely to eliminate the need for other forms of intervention such as those based on psychological principles. Indeed the pharmacological and psychological interventions are far more sensibly regarded as complementary rather than contradictory.

A number of psychological approaches to the amelioration of functional impairments in Alzheimer type dementia have been outlined. What emerges from this work is that some techniques have been developed which can produce beneficial improvements although these are small and, as yet, certainly do not lead to major improvements in the way that afflicted individuals can manage to live more independent and fulfilling lives. Nevertheless, they do represent some gain and offer a base on which further and, it is hoped, more effective methods of intervention can be developed.

References

Alfrey, A.C., LeGendre, G.R., & Kaehny, W.D. (1976). The dialysis encephalopathy syndrome. Possible aluminium intoxications. *New England Journal of Medicine*, **294**, 184-189.

Ankus, M., & Quarrington, B., (1972). Operant behavior in the memory disordered. *Journal of Gerontology*, **27**, 500-510.

Baines, S., Saxby, P., & Ehlert, K., (1987). Reality orientation and reminiscence therapy: A controlled crossover study of elderly confused people. *British Journal of Psychiatry*, **151**, 222-231.

Benton, A., Varney, N.R., & Hamsher, K. (1978). Visuospatial judgment: A clinical test. *Archives of Neurology*, **35**, 364-367.

Birchall, J.D., & Chappell, J.S. (1989). Aluminium, water chemistry and Alzheimer's disease. *Lancet*, **1**, 953.

Bleathman, C., & Morton, I. (1988). Validation therapy with the demented elderly. *Journal of Advanced Nursing*, **13**, 511-514.

Burgio, L., Engle, B.T., McCormick, K., Hawkings, A., & Scheve, A. (1988). Behavioural treatment for urinary incontinence in elderly inpatients: Initial attempts to modify prompting and toileting procedures. *Behaviour Therapy*, **19**, 345-358.

Butler, R.N. (1963). The life review: An interpretation of reminiscence in the aged. *Psychiatry*, **26**, 65-76.

Downs, A.F.D., Rosenthal, T.L., & Lichstein, K.L. (1988). Modeling therapies reduce avoidance of bath-time by the institutionalized elderly. *Behaviour Therapy*, **19**, 359-368.

Eslinger, P., & Damasio, A.R. (1986). Preserved motor learning in Alzheimer's disease: implications for anatomy and behaviour. *Journal of Neuroscience*, **6**, 3006-3009.

Feil, N. (1982). *Validation: The Feil Method*. Cleveland, Ohio: Edward Feil Productions.

Folsom, J.C. (1968). Reality orientation for the elderly patient. *Journal of Geriatric Psychiatry*, **1**, 291-307.

Gronwall, D. & Wrightson, P., (1974). Recovery after minor head injury. *Lancet*, **2**, 1452.

Hanley, I.G., McGuire, R.J., & Boyd, W.D. (1981). Reality orientation and dementia: a controlled trial of two approaches. *British Journal of Psychiatry*, **138**, 10-14.

Harris, J. (1980). Memory aids people use: Two interview studies. *Memory & Cognition*, **8**, 31-38.

Head, D.M., Portnoy, S., & Woods, R.T., (1990). The impact of reminiscence groups in two different settings. *International Journal of Geriatric Psychiatry*, **5**, 295-302.

Hill R.D., Evankovich, K.D., Sheikh, J.I., & Yesavage, J.A., (1987). Imagery mnemonic training in a patient with primary degenerative dementia. *Psychology and Aging*, **2**, 201-205.

Holden, UP., & Woods, R.T., (1987). *Reality orientation: Psychological approaches to the 'confused' elderly.* Edinburgh: Churchill Livingstone.

Hughes, J.T., (1989). Aluminium encephalopathy and Alzheimer's disease. *Lancet*, **1**, 490-491.

Kay, D.W.K., & Bergmann, K., (1980). Epidemiology of mental disorder among the aged in the community. In J.E. Birren & R.B. Sloane, (Eds.) *Handbook of mental health and aging* (pp. 34-56). Englewood Cliffs, N. J.,: Prentice Hall.

Lezak, M.D., (1976). *Neuropsychological assessment.* New York: Oxford University Press.

McLachlan, D.R.C., (1986). Aluminium and Alzheimer's disease: A review. *Neurobiology of Ageing*, **7**, 525-532.

Martyn, C.N., Barker, D.J.P., Osmond, D., Harris, E.C., Edwardson, J.A., & Lacey, R.F. (1989). Geographical relation between Alzheimer's disease and aluminium in drinking water. *Lancet*, **1**, 59-62.

Miller, E. (1971). On the nature of the memory disorder in presenile dementia. *Neuropsychologia*, **9**, 75-81.

Miller, E. (1987). Reality orientation with psychogeriatric patients: The limitations. *Clinical Rehabilitatiion*, **1**, 231-233.

Miller, E. (1992). Psychological approaches to the management of memory impairments. *British Journal of Psychiatry*, **160**, 1-6.

Morris, E. (1992). Psychological approaches to the management of memory impairments. *British Journal of Psychiatry*, **160**, 1-6.

Morris, R.G., & Kopelman, M.D., (1986). The memory deficits in Alzheimer-type dementia: A review. *Quarterly Journal of Experimental Psychology*, 38A, 575-602.

Powell-Proctor, L. & Miller, E., (1982). Reality orientation: A critical appraisal. British Journal of Psychiatry. 140, 457-463.

Reitan, R.M. (1958). Validity of the trail making test as an indicator of organic brain damage. *Perceptual and Motor Skills*, **8**, 271-276.

Rifat, S.L., Eastwoon, M.R., Crapper McLachlan, D.R., & Correy, P.N., (190). Effect of exposure of miners to aluminium powder. *Lancet*, **2**, 1162-1165.

Rinke, C.L., Williams, J.J., Lloyd, K.E. & Smith-Scott, W., (1978). The effects of prompting and reinforcement on self-bathing by elderly residents of a nursing home. *Behaviour Therapy*, **9**, 873-881.

Rossor, M., (1987). The neurochemistry of cortical dementias. In S.M. Stahl, S.D., Iverson & E.C. Goodman (Eds.), *Cognitive Neurochemistry*. Oxford: Oxford University Press.

Schnelle, J.F., Traughber, B., Morgan, D.B., Embry, J.E., Binion, A.F., & Coleman, A., (1983). Management of geriatric incontinence in nursing homes. *Journal of Behavior Analysis*. **16**, 235-241.

Solyom, L. & Barik, H.C., (1965). Conditioning in senescence and senility. *Journal of Gerontology*, **20**, 483-488.

Sommer, R. & Ross, H. (1958). Social interaction on a geriatric ward. *International Journal of Social Psychiatry*, **4**, 128-133.

Tomlinson, B.E., Blessed, G., & Roth, M., (1970). Observations on the brains of demented old people. *Journal of Neurological Science*, **7**, 205-242.

4 The burdens women carry

C. Rayner

One of the particular reasons I'm here this afternoon is that agony aunt 'hat'. I want to make it clear that what I've got to say and much of what I think, some of you will say, as my mother used to, is 'teaching my grandmother to suck eggs'. Apart from what people have told me, I've been dealing with, on average, over the last 25 to 30 years about 1,000 letters a week. I'm still dealing with about 500 a week, a lot of people with all sorts of problems. They are not, 'my heart goes pit a pat, I did not know what he really meant', you know, nor is it 'which boy should I choose', nor is it deep and dark secrets about their sex lives, though I get those as well, most of it rather dull. It also includes a lot of anguish and very real pain, and a great deal about what we are here to talk about this afternoon.

I have been given a precise briefing for what I had to say to you, 'the aim of the Conference' I was told is 'to present, discuss and promote mental health as a distinct and separate concept rather than a euphemism for mental illness' and I think that is a very important difference to talk about. Preventing mental illness and being positive about mental health is not the same as talking about what you do about people who are already ill. That is an important subject as well, but the main function of my talk this afternoon was the promotion of mental health. Now I have to say that it is a very difficult thing to do because first you have to define what you are talking about. Long ago, when I was a student nurse my tutor set us all the task of defining what good health is and the best we could come up with, and it took us all day I remember, it is 'not being ill'. I presume this is a negative concept; the World Health Organisation has a definition which tries to be positive which says 'that health is a state of complete physical, mental and social well being and not merely the absence of disease or infirmity', that pleased me because other people saw the definition as the absence of illness. So it's a positive thing, the complete physical, mental and social well-being, but that begs the question. What is the state of complete mental well-being that we are here to discuss? I don't think I can outline that, the only way I can reach any sort of answer is to go back to those negatives, the factors that seem to me to make it harder for women in particular to enjoy complete mental health.

I was told to speak to the burdens women carry! So what are those factors? Well, the WHO definition makes it clear to me anyway that you can't look at one sort of well-being with out taking account of the other sort. And social well-being is very important indeed to women, and I think more so than to men. There is an obvious reason, women bear the brunt of responsibility for human reproduction, I mean we don't just give our bodies a good old battering when we carry a baby to term and, by the way, I can assure any man here that you are left shattered in more ways than one. We are also far more likely to carry the responsibility of caring for the babies as well as bearing them. I think it is one of the great natural injustices that for a chap to pass his genes on down the sands of time and all that 'stuff' is ten minutes if he is lucky, alright half an hour! For us women for every baby you are going to invest a good year of your life and probably more and you are going to do it with marked damage to yourself. I did the sums once, assuming that a man could fertilise a woman with every act, every emission of sperm, he would produce something like 6,000 infants. Quite a lot actually when you think of a life time and it would not do you any harm whatsoever. It makes you bright eyed and bushy tailed. A woman on the other hand, if she fulfilled her full biological function, if she had a baby as often as she could throughout her reproductive life (allowing for the possibility of twinning) which is common the more babies you have, she might manage 30. She would not be bright eyed and bushy tailed! So taking all that into account we have to look at the fact that women carry the brunt of reproductive function and we are far more likely to carry the responsibility for caring for the babies. Some of us are lucky and get the support of the baby's father. A great many more have not and that means that women's social needs are more pressing than those of men; we need safe warm clean housing more than men do because we have to look after our children. We need money to enable us to do our child caring job properly and yet because we are doing it we are prevented from going out and earning it for ourselves, the original 'double bind'. That is a very painful and unhealthy situation to be in and of course we do need opportunities for personal satisfaction and contact with other people because caring for babies and children is such hard work. With-out such possibilities, we are more likely to collapse under pressure. Add all that together and it is obvious that our social needs are greater and more complex than those of the average man. Now, he might like to have clean warm housing, social contacts and freedom from poverty, but he needs such things primarily for himself, not for his babies. Yes, I know there are some men who are one parent families and they carry all these burdens just as women do. But, that does not alter the truth of my argument, it just means that such men are frankly honorary women and more vulnerable as a result. Men with partners who care for the children are by and large free in a way that women with partners can never be. However reconstructed a man he is, she will carry the brunt. So let's get on, that's the social well-being.

Let us look at the physical factors! Well, if such physical well-being is past the definition of good health you have to look at ways in which women are extra vulnerable in the bodily sense, and guess what? surprise! surprise!! It's the same area they are socially vulnerable and that is the reproductive function. Now I don't want to play 'snap cancer of breast, that's cancelled the prostrate', matching male/female risks because of their different biological structures. But I have to say, women are generally more likely to experience illness, pain and disability as a direct result of their reproduction function than are men; from the minor tiredness and painful periods, and they are only minor if you are not suffering from them, to the major handicap of being in an advanced state of pregnancy. Anyone who has been in an advanced state of pregnancy knows what a handicap it is! Women are lumbered with all those extra physical problems. All of which may and often do detract from mental well-being. I mean, premenstrual syndrome may sound like a newly fashionable complaint, unless you suffer from it! The menopause may be regarded as a normal physiological event, nothing to make a fuss about, quite funny really, unless you are one of those women who have debilitating flushes and headaches, aches and pains, sweating and depression and all the rest of it. The risks of child birth and damage to the bladder and rectum resulting in constant dragging and nagging pain, possible incontinence (lovely thought!) and a sense of deep and biting embarrassment may seem unimportant, unless you are one of those women who daren't go more than a few yards from home or get involved in any activity that takes you far from a loo, because you don't have that very handy gadget that chaps have that makes it convenient for them. All this adds up to very formidable total and if you do add all these together and many women suffer from **all of them** and all women suffer from some of them, it will be clear that our opportunities for life long physical well-being i.e. health, are undoubtedly reduced.

So with that in mind, let's look at the mental aspect, which is the core of our case; as far as today's conference is concerned anyway! Let's assume that the woman has perfect housing, an adequate and safe income, a caring partner and other relations, lots of friends, lots of social contact, every chance to fulfil her personal needs and interests in an agreeable setting. Let us assume that she is that rare creature who never has a moment's discomfort from her periods, who conceives easily, has a totally trouble free pregnancy, gives birth without pain with no damage whatsoever to any of her adjoining body structures, without a hint of postnatal depression or later menopausal problems! None of that. Are there any other burdens a woman carries which might predispose a woman's failure of her mental health?

I think that there are. The fact is that it is women themselves who often subscribe to the pressures they experience, but that does not make it any the less onerous. In fact, it can make the pressure heavier because shame is added on to the initial problem. Image consciousness puts the heaviest burden on women. Because of the way the society has grown and structured itself, particularly over the last century or so, women have come to demand perfection of themselves in a number of roles. It is no longer good enough to attract a man until you can make babies. You have got to go on being attractive until long, long afterwards! The novel 'Pride and Prejudice' stops when the five daughters get married; that's all they have to do, get themselves married. After that they can relax. It ain't like that any more. There has been for sometime now, at least 70 years, a fashion for us all to look like pre-maternal women, (sexy virgins) and this image projected at those who are still young and actually are still partner hunting causes an enormous amount of anguish because a very limited number have the right sort of appearance for the dictates of fashion. I mean many girls look at themselves and they breathe deeply, because they have breasts that are too big, or too small, slightly different in size or they stick up or they don't stick up, or because they have buttocks and hips or they don't have buttocks and hips, or they don't have them in the right style. They literally weep, they break their hearts over every aspect of themselves eyes, skin, teeth, nose shape, hair in the right place (the scalp) where it's got to be thick and glossy and shapely and beautifully coloured and all that; hair in the wrong place, breasts upper lips and bellies and arms and legs where it's got to be totally absent. In fact they grieve unless they look like perfect cupy dolls which of course never, never sweat! Now that may sound extreme to you but I honestly have to tell you there are thousands and thousands of women who fret themselves into a state of near despair because of some aspect of their appearance. Now, all this would be bad enough if at least it lost its power once the young had found the sexual partner; could stop competing in the open market like the Bennett girls in 'Pride and Prejudice; but it does not stop women who, settled happily in long term relationships in spite of these hangups about aspects of their appearance, will still grieve and weep over what they look like; about the shape of breasts and buttocks and so on, and particularly when their bodies have been changed by having babies. Now, for years my mail has carried a really wide load of anguish carried by women because their breasts after feeding no longer look like virgin breasts; they have a few stretch marks and it's not just that, these women are not just a little fat, with the changes in their life they sit around saying 'when I was young'. I mean we all do that, it's quite a pleasant thing to do! No, these women are much more affected, they are desperately anxious and depressed and often agoraphobic as a result. They can't go out of the house, they write 'I am so selfconcious' about whatever it is. 'I would love to take the children swimming but I couldn't possibly be seen in a swimsuit'. Now, these women you could say, are being very silly. I don't think they are. They don't do it because they are stupid or because they are silly, they react like this because of the pressures that are put on them from all directions to look right. They are obsessed, no question about it! Let's face it, there is no reason why they shouldn't be. Look down any street, posters, television, newspapers, magazines everywhere! You look! The emphasis is constantly on what women look like. To a lesser degree now it is happening to men and I don't think you like it very much do you? No, well we have been putting up with it for centuries and its pressure is constant and we don't just get it from the advertising of course! We get it from each other. The awful thing is our mothers do it to us when we are infants; worrying from the word go what their little girl looks like, in a way they never worry about their little boys appearance and so it goes on. Women even put themselves at risk of life threatening disease and premature death with bulimia and anorexia nervosa because of their obsession with appearance and, although the many experts on these conditions will maintain that the behaviours of self starving and purging and vomiting are due to more complex issues than being concerned about appearance, I have to say from my experience of women with these problems, the role that image pressures play is enormously high.

That is what makes it certainly the worst part of it but, it's not just physical image matters. Let's just put that on one side, let's assume that they are absolutely gorgeous to look at, no problems in that area. Women

51

are also now expected to be achievers in every other way, we are supposed to be clever, to take a vital and active interest in every aspect of modern life, and what of the one's who don't do so and opt to stay at home? That is if they can afford to do it, (an important point), they are dismissed as only housewives. Very small value now is put on traditional female tasks linked with the primary burden of child bearing and caring. Modern Women are expected to do all that and also be honorary men, in terms of social, intellectual and commercial achievement. 'Having it all,' that was the goal that was held out to us and it's still there. It gleams seductively just out of our reach. We have got to be, not just wives and mothers, we have got to be beautiful and clever, and successful and high earning and wives and mothers and sexy with it. Now it's an old complaint, there is nothing new about this, it's been made over and over again; books, newspaper articles, women, sensible women have been going on about it forever. Well, I wrote articles on this theme back in the 60's in Women's magazines telling readers that it was alright to settle for 'who you are' and 'what you are' you don't have to be all the things fashion demands, you don't have to feel inadequate and deprived because you are not a standard beauty or a standard dress size or a standard sexual olympic gold medallist or anything else. But it doesn't make any difference however long we have been saying it, it makes no difference at all! Women still feel this pressure on them to be all these things. And something else as well, happy. These women who somehow pulled out every atom of energy they have got, and every atom of ability, and created this perfect image, the ideal home to the adoring husband and children and the high income and the whey ho! in bed every night and they are then amazed and angry to discover that they are not after all blissfully content; that adds even more to their burden because they feel guilty because they are not happy!

It happens to all of us. It does not matter how sensible you are, it doesn't matter how hard you try. I mean, I have been fighting this battle personally for years and I now feel, 'O God, I'm getting older, what good am I now.' I have to work quite hard not to allow myself to be swamped by that attitude that older women are worth even less than younger ones, and that's little enough. All of that leads, as I say, to guilt. You feel ashamed of your feelings, you feel guilty because you are being so 'silly', and yet you still do it. That defines the next major burden that I think women carry. We have, in my experience an amazing capacity for guilt and self blame. I remember a distraught mother when I was running a children's out- patient department, this young mother, she ran in cuddling this child, he was barely 2, screaming his head off, really quite ill. He was feverish and covered in very big very unpleasant spots, and she begged me, 'What have I done, What have I done, what did I do, to do this to him?' The poor little scrap had chicken pox. Now this wasn't her fault, it couldn't be her fault, there was an epidemic going on out there, but as far as she was concerned her first reaction was to blame herself, 'what have I done?' Now have to tell you, at that time I was 24, I had not yet had children. I was, I have to confess more, than a little scornful inside. I do hope I didn't show it. But I thought 'silly woman', I mean, how could she possibly blame herself because the child has got chicken pox. About 4 or 5 years later, I now had children and when one of mine had a rubella rash, my first reaction, and I'm an informed and educated nurse, a woman who knew, my first reaction was to check on the soap powder had I been using. 'What had I done, to do this terrible thing to my poor little infant,' he had German Measles. I mean it's there, it's built into us and I think its programmed in some ways I think from the moment we push our babies out into the open air from the safe havens within our bodies. We are consumed by it, we have made it more difficult for our children because we haven't held on to them. And it goes on to colour every aspect of our lives; if she doesn't pass her exams at school, he shows more interest in boys than girls, she still isn't married at 25, he hasn't got a decent job at 30. Oh! 'where did I go wrong'. I mean you can hear this in mothers all over the country. Now add this guilt, which is an occupational hazard of motherhood, to the guilt that women pile on themselves because they are not beautiful, or not clever or not sexy, or, the latest, not sufficiently liberated and feminist. You have got a very heavy load of distress indeed and all that leads to the third major stress for women and that is lack of self esteem. There are women who feel themselves so worthless, so useless so altogether a blot on the face of the earth, they lose all their ability to cope with the stresses of adult life. A lot of this stems from our own child rearing practices, the very women who are suffering this lack of self esteem are passing it on to their children. We bring up our children in this country by putting them down. We don't say to them, 'please don't do that I don't like it', or 'I don't like what you are doing', or 'don't do that I hate it when you do that'. We say 'don't do that, you are a naughty boy', 'you are a bad person, you are a bad child, a bad girl'.

In this room right now, somewhere inside all of you adults is a baby cringing, terrified that she/he might walk on mummy's newly scrubbed floor. 'I create trouble for mummy'. This is something that is done to us from the word go. Is it any wonder that so many people emerge into adult life already carrying a lack of self worth as part of their luggage. And the other thing of course is that I think so many mothers seem to spend the first 2 years of their children's lives teaching them how to speak and the next

10 telling them to shut up. But the result of this is an adult who feels they have no right to help when they have a problem. They don't seek it when they need it because, if they think of the Doctor, well, 'I can't go to the Doctor, he's too busy dealing with real illness to be bothered with me'. The Doctors sometimes actually confirm that opinion, if they do have the courage to go. They don't always know where else they can go, a lot of them write to me or my colleagues or people like me. Because we are seen as accessible, we are often the only comfort they will allow themselves. We are anonymous in the sense that they know us and we don't know them. And there is no risk of us passing them in the street and giving them a withering look that confirms them in their lack of self-esteem. So they write and tell us what it's all about. And they add guilt about the fact that they have written a letter to the other guilt they already had. The end of the letter, 'I feel better writing this but I am so ashamed, Claire', it's heart breaking, it really is!

So these are just some of the burdens that women carry that men don't. And of course, they carry the same ones as men. One of the current ones, a very major one for me is anxiety about the world in which we live. I'm getting more and more letters from people about this. Women in particular who worry about the state of the planet. About the risk of war and about the loss of status and money and security. Again, to quote personal experience I do remember vividly when the Berlin wall went up I had a 10 month old daughter. I had always been interested in world affairs. At the time of Suez I sat round in coffee bars with everyone deciding how we were going to put the world to rights. But when the Berlin wall went up, all I felt was cold sick terror and fear that something terrible was going to happen to the world into which I had brought this baby. Having babies does alter your perception to an incredible degree, of who you are and what you are and what your worth is. Of course the fear of loss of status and loss of money and loss of security, and loss of home is even more poignant if you are not just facing it for yourself but for your children. Of course some men worry about the future and they worry about the future welfare of their children. We know they do, but in my experience it is women who worry most and suffer in a most acutely poignant way. The recent wars in the Gulf and Yugoslavia and the famine in Somalia have brought me a great flurry of letters from women with children. All of them finding the anxiety about these matters hugely increased, because they have children, they find it even more painful to deal with. I sometimes feel it is as though childbirth strips several layers of skin from us and makes us suffer more pain more quickly whenever the cold winds blow. So back to our mums as it were, with all this awareness

54

of the burdens women carry. What can we do to promote mental health for them? Because it is necessary to do so, it is undoubted that more women break down into depression and into eating illnesses and phobic and chronic anxiety states than do men. We all know that women are the prime users of the mental health services. We all know that most women who turn up at their doctors surgeries, even if they present with physical problems, very often have a massive overlay of psychological disorder, and anxiety difficulties of this sort. How are we to take these burdens from womens shoulders or at least, make it easier for them to carry them? I mean, if I knew the answer to that, I would be a very happy and successful woman. I don't know the answers, I think that's why this conference is happening. I am hoping that you can help find the answers. And who knows, what you might come up with in the next few days; by Wednesday evening we may have a very simple, clear account of what we have to do to help women in particular to cope with the very severe burdens that they carry, which may make them so vulnerable, and I for one, look forward very eagerly indeed to hearing what you think the answers might be, because as a woman myself I wouldn't mind a bit of help carrying my load, thanks! So I leave that to you!!

5   Guest speaker presentation

D. Rowe

What I am going to talk about today, is part of the theme from my last book called 'Wanting everything' which my publishers with great foresight and planning, have not managed to get here. It came out in hardback a year ago and in paperback this week. It is a very big book and I don't intend to inflict it all on you. I just want to look at the main theme of the book and relate it to some of the things in mental health. I have take as the title something that I heard Adrian Love say back in the days when he used to be on Radio Two with 'Love in the Afternoon' he now has 'Love in the Afternoon' on Classic FM. I heard him say 'If ignorance is bliss why aren't there more happy people?' True!

There aren't many happy people. When we look around us we see an enormous amount of suffering. I was listening to Radio 4 on my way here driving up the motorway, and more and more terrible news coming out of Bosnia and such other stupidity. If you've been to Yugoslavia you will know what a beautiful country it is. They could have organised themselves into the greatest tourist country in the world, and just bled us dry, instead they've just destroyed everything they have got, really stupid. When you look at the amount of suffering in the world, present and throughout history, the amount of suffering that is caused by natural causes, changes in the climate, or in our body that amount of suffering is really quite small. By far the most of our suffering, 99.999% of our suffering comes from what we do to one another and what we do to ourselves. Curiously we do not seem to have any interest in finding out why. If you watch television you see lots of excellent programmes explaining to us what happens, you know John Pilger's programmes of investigating programmes, Cambodia, or on Saturday evening on Channel 4, Sheila MacDonald presents a wonderful programme called 'This Week'. But, when these programmes look behind, you know, why are these terrible things happening. They don't come up with answers like, this particular country wants to take over that country. Or this particular group of people want to dominate in that particular place. That's where they stop, they never go any further and say why? Now why do they feel like this? Why are the Serbs still fighting a battle which was fought back in 1941? and the battle against the Muslims which has been going on since the 6th century. Why are they still doing that? Those questions aren't asked, there is no interest in finding out the reasons that lie behind what we do. People will come up with explanations, but particularly stupid explanations: they really explain nothing. It seems to me that perhaps we could think about this in terms of there being two kinds of intelligence, because on the one hand as a species we are remarkably clever in understanding objects. We understand how objects work, it's not just western cultures that produced science and technology. All cultures, all societies produce a technology and a science appropriate to that culture's need and the situation that it's in. We are quite good at understanding people when we treat them as objects, we know quite well how to take a nice kind young man and turn him into a paid killer. An interesting television series now called 'Civvies', which the army denies's, but, the army officers, the whole military complex, are very efficient in understanding people when they treat people as objects. But in understanding ourselves, we show very little interest, very little improvement. The kinds of things that people discover in therapy, are just the kinds of things everybody has known forever. It is simply that people are discovering fairly late in life what they should haven know early on, somebody should have told them. In Psychology, a great deal of all the psychology that is done, is to discover things which everybody knew.

But we haven't made any great advances in understanding ourselves. Another curious part of this, is that anybody who has a high degree of the kind of intelligence for understanding objects, is praised and rewarded. But, anybody who is good at understanding ourselves, anybody who even shows an interest in understanding ourselves is not rewarded and in many cases is punished and persecuted. In the Health Service high tech stuff gets money, mental health does not. So, it seems like we do not even want to understand ourselves. Now it might be possible that we are actually born like this, that we do have two kinds of intelligence and not understanding ourselves is just one of those genetic deficits. Perhaps another species might come along after we manage to wipe ourselves out, and another species might have that intelligence in understanding them-selves. But, I do not think that is the case, I know that when I was training for coming into psychology as an undergraduate I was taught that we were each born with our specific lump of intelligence and you could measure it, and get an IQ, but no psychologist believes that now. We know that intelligence is simply a potentiality which is drawn out of us, or not, by the environment we are born into. So perhaps, there is something which happens to this second kind of intelligence.

Another thing that suggests that we are born with the intelligence to understand ourselves, is that it simply seems that babies have an ability to understand their mothers, they don't have the range of concepts to be able to explain to themselves why their mothers are doing feeding and such things, but they are able to make that imaginative link of empathy to be able to hone into what their mother is thinking and feeling. So it does seem as if we are born with that ability and we lose it. The reason that we lose it is that the adults engaged in educating us set about a deliberate policy of bamboozling us, of not telling us the truth. They withhold from us the necessary tools of understanding. We are not given them, when we are small children we are given the tools for understanding the world, tools like reading and writing and arithmetic and we learn and get the tools of understanding how you play games or make music, but we are not given the tools for understanding ourselves.

Now to describe how this comes about, just a general pattern. What seems pretty clear now is that in the womb, we start making sense of things. When I was an undergraduate we were taught that a new born baby had around him nothing but a 'booming buzzing confusion', as William James described it (William James we now know was wrong). We know that babies are born being able to identify faces, and prefer to look at faces, and we know that babies in the womb can hear and they can connect up one event with another, and when they realise that the first event has occurred then they expect the second. We have lots of babies being born who already recognise the music of 'Neighbours' and look towards the television with pleasure, new born babies, because in the womb mum always had a rest when that music came on.

So we know that in the womb babies form a whole lot of expectations and I would guess that one of the expectations that we had formed when we were in the womb was that if you wanted something you got it. Because in the womb that was it, if you were hungry you were fed. So there was this expectation that when we wanted something we got it. But of course within minutes of being born we discovered that the world was not like that, and we discovered loss. Now we complained about it very much that

59

we weren't being fed when we were hungry, we weren't being held when we were lonely, and the adults around us would be in some way explaining to us why we couldn't have something, and gradually as we came to understand more and more of language and what parents were communicating, we would be getting explanations as to why we suffered loss. Now if you look at the reasons why you can't have something these reasons fall into two categories. If I call them category 1 and category 2. Category 1 are the reasons you can't have something simply because of the way you or somebody else has chosen to define things. You're a little girl and you can't play rough games and get dirty because little girls don't do that. Now that's just a definition, little girls can do it. Little girls want to do it, but somebody has defined how little girls should behave and so all of us women in this room suffered a lot of loss in our childhood, all the things we weren't allowed to do because that was the way femininity was defined. And of course, all the men in this room suffered a different kind of loss because of the way masculinity was defined. Those of us who have lived long enough have seen those definitions change over the last three decades. So that's category 1. In category 2 are the things that we suffer loss of because of something like the nature of life, you can't go back in time. That is one of the main things, if you have missed out on something you have missed out. When you have chosen to follow one path, all other paths are then excluded, in the way time and space operate for us in the kind of world that we live in. So category 1 are definitions and category 2 have a certain absolute nature that relates to some of the physical facts of our lives.

But what happens to us as children, is that the adults around us explain category one losses as if they are category two. They make out that we have been born into a world where there are absolute rules, laws of the universe, and you can't do certain things because of these absolute laws. There is an absolute law of the universe, that feminine women never get angry, nice women never get angry, any woman who gets angry is challenging the laws of the universe, and will be punished by the universe. You know how those sorts of things were presented to you, by your parents; your parents were representing the state and the church. These were the absolute rules and you had to follow them, and if you didn't follow them you were wicked.

Now parents and teachers had a very good reason for doing this, first of all it was the way they had been given to understand life. That life was full of all these absolute laws, and secondly that it was a way of making us be obedient and stop arguing. Stop expecting that our point of view be taken seriously. When I was in Australia last Christmas, I was talking to a young woman, she was telling me just something, chatting about her parents, and she just said in passing, 'You know what it's like as a child'; and she's talking about an Australian society where everybody has a car, at least one car per family, if not two. 'You know what it's like as a child, when your parents sit in the front seat of the car and you sit in the back, and everything they say is right, and everything you say is wrong'. Yes that sums it up, that's childhood, everything you say is wrong. While we are learning all of this, having all of this presented to us, that we are wrong because we are children and adults are right because they are adults and they know what the world is about, we are actively being prevented from understanding our own nature and the nature of the world we live in. We are being told that the world is fixed and real, and what we see is real and what we hear is real. It's not explained to us that what we see and hear, our whole understanding, our whole perception of what's going on, is a very strange physiological trick that our bodies and ourselves use. That as I'm standing here talking to you I feel that I'm here and you're out there, in my external reality, well I think you're out there in my external reality. I act as if you are. But, what I am actually seeing, and hearing, goes on inside the box inside my head. You're not, as far as I am concerned, you are not out there you're in here, and you're sitting there thinking I'm over here. But, what you are actually seeing and hearing, are the structures you are making inside yourselves. You are only seeing structures that you have created, you are not really seeing what is happening. If we could see what was happening, the world would not look the way it does to us. The way we process everything inside that box inside our head, is that we simplify, we cannot see everything that exists, so as I stand here I see separate things, different people, chairs, lights. But, what is actually there is possibly like the physicists describe, if I could see reality what I would be seeing would be a whole mass of sub-nuclear particles whizzing round. Every so often clumping into a human shape clump and then whizzing off again. But, we don't see that because we can't see, we cannot be directly in touch with reality. All we every know are the structures that we create about it. Now if you have never come across that kind of understanding, it sounds really bizarre, and it takes a long while to accept it and understand it, and I write about that, in every article and every book I write I keep trying to find ways of describing it. But, if we had been given that kind of understanding when we were children, just gradually built up that understanding from our earliest days it wouldn't be bizarre, we would understand, we would know a lot more about it, and I wouldn't have to go around trying to describe it to people and say 'what you see is not what's really there, what you see are the meanings that you have created'.

Now the reasons we are not taught that, is because, no two people create the same set of meanings. Each person has their own way of seeing things, and we cannot do otherwise. It is not that we have a right to see things in our own way. We just can't do anything else, we have no other way of operating. We can only create our own world of meanings. No two people do it in the same way, because, all of us have different experiences. We have some sort of overlap, if we didn't have some kind of overlap we wouldn't communicate, but then we don't communicate very well, do we. So we have to interpret other people, and our interpretations of what other people do are different from other people's interpretations of what they do, that's why communications fail. But the reason that isn't taught to us when we are children is because, that would simply reinforce what children believe. Children believe that they have their own point of view and that they have a right to present it and for it to be taken seriously. Any child that is allowed to grow up like that, I know that some of my friends are letting their children grow up like that, it gets them into endless discussions with their children, they have to be forever justifying why it's time to go to bed. Instead of giving the child a clip round the ear and sending them off and telling them 'You'll do what I tell you because I'm your father, and not another word out of you, go' or 'I'll give you a good hiding'. It's much easier just to terrify kids into obedience and make them believe that what they know is their own truth isn't true.

Well, at least that keeps us all in business, we would have no mental health problems if we weren't taught as children that our truths weren't truths at all they were just silly and childish and we had to learn to think the way adults wanted us to think. Now, the fact that we get these faults, explanations as to why we can't have things, when we are children, does not stop us from wanting. We all want everything, I know there are some very good people who say they don't want everything. We always want everything, we want the world to be the way we want it to be. As we get older we might change in the way we define everything, but we all do want everything and we try to get it, by a number of strategies. Now the reason my book 'Wanting Everything' is so large, is because in the bulk of the book I look at the different strategies we use in an effort to get everything. There are the up front open strategies where people show that they want everything and these are the strategies of trying to get power, or being greedy, or being selfish. But then there are a lot of people who, while wanting everything, wish to appear to be good, so they adopt strategies which present them as not wanting everything, but as being tremendously unselfish. As taking responsibility for other people. Putting

62

aside their own needs in order to be responsible for the world and being very expert in feeling guilty. Now feeling responsible for other people and the world is a wonderful power ploy. Because when you say 'I feel very guilty because my family isn't very happy,' 'I ought to have made my family happy', or 'I feel very guilty about the amount of poverty in the world, I ought to do something and make the world right'. That's based on the wonderful notion that you actually have the capacity to make your family entirely happy. That is, control the entire universe, to ensure that your family is entirely happy. Or that you have the power and the wisdom to enable you to control the entire universe and make everybody in it happy, so it's a wonderful statement of pride, being responsible for other people. You can't be responsible for other people in the way that they interpret the world. Because the people make their own interpretations the only thing you are totally responsible for are the interpretations that you make. You are not responsible for everything that happens to you but your are responsible for how you interpret it. So, I examine these different strategies and then go on to show why they all fail. And they fail because we don't understand we are meaning creating creatures, and that everything in the world is connected to everything else. We see the world as being divided into sections but actually everything is connected to everything else and because we don't understand that when we try to get everything for ourselves we fail.

I would just like to look at some of the mistakes we make in the mental health field because we don't understand ourselves, because we don't apply the two tools we need to understand ourselves. What we need to understand ourselves, we need to understand first that although the world looks like it's divided into different sections actually everything is connected to everything else, and secondly that we are meaning creating creatures, we are always in the business of creating meaning.

Everything that we know is what we have interpreted: we know our interpretations, we don't know what actually happened. Now if we understood that, we would not have spent such a vast amount of time and effort, and inflicted so much suffering on people, by believing that there are such things as mental illnesses with physical causes. We would understand that while certain things in our bodies are happening all the time, what we know are the ways we interpret it. So whether we have got a physical change like a broken leg or a physical change like a change in the biochemistry of the brain, we don't know that, all we know is our interpretation of it, and these interpretations come only from our past experience. All the meanings that we create come out of the past meanings that we have created, we haven't got anything else. As an example, very straight forward, when one of the ideas we carry round all the time is the notion 'my body functioning OK'. You know, a sort of sense you don't often bring to mind, but 'I feel OK, there is nothing wrong with my body.' I think what most of us do first thing in the morning, just as we are waking up, is, we run this bit of meaning over ourselves, you do a kind of spot check, as you are waking up, and if there is no discrepancy between this meaning 'I'm physically OK' and what we are actually feeling, then we move on to other things to worry about, like, 'what's going to happen today?'

But, suppose when waking up you notice a discrepancy between 'I feel OK' and something in your body, you immediately have to give it a meaning, and you might lie there thinking 'Oh God, I'm hung over, I shouldn't have drunk so much last night', or ' I'm tired, I need another couple of hours in bed'. Or you might say 'somebody's pointed the bone at me', you know 'there's a witch doctor out there, who's out to get me', or you might say to yourself 'I feel sick'. Now suppose you choose, this one 'I feel sick', what you do next depends on how you construe yourself. If you value and accept yourself, you immediately move into the nurturing mode. 'I'll stay in bed today, I won't go to work', 'I'll get my partner to bring me breakfast in bed', 'I'll get her to ring the office and say I can't come in'. If you feel worse, 'I'll get the doctor to come'. You will do all those nurturing 'looking after' things for yourself because you care about yourself. But, if you don't like yourself, if you feel guilty because you exist then as soon as you discover you feel sick you move into the 'I am in danger' mode. 'I cannot ask anyone for any help' mode, and so you drag yourself out of bed, 'can't go and see the doctor, can't go and see him again, must get myself to work because if I don't they will discover how useless I am', and so on, and so on. So even we have got quite a clear, apparently clear physical change in our body, how we interpret that change determines the course of action. Of course, once you move, go off and consult the doctor, your interpretation may then be in conflict with the doctor's interpretation. You think you have got a physical illness, he knows that you are malingering, and then it is a battle as to whose interpretation shall win. The question is, why is it that some people supposedly having endogenous depression can produce all these terrible thoughts? The reason is they were there before, the potentiality was there, that's how they are interpreting what's happening in their lives. Another thing we would not wasted time on is looking for simple linear causes. There is a gene which causes biochemical change which produces schizophrenia, that's a nice linear cause why A leads to B and B leads to C. Causation is not like that, that is the very rare case of linear cause, because we live in a universe where everything is connected to everything else, everything that happens arises out of a vast network of causes. Now the ancient Chinese understood that or a great deal of their scientific work is based on that notion. But if we had understood that we would have got much more quickly to the kind of mathematic thought of being used now, in things like chaos theory. But we will spend an awful lot of time believing that there is such a thing as linear cause in all sorts of complex things, and there just isn't.

Knowing that everything is connected to everything else, and looking at that, we would realise that everything that happens in this world has good implications and bad implications. We wouldn't waste any time thinking about making everything perfect. Everything that happens has good implications and bad implications. What's been happening in Northern Ireland, lots of bad implications: but for a flaw in a setting up a bomb a lot of people would have died last night, apparently. One good implication in Northern Ireland is that they have advanced the cause of curing a head injury enormously. If you have a head injury on your way home tonight you will get much better looked after because of the terrible things that have happened in Northern Ireland. The same things apply to all the meanings we create. Every meaning that you create has good implications and bad implications. There is no way of seeing the world which will ensure that you live securely, freely and happily. Every meaning that you hold has good implications and bad implications. And this is something that needs to be looked at in therapy because quite often when people are resisting changing, the reason they are resisting is that, OK they can see that if they change then all sorts of great things will happen, like, 'If I stop being depressed, I'll be much happier and be able to do lots of things, but if I do that my husband will find that very threatening, and my mother will have to look at what she's done to me and that's going to be pretty awful, so perhaps I had better stay depressed'.

What we need to understand, is that we don't live in a world where there are absolute laws. There are no absolute laws, and that can only be a conditional statement. There could be some absolute laws, but we could never know them because what we are, the kind of meaning creating creatures that we are, we could never tell that an absolute law was absolute law. All we can ever know are the meanings that we have created.

6   Guest speaker presentation

Judge S. Tumim

Mental Health promotion improvements. Well, the first thing you have to ask about that is, 'what are these improvements for?' because in any question looking at prisons you have to ask that question. When I go about and inspect them and trudge the endless landings and so on again I'm saying, 'what are we trying to do?' That, I think, is the first question with any prison and although acres of libraries have been written on this paralysing subject, in actual fact there is a very simple answer to it. Its written up in a large statement of purpose in every prison in the country and I think it's pretty good. It says this 'HM Prisons service serves the public by keeping in custody those committed by the courts,' well that means that you have got to hold them there, you have to be secure or else it is not a prison, it may be a college, it may be a hospital, but it's not a prison. Second, 'Our duty is to look after them with humanity, care, and to help them to lead law abiding and useful lives, in custody and after release.' (Preparation for going out again.) Full stop there, end of statement. Nothing about punishment, punishment is not for the prison service, it is a matter for judges and the courts. They decide on punishment, and when they deprive you of your liberty they are punishing you. It then goes over to the prison service and their job is to hold you so you can't escape, to look after you with humanity and behavioural care, and thirdly to prepare you to come out again. If they did their job really marvellously well and successfully, particularly the third one, the prisons would rapidly empty and they would be out of a job. Because you wouldn't have the cynicism, you wouldn't have people coming back again, because they would have been prepared for a law abiding and useful life. But like all statements of purpose, it is what is called happily in the Home Office, 'aspiratory', and they do what they can.

Well now, in these prisons where you are preparing them for release you have, or used to have a prison medical service. You don't have it any more because, a few months ago they ceased to exist and were replaced by something called 'a health care service for prisoners' which is of course, quite different. It's administered by the same people, same doctors, same places, same hospitals, same surgeries, but it's a different idea. What does it mean? If you ask them they are a little embarrassed about it in the Home Office, because I keep saying 'how splendid to have a health care service. It means that I am now going to have allies who complain about the diet, who complain about the lack of physical exercise, not enough time out of cell, and what about the possibility of self harm.' Well, all these splendid either full time or part time medical men and women who are working, and thought they were working in a prison medical service, now have a duty of preventative medicine and they have taken upon themselves that splendid and valuable title. I am sure they are going to be very helpful to those like myself who have to advise ministers, and indeed they have brought in no less a person than Sir Donald Atkinson, formerly from the Department of Health, to advise them. So I look for a great deal of assistance, no longer at Brixton will 1,000 unconvicted young men not have a gym, because it's an insecure area, because now I have got an ally in the health care service for prisoners and they are going to come along and complain about it, I hope.

May I look at the position as far as mental health is concerned, because I have talked so far wholly in general terms. The Act, The Mental Health Act of 1983, provided in general terms for transfer of those who need it from prison to mental Hospital or RSU, whatever, and back again when they are better. The sections are all there, but very often it's creaky and doesn't work very well. The transfer depends very largely, in my experience, on the personalities involved between the prison and the hospital. But let us look for one moment at what is the problem of mental health and the size of it. I used to think that when the mental hospitals were closing, the old ones in the early 80's, that we were going to have an enormous number of prisoners with psychiatric problems, a vast increase, and indeed that was, I think, a general expectation. But it hasn't worked quite like that in fact, and there has been a report, as I am sure you are all familiar, by Prof. John Gunn taking a pretty large sample of prisons. He looked at I think, 16 prisons for adults, and 9 institutions for the young. The results that he came up with were that 37% of the male prisoners whom he saw had psychiatric symptoms actually diagnosed. Only 8%

were organic disorders, and there was a neurosis somewhat higher at 10%, psychoses at 6%, and the personality disorders were quite a high percentage. He concluded that from the symptoms the prison population included, out of about 50,000 people in prison, some 700 men who were psychotic and around 1100 who would warrant transfer to hospital for psychiatric treatment. Provision of secure treatment facilities and long term medium secure units needed to be improved and the service, both in the prison service and health service was in need of detailed and particular improvements. However, the figures taken generally are not as overwhelmingly depressiing as we thought at one stage thye might be.

So let us look for one moment at what ought to happen within the prisons. What is a prisoner entitled to by way of expectations, by way of treatment, for mental disorders? I think it is worth looking at that really quite basically. The prisoner with minor mental disorder, the neurosis and the mild depression, he ought to have, should he not, ready access to a doctor with good practitioner skills. He is entitled, secondly, to confidentiality. Thirdly, to a professional relationship with the caring agents, and access to psychological therapists. From a psychologist, or social worker, he ought to be able, if necessary, to have the advantages of behavioural therapy or group therapy. If he has got a major mental illness, if he is schizophrenic or severely depressed or suffering from mania or something of that sort, then what he needs is access to a specialist psychiatrist for an opinion and for treatment. Well, he doesn't always get what you or I would call 'ready access'. He needs ready transfer to specialist facilities, that is, to a psychiatric hospital, as needed. He may need to be moved very rapidly. He needs appropriate standards of care and a prison hospital. Let me pause for one moment and say that a prison hospital is very often like a school sick bay, or ship's sick bay. Perfectly reasonably, if you have got a modest sized prison, you have got, say, 150 healthy young burglars, you don't need to have much else, particularly if you've got a good local hospital and they are not a tremendous security risk. If they have a sudden appendicitis you whizz them down the road. If that's so, there's no need for anything unduly elaborate. But coming back to the psychiatric conditions there you do need, I think, very careful nursing access and psychiatric provision.

The expectation of suicidal patients, what are they entitled to? Well firstly it seems to me they are entitled to diagnosis. When they arrive they come into reception and they are examined, usually by a hospital doctor. Sometimes they have to wait for hours and hours, sometimes the reception is a very short one, so nobody comes, or somebody comes, and they are interviewed for a very short while. But it's not altogether easy to diagnose, it seems to me, in only a very short while. Some of the questions put to them are questions like 'Are you suicidal?', well I don't know, I am told in fact it's quite a good question. Distinguished psychiatrists say it's quite a good question to ask, and you get some very interesting answers. But, certainly that seems to me, something you have got to look at very carefully, and there where the hospital officer or interviewing doctor sees somebody and is not sure must be provision for intermediate holding them, when it is not obvious one way or the other. What should they do if they are thinking that maybe he is suicidal? Well, the first thing you must not do is, obviously, leave him to his own devices. He's got to be got into, preferably, a ward with all round vision, where he can be watched thoroughly and properly. If he goes to a cell, and if he is not regarded as too serious, there is certainly a case for that cell to have more than one prisoner in it. Because although one does not want to use other prisoners as additional nurses, suicide is a problem in prisons which everybody, not just the medical officer, must get accustomed to. So I think that if you have, in addition to that, patients with addictions, they are entitled also to be diagnosed pretty fast, and pretty regularly.

How do they move on from there? One of the problems we have had with prison medicine, one of the most grave problems over the last few years, has been the substantial increase in suicide and self harm in prisons. There was an argument for a long time in the profession that the physical conditions, grey and dreary very often, in which prisoners live, makes very little difference to their state of depression because they apparently don't notice. I must say I do not go along with that, because if you go to a prison that is efficient, caring and active when they are doing things, you get a far lower rate of self harm, if any than you do if you go to one of our urban modern monsters. If you go to Leeds or Birmingham or Liverpool, Wandsworth, Pentonville or Brixton, there is a high rate of suicide, attempted suicide and self harm. Very often the figures and statistics do not support the reality because a lot depends on how these incidents are recorded and the different view taken of that. But having said that, one does, I think, immediately have a view that the grey prison is where the real trouble lies and where the real trouble, in the sense of depression, lies more than anywhere else. Where you get the big urban local prisons the prison which to ordinary senses seems somewhat soulless.

At any rate, because of the increase in suicide, and particularly in one or two prisons, I was asked two years ago to report to ministers on the position, and I prepared a report with a team including the a distinguished consultant forensic psychiatrist, as to what really emerged from our inspections. What we found ourselves doing in the end was really preparing an advisory sheet as to how you could reduce the state of anxiety in prisons, in particular for prisoners who hadn't been inside before, and in particular without spending too much money, which I thought we weren't going to succeed in getting the Home Office to do. So we produced a document designed to lower the anxiety level. I am afraid I rather increased it in the Home Office I think, although we may have lowered it amongst prisoners, because we made 103 recommendations, each of them comparatively small and comparatively cheap, for example in prisons where the cells had no internal sanitation, we said that when the bell was pressed it ought to be answered by a Prison Officer at night. Frequently when I have been round prisons where it's not answered and you say 'Why don't you answer it more quickly' the Officer will say 'Oh! he's only showing off'. This seems to me to be classic, and it's the sort of thing we were attempting to remedy.

When one looks at these recommendations I am happy to say I am not going to go through 103 of them with you. But they included recommendations such as, that inmates should be involved in suicide prevention. They included a very strong recommendation, I think, that self inflicted death should not be treated as exclusively a medical problem. There is far too much of 'Oh! well if he's mad the doctors will find it out'. The doctors in prisons are not necessarily highly qualified in psychiatric matters, it should matter to everybody. Greater priority should be given to the quality of care in receiving people into prisons. The reception where you go into is very often the lowest and most depressing of buildings and of rooms. and if you put yourself in the position of the young person coming in for the first time, it is in itself enough to give very suicidal thoughts, and it is no better in the women's prisons than it is in the male ones. Links between medical Officers and local GPs should be improved. One of the difficulties with our healthcare service for prisoners is that it is staffed of course partly by medical officers who are full time and partly by local groups of General practitioners. When you think of prisons in terms of, say, a local school which is not a bad way of thinking about it, you think it would be better, surely, if they are all done or mostly done by local medical practices. So that when somebody comes in who is accustomed to dealing with patients from outside, it is, after all, only a bizarre form of general practice in prisons. We don't have any small children, thank goodness, and you don't have much by way of old people, so that you are dealing with limited general practice. The difficulty about that is that some prisons are going to be too big to be able to cope, and you need to have full time medical Officers just as a reality.

Sometimes there is a combination where you have a full time medical

71

officer but the surgeries always seem to be taken by doctors who come in for a time. This is something which I also notice as one goes round; there is, in other words a total mixture but there is no requirement that the senior medical Officer of a prison should have any psychiatric qualifications. One then looks at the position with regard to nursing and hospital officers. I have referred to hospital officers before, they are often described to me by inmates as prison officers in a white coat and of course they are essentially, many of them, most of them prison officers who are training for a few months in nursing. They have seen a lot, and a lot of them do immensely good work, but it is right to say there are a very low percentage of trained mental nurses working within the prison.

So one begins with that general picture, in the report there is a chapter, which I think is a very interesting chapter, comparing the position for patients between the NHS mental hospital and the prison hospital. Obviously, it generalises, it must, but this was done with great care with the assistance of forensic psychiatrists with great experience and I think it has not been criticized as factually incorrect in any way. But if you compare them in any sense, outside in the NHS if you are thought to be ill you are diagnosed by a GP and a consultant psychiatrist. In the prison where you are more likely, I would have thought it common sense, to be depressed than in Keele University, you are looked at by a GP and then by the Prison Medical Officer, but a Psychiatrist will only brought in, in the ordinary way, if he's sent for, so to speak, and that takes time. The outpatient psychiatric care outside is done by the consultant or trainee psychiatrist or by a community nurse; here it is done on the main wing by the Prison Medical Officer and the Medical Officer who I have said is essentially a prison officer. For inpatient care outside, there is a consultant in charge and in prison there is a prison medical officer in charge. He has access to consultant advice and he can of course, work very well but it is lower provision and all the way through that seems to me to be continuous. The suicidal patient in an ordinary hospital is observed normally by a form of continuous observation whether he's on association with other patients or in a secure room, but in a cell he's not in continuous observation; there is a 15 minute look through the door, but it is not a very satisfactory or well timed matter, nor is it adequate. Continuous observation in prison only happens if he happens to be in a ward or dormitory and otherwise it is intermittent observation and that is only for the more disturbed, and there is an hour when there are not enough officers on duty, so there are problems of comparison. At the end of the day what it comes to is that the provision within the prisons for the mentally disordered patient is not as good in general as it is within the National Health

72

Service, and whatever may be said of titles and Health care Services and everything else one comes back to that problem, which is a problem of staffing, of nurses and of doctors. What we now need to do is to consider very carefully whether we should not be getting a great deal more of the prisoners into mental hospital where they could be better looked after.

When I last inspected Brixton Prison, which is the biggest remand centre in Europe, that is for prisoners who are not convicted, there was, (this is now two or three years ago) F wing. This was the hospital wing, and it was very worrying and a source of great concern to my medical advisors, indeed to all of us who saw and heard what was happening, and our recommendation was that it should be raised to NHS standards and possibly run by the Department of Health. That did not go down very well, and has not been followed up. The hospital wing has been greatly improved, but it is still in a position where there are many inmates who shouldn't be there. Those who should be coming within Prof Gunn's rules should be transferred. One of the problems, I think, are passages in the 1983 Act 'the remand prisoner can be moved only', in the wording of the section 48 of the 1983 Act 'if he is in urgent need of hospital treatment, alternative of which he cannot be given in prison'. 'Urgent need', well it is a very difficult phrase to deal with; you could say 'well he's schizophrenic, but there is nothing desperately urgent', 'Well he's psychotic but he is not florid he's not in great urgent need', all sorts of ways out of problems. That is why I say I think it depends a great deal on personalities as well as activities. But coming back to my recommendations, they were essentially, comparing the facilities and making recommendations, as I have said, to reduce the troubles in prison, to allay anxiety. They summarised one passage in this way 'it is essential that steps are taken to confirm the dignity of the individual, especially where his esteem is most threatened. Every inmate should have the right to expect some fundamental standards'. This caused concern at the Home Office. A clean bed with clean, waterproof mattress covers, and sufficient space in which to live. Access to a toilet and washbasin at all times, with a daily shower. A reasonable degree of privacy, clean, presentable and properly fitting clothing, healthy food, a varied diet, careful medical attention. which should provide standards equivalent to those in the community. The opportunity to communicate by way of visits, letters and telephone calls, that, I must say, has improved considerably in the last year or so. The opportunity to receive assistance about personal problems, and preparations for release.

Well then that is my summary, you may think that they are wild, Butlin's Holiday Camp like pro-positions, but it seems to me that they are the absolute minimum which you can offer any human being. It is rather interesting, I think, when you look at the provision of mental health in prisons, one thing which we have totally ignored to provide, just cast your mind as to what goes on in a prison, at about four or five o'clock the prisoner is normally locked up in his cell, he is very likely on his own in the cell, he may have to share it with somebody else or two people, it may be that he gets out for an hour of 'association' that is chit chat on the landing, or whatever, in the course of the early evening. May be he does not, more often he does not. Then by 8 or so, finish, back in the cell, end of story until 7 or 8 the next morning. So, he is in a cupboard, a room, a cell for a minimum of 12 hours at night, very often, as I have to say, in a number of prisons he is in his prison cell for something like 20 or 22 hours in the 24. Certainly they are there for a very long time. Well then, one asks, if you are going to preserve his mental health, surely there is one very obvious thing, that is to provide him with a television set. Television may be a bore to everybody else, but it seems to me ideally suited either for the sick, the ill, or for prisoners. It keeps them in touch with the world to some extent, although perhaps an eccentric world, it keeps them up with current practices, News, sport. If you think it is unseemly, prison officers can turn it off if a particular programme is wrong. Why shouldn't he have a television set? He's allowed to have a radio, but on the whole, except for one or two experiments, he is not allowed to have a television set. The idea is that he will have to read and improve his mind. Well, how far that is from reality! I don't know how many of us would set ourselves, and stick to, a proper course of reading, if locked in a cell for 22 hours a day. Perhaps we would, but, certainly that is quite beyond the capacity of the average young burglar in his 20's, and he is not going to, so why shouldn't he have a television set?

There is one thing worse than an ordinary television set, in the views of the leader writers of some of the newspapers, and that is something called a 'colour television set'. That is infinitely wicked and depraved, and turns the cell into a Butlin's Holiday Camp; so that is bad news and when the prison service has experimented, in providing a television, or allowing it, there are two extraordinary barriers. First there is no provision put in for mains electricity. Although he has enough for electric light, very often cells do not have enough to provide, without conversion, for a television set. So he has to provide, out of his pocket money, batteries. Batteries don't last long in a television set, and he's limited to an income of something around £5 per week, £6 a week, even £3 a week, depending what he does. So that really makes a television pretty ineffective for him, if it were allowed. Secondly, our great glorious system of government provides

74

that everybody should have a television licence, and whereas if you stay in a hotel and you have got a television in your room nobody seems to worry about it, I don't know who pays the licence but you don't. Nevertheless, a prisoner going in for a few months has been informed by the Home Office that he is expected to pay a year's licence fee. I don't know, there may be some prisoners whose families could bring them the money, or something of that sort. It is just an absurd situation, and prisoners rightfully say that proposals for television are not serious ones.

What I said in the report we gave ministers last year, is that we favour an approach to inmates which, wherever possible, encourages constructive physical and mental activity. We see this as the most effective means of preventing deterioration. Even when the cell door is closed hobbies can be pursued or books read. But we realise that, by not being allowed television in cells, inmates are deprived of one of the most effective modern systems of distraction, information and entertainment. A strong argument against television in cells is that it may make prisoners less likely to pursue educational or other active interests, but in our judgement the argument is in favour of encouraging personal choice. That argument is healthier and stronger that television is likely to keep distracted minds occupied, and reduce incidents of self harm and possible suicide. In our view people held on remand should have television paid for possibly by public funds, while the convicted prisoners should be expected to contribute towards its cost. It is time also to introduce low voltage electricity into cells, for television and other approved electrical equipment to be used without depending upon expensive batteries. Then I go on to snort a bit about the licence fees.

So that seems to me one simple method by which you could reduce the likelihood of possibilities of depression in prison. It is a very odd state of affairs, government seems passionately opposed to colour television. It's always this word 'colour', which worries me slightly. But the problem largely with that background is a fear, I think by the Home Office and by Government that if they give in to this they will be open to comments in the public prints. An odd position with television, because it would make controls of staff a great deal easier. If you have got everyone watching 'Between the lines' or one of these programmes about the police, or about something like that, or even watching sport, it seems to me life for prison officers on the wing is going to be easier and not more difficult. It might even be, although I wouldn't push this too far, they might even derive some educational benefit from what they see. But at any rate there is an opposition.

I think that opposition goes to something very fundamental in public attitudes. We do have some extremely bad prisons, it could be said we have some of the best and some of the worst penal provision in Western Europe. Certainly some of our big open prisons are a scandal and some of the others are very good. But what we have is, I suspect, largely due to the sentimentality of the public in relation to prisons. We keep asking the wrong questions, 'is it too nice?' 'is it wet?' 'is it like a Holiday Camp?' We have a great thing about holiday camps, 'is it like a holiday camp?' is a very common question. Or is it too vile or nasty, too dank, too medieval in its dungeonry. They are the questions we ask, and they are the wrong questions. If you go round a lot of Europe and a lot of European prisons they are asking the questions 'are we keeping them busy enough, is it active enough?' and that, in my view, is the right question. 'Is the regime good enough; the way of life, are they actually getting on with something?' I went not long ago to a young offenders institution, and I was puzzled by what I found, because they were all on remand and they hadn't been convicted. I said to the governor 'How do you get them all running about so much? They are always digging potatoes, or learning maths or studying something or doing some work. They have not been convicted, you can't make them do anything.' 'Oh! we don't tell them that they have not been convicted, we tell them to go and attend a class'. It seems to me that there is quite a lot in that. I have never understood something very fundamental about our prison thinking. Education, which must be vital if we are going to prepare prisoners to come out into the outside world, is something which stops, according to prison service views, at 16, because you can't have compulsory prison after 16. Although it is provided after that, there is no possible pressure after that to attend classes. If you can say 'you have got to go and do some work in the workshop', if you can say 'you have got to go to the gym, you have got to do this', why on earth can't you say 'you have also got to go to a class and learn something'. Or you could put it another way you can do it by good old fashioned bribery, which is quite a good way of doing it.

In the state of Tennesee, I think it was, the practice there is to pay prisoners quite well if they work in the workshops , but you can't work in the workshops until you can produce a certificate of basic education. To get your certificate of basic education you have to go to the prison class rooms, and pass some very simple sort of exams and get your certificate of reading writing and arithmetic, and then you can go and earn money. This is quite an effective system of bribery. Again, if I may produce one other form of an idea like this. In France instead of earning the £5 a week or so which you can earn in English prisons, you earn about £30 a week if you work in a workshop, and if you earn your £30 a week you can hire a television set, or do it jointly if the cell has other people. A certain percentage has to be sent back to your family and a certain percentage is saved up so that when you come out of prison you have a bit of a nest egg and not just two weeks' social security money, which is what we do. There is more time for you to find a job, with having some money meanwhile. The idea of sending money home to the family is a very interesting one, because it is obvious there are social security complications if the family is on social security. On the other hand in England you are allowed, you may not know this, your family can send you in £2 a week, approximately, and there is a lot of pressure on the family from 'Charlie' in the nick to give the £2 a week although the family may not be able to afford it after scraping along with the wage earner inside. I rather fancy the French idea whereby the prisoner is actually pushing money the other way. It may be a very small sum, but money going to his family rather than coming in by way of private cash. The other advantage of course of doing it that way is that it helps to support what we really have got to do a lot more about in next few years, which are family links. You are not going to get prisoners avoiding returning in large numbers; you are not going to get them to prepare themselves for life in the outside world; you are not going to help them lead law abiding and useful lives after release unless, I generalise, you can improve their relationships with their families. One of the essential background problems, with prisons is that the prisoner tends to be a young man aged somewhere between 18 and 30; a man rather than a woman; he tends to be young rather than old; he tends not to be a maniac, a terrorist, a murderer, or a rapist, but rather an ignorant, slightly yobbish young burglar. Over 50% are in that sort of category. Now, he has failed at school or school has failed him, it hasn't worked. He needs some basic, very often remedial, education. He has failed in relationships more often than not, his relationships with women and particularly his relationship with his family.

When Lord Wolfe and I produced the report on the future of prisons, we recommended community prisons, by which we meant as far as possible getting the prisoner within reach of his family, so they communicate. Prison ought to be a place not only where you don't sit with a blank room and a blank wall with nothing to do, but it ought to be a place where you can improve the links with your family, and not let them get worse. So again, I think the money side comes into it. The family that has to produce £2 a week for you will get pretty fed up. That has got to be got over, so I would say that in Health Care, our new service in prisons, the Health Care Officers, which is my new invention for medical officers, have got to really look very carefully at how the regime is going in prisons, and how all this is starting.

There have been one or two recent and extremely helpful publications, 'Treatment, Care and Security: Working for change' published by MIND in July of this year, produces some extremely good ideas ready for the Reed Committee to report. Then there has been a best practice and advisory group report on mentally disordered offenders, which is published by the Lord Chancellor's Department, again in July. There is quite a lot coming out, but having looked at it like that, you still come to the final statement, which I think appears in an earlier report, the Dell report, on mentally disordered. Remands in custody are an inefficient and inhumane way of securing psychiatric assessment treatment and it is particularly with those who have not yet been convicted but are going to have to wait around, that the problem of mentally disordered prisoners stands. We have had, as you know, various attempts at bringing psychiatrists to magistrates courts for on the spot assessment. Very interesting schemes which can work in an absolute tight urban world, not elsewhere. At the end of the day it seems to me that you have got an essential problem in the relationship between medical matters and the law, and this is something that is very difficult to solve and may ultimately, a very dreadful thing to say, be insoluble.

When I was president of a mental health tribunal and used to go to Broadmoor and the special hospitals, and consider discharge and release, I remember having a number of cases that were really all the same case. They were the case basically of the man who, in a fit of depression, has murdered his wife, whom he was fond of. He had been found unfit to plead, sent to Broadmoor. I am thinking of three cases all of which fall within this. He was got on to proper medication within a matter of a few weeks. There was every reason to think he would take his medication regularly, it wasn't a question of irresponsibility,and while he took his medicine the psychiatrist's evidence was overwhelming that he was perfectly alright. So there was in practical reality terms, absolutely no case for holding him. What do you do? It is only six months since the national press was zooming about on the murder, it is all known locally where he lives and where he comes from. The hospital is not meant to be a prison, Broadmoor is a hospital. What should you do? Should you let him straight out? This is where the diagnostic difference between the law and the newspapers and public opinion would say 'You can't let him out', 'he's killed his wife, otherwise he will be getting away with it'. and the simple medical psychiatric answer, 'he was depressed at the time, he wasn't responsible, but now he is alright, and we have got his medication right and it won't happen again'. Well, its a difficult problem and in the end, as with so much, people end up with compromise. He is held a little longer, and gradually released, and whether that's right or not I don't know. It seems to me that where you are looking at the promotion of mental health one has to accept that there are very difficult problems of communication between doctors and the people who run prisons. I would need more psychiatric help actually around and within the available, that marvellous phrase 'within the available'. I would need to see, or would like to see, considerable improvement within the nursing provision in hospitals, and many more professionally trained mental nurses.

At the end of the day it could said 'well, should we be improving the provision of mental health in prisons? Because if we do, and we have a smashing mental hospital in Brixton or Wandsworth, are not the courts going to send to prison, people who they should be putting into a hospital?' It is an argument being put forward by Government, it has been put forward publicly and it has been put forward to me from time to time. I think it's a lousy argument I should think at the end of the day you have to provide for the people you contain, forcibly contain, as near as appropriate treatment as you can. If they are too ill to be in prison they shouldn't be in prison, they should be transferred. But if they are on the border lines or within the limits where they can be held in prison, then they must be provided with the best possible mental care which is comparable with what they get outside.

Against that background there is a long way to go. Although I make somewhat cynical observations about it, I do think the possibility of a healthcare service for prisoners is a very good one, because it brings into prisons for the first time something which they cry out for, which is the introduction of preventative medicine on a substantial line, and it is that line that I think, more than anything else, we should be pursuing within the prisons.

7   Guest speaker presentation

T. Yeo

This conference today on the Promotion of Mental Health is extremely timely, because in the UK we are recognising that successful treatment of disease and its ultimate reduction lies within the wider context of good health, that is positive good health for everyone, not just the absence of ill health. This reorientation of priorities has its origin in the World Health Organisation's global strategy for Health for All by the year 2000.

In England the need to concentrate on health promotion as much as health care, culminated in our White Paper published in July 'The Health of the Nation', for the first time since the formation of the NHS this country has an explicit strategy for health which provides the context within which the health service can operate, it also focuses attention on the broader health issues which extend well beyond the responsibilities of the NHS.

As you will all know, 'The Health of the Nation' identifies mental illness as one of five key areas and the inclusion of mental illness within those key areas demonstrates, very powerfully, the importance which we in Government attach to reducing the burden of mental ill health and of achieving optimum health throughout the country. Now the reason why mental illness was chosen as a key area really comes under three headings. Firstly prevalence; six million people in the UK suffer from some form of mental illness in the course of the year, that is one in ten of the population. Mental illness is as common as heart disease and three times as common as cancer, it is also a leading cause of illness and disability. The second reason was cost, mental illness accounts for about 14% of National Health

Service in-patient costs, and no less than 23% of NHS drug costs. So that the financial burden actually extends much wider than the National Health Service. 14% of absence from work is due to mental ill health, the cost in human misery, the suffering to both individuals and family, of course can not be reckoned in purely financial terms. The Third reason why we chose mental illness as a key area was effective intervention. Mental illness can be successfully treated, its impact can be alleviated and there are some means of prevention which are demonstrably successful. So prevalence, costs and scope for intervention are the three factors which won key area status for mental illness, the visible proof of the Government's commitment to effectively promoting mental health and preventing and successfully treating mental illness. The key area status ensures that mental illness is at the fore front of the National Health Service agenda, and despite now being a priority care subject, never before has mental illness been identified as warranting a nationwide effort to achieve specific targets by specified dates, This isn't just a one-off attempt; it's going to be concerted action from now on to improve services, with the targets adjusted as progress is made.

Our main objective in the White Paper is to improve the health and the social functioning of mentally ill people. We will realise that by setting targets, and measuring progress towards those targets. At the moment the only feasible quantitative target is in respect of mortality, in other words suicide, and in 'The Health of the Nation' we have set, firstly, an aim of reducing the overall suicide rate, by at least 15% by the end of the century, and secondly to reduce the suicide rate of severely mentally ill people by at least a third by the year 2000. Achieving those two targets will involve measures ranging from reducing access to methods of suicide, to improved supervision of care in the community, through proper and comprehensive application of the care programme approach. A misconception about suicide, is that if they want to do it they will do it anyway. We know that is not actually the case, availability of means is important, as illustrated by the drop in suicide rates when coal gas was replaced by non toxic North Sea gas. The introduction of catalytic converters to all new cars from next year, may also have an effect on the rising rate of suicides in young men from exhaust gas poisoning. The development necessary to realise the suicide targets, should be beneficial to the health and social functioning of all mentally ill people.

The suicide targets are concerned with reducing mortality but of course, morbidity is the main burden of mental illness. It was not possible to set quantitative targets for morbidity because of the basic lack of statistical information, but the Government does intend to set targets, and efforts are therefore being made to ensure that the necessary knowledge base is developed. So that Services can be properly focused we need to know how many mentally ill people there are. Where they are, and the specialist needs and requirements of particular groups. At a National level, we are planning a survey of psychiatric morbidity and pilot trials are due to take place this Autumn. At local level both health and local authorities are required to assess needs. That implies systematic quantification and the building up of user centred information bases, which will in turn allow services to be framed to meet identified needs. It is also intended that providers of psychiatric services periodically assess on a sample basis, symptom state, social disability, and quality of life. To do this the Government is already working with the Royal College of Psychiatrists to develop brief standardised assessment scales with a view to them being introduced nationally in 1994.

If the overall objective of improving the health and social functioning of mentally ill people is to be achieved, there needs to be continued development and improvements in local services to ensure that they are both comprehensive, and community based. The provision of community based mental health services will need to be both varied and extensive, ranging from simple domiciliary services through different types of day time facilities and residential services, to ultimately in-patient provision. The exact proportion of these components is a matter of local decision. But one thing is clear there is no room for those obsolete Victorian institutions which in the past too often dominated the local psychiatric service. They consumed resources, almost half of what the National Health Service spent on mental health services, and where their presence continues it can inhibit the development of modern adequately resources community based services. A mental health task force is now in operation to expedite the development of community health services and the corresponding demise of the old institutions. Under the National Health Service and Community Care Act of 1990 local authorities are required to consult health authorities and relevant voluntary organisations in drawing up plans for community care services. The Health of the Nation builds on this process. Not just joint planning, but joint purchasing, is now our goal. Joint purchasing by District Health Authorities, Family Health Service Authorities, Local Authorities and the relevant Voluntary bodies, can provide continuity of Health and Social Care. The mechanics for achieving this are already being hammered out and the task is complex, but the aim is for each district to plan for mental health services with the cooperation of all concerned and based on quantified need leading to joint purchasing of services to provide a good quality mental health service.

This is a vision about which the Government is both sincere and explicit. I am determined that it will succeed. Now I am well aware that there is concern about the community care changes due to occur next April. As you will know resources are to transfer to local authorities from the Department of Social Security. This will mean that they can be allocated to assessed need rather than as previously being tied to exclusively residential provision. That is in my view a major step forward. It will enable more people to remain in their own homes if they so wish. It is also important to stress that the calculations involved are taking into account the need to include provision for, among other groups, people with mental illness presently inappropriately placed in mental hospitals, who are unlikely to be discharged in the future. Further resources have been provided by the Mental Illness Specific Grant. This grant is payable to local authorities, to enable them to improve social care for mentally ill people. In the current year the grant is 31.4 million pounds, and as recipients of the grant, local authority recipients are required to make a contribution as well, the total expenditure supported by the grant will actually be over 43 million pounds this year. That money is specifically targeted to improving existing social care services and to developing new services. It is another sign of our determination that mental health services should improve and should improve rapidly.

One aspect of service provision which is particularly important, is respite care. In the context of good practice the White Paper specifically mentions as a high priority the importance of education, and support for carers of people with a severe mental illness. This support will derive both from the secondary care teams and the voluntary organisation, additionally the White Paper indicates that the voluntary organisation themselves are to receive local support so as to strengthen their contribution. Carers are by far the greatest natural resource that the National Health Service has in terms of caring for mentally ill people, after all the vast majority of mentally ill people are cared for outside the specialist psychiatric services, and as with other resources the carers themselves need to be looked after. Care for the carers, is most usually manifested in pleas for respite care, and respite can, quite literally in some cases, enable carers who have been providing for 24 hour care for years to take a holiday, or even just to get out to the shops without worrying, and without having to return as quickly as possible. Forms of respite care vary from in-patient provision to domiciliary sitters, who will hold the fort for an hour or two. Apart from the advantages for the carer there are potential clinical advantages to the patient in terms of assessment and a fresh environment, the opportunity to learn skills to enable them to cope away from home. Adequate provision of respite care is essential for proper maintenance of the large voluntary caring force, it is directly a means of promoting mental health. Respite care also has considerable potential for increasing the scope for care in the community. If carers are assured that respite care is available when required, then they will be more prepared to look after patients at home. Adequacy of respite care provides a yard stick against which the quality of a mental health service can be measured.

The auditing of suicides of mentally ill people, which some services now do, can also indicate improvements which may be made in professional practice and in service provision. Accordingly the White Paper states that health authorities should specify in contracts from 1993 onwards that mental health teams should introduce local multidisciplinary audits of suicides and of undetermined deaths of mentally ill people in contact with specialist mental health services. These audits will be supported by the confidential inquiry into deaths by homicide or suicide by mentally ill people which the Royal College of Psychiatrists is carrying forward by a multi-disciplinary steering committee at the request of the Secretary of the State for Health. In line with the aim of reducing the overall suicide rate we intend that eventually suicide for people who are not in touch with the specialist mental health teams should be audited by the Primary Care Team.

Let me now stress the importance of one improvement in service provision which is actually in the power of some of you here today to take forward immediately. I refer to the care programme approach, which came into force on the 1st April last year. We acknowledge that its implementation has been rather patchy and rather selective. Its main features are, firstly, that it applies for all patients being considered for discharge and all new patients accepted by the specialist psychiatric services including children and adolescents, secondly, each patient has an individual care programme which is drawn up in conjunction with all concerned professionals and in consultation with the patient, and if appropriate his or her carer. Thirdly a key worker is nominated to keep in close touch with the patient and to monitor that the agreed care is in fact delivered. In the case of the more severely mentally ill patients the key worker will normally be a Community Psychiatric Nurse or a Social Worker; for patients whose needs can be adequately met within the out-patients' setting the consultant may be the appropriate key worker. Full and proper implementation of the care programme approach would directly result in an improvement of mental health service provision. Its relevance to the reduction in suicide targets is obvious. Furthermore, full implementation will necessitate an effective and up to date record keeping system, so as to ensure that everybody who should be involved is involved and to ensure that patients do not fall through the care network. This approach complements The Health of the Nation information targets, that all provider units should have effective systems for collecting and using data about various contacts by 1995.

So far I have spoken about the necessity for improved statistics to enable us to set qualified mental health morbidity targets, and the development of comprehensive local services to assist in improving the health and social functioning of mentally ill people. A further area of development in the White Paper, to improve health and social functioning, is that of good practice, which the Government in conjunction with professional, voluntary and other bodies will work to identify and promote.

Good practice includes guidelines for the assessment and management of common psychiatric conditions; it also includes training of primary care teams to help them improve their recognition and assessment of depression, anxiety, and suicidal risk. One important aspect of this, mental health at work, will be covered this afternoon by Dr Jenkins from my Department.

Another area where there is scope for improvement in current practice concerns women and mental health. And in this connection I must mention MIND's current 'Stress on Women' campaign. I will leave it to Judi Clements to describe the campaign to you in detail but I welcome its aim to engender a heightened awareness of women's particular mental health needs. The campaign will strike a chord with many people, with its call for an end to the sexual harassment of many women in mental hospitals, or indeed in other health settings, and for the right of women with mental illness to choose a woman to be their care manager or key worker.

Choice for women in the provision of health services is in fact consistent with the general theme that we are supporting, for example in relation to choice of General Practitioner, or Hospital Clinician and in the provision of Maternity Services. The provision of women only wards does need to be balanced with the development of smaller, locally based units. But mental health services will wish to give active consideration to having space, particularly around sleeping areas which, is for women only. Offering the choice of a female key worker also seems appropriate, as does highlighting in training courses the particular needs of women and how a professional can appropriately respond to them. With regard to gender monitoring we are moving towards more uniform patient based information systems in which analyses of personal characteristics such as age, gender, ethnic origin, will be more important components of improved management data, and more responsive service provision. Women are of course, majority users of mental health services. They have a particular interest in our aim under the new community care arrangements to put the consumer at the centre. Section 46 of the NHS and Community Care Act makes clear that in drawing up community care plans local authorities must consult representatives and users and their carers. Assessment of individual care needs underpins the policy and will ensure that services are tailored to need rather than need to services. Our policy guidance makes clear that individual users and their carers should be involved throughout the assessment and care management process and that they should feel the process is aimed at meeting their wishes.

The Department of Health is currently in touch with MIND Link and the National Advocacy Network to consider how we might help to advance the cause of Advocacy in the mental health field through grant aided projects. I would also like to draw attention to the fact that since the introduction to new complaints procedures in April last year, users or carers can now complain to the local authorities concerned if they are dissatisfied with the services provided. If the complainant is not satisfied with the local authoritys response he or she can ask for the complain to be considered by a panel including at least one independent member. In relation to National Health Services patients have had the right, since the 1st April this year under the Patients' Charter, to have any complaint about services investigated and to receive a full and prompt written reply from the Chief Executive or General Manager. This is all part of the progress we are making towards real choice for users. Responsiveness to their needs, and it should spur on the drive for a better quality service. In addressing the health needs of people in specific groups of the population The Health of the Nation emphasises that the needs of women should be considered in relation to each of the five key areas. Finally as announced in the Health of the Nation a handbook is being prepared which will provide guidance and information to assist the National Health Service and Personal Social Services Managers to achieve the set targets. It is being developed by a group which includes the users of services, managers and professionals, and it will be available at the beginning of next year. That is the Governments plan for promoting mental health. Your involvement and your cooperation are essential if we are to succeed in improving the health and social functioning of mentally ill people. So I wish your conference today every success.

Section Two
THE PRESENTATIONS

8 Television literacy and young children's mental health promotion

M.R. Afzalnia

Abstract

In order to explain the cognitive importance of televiewing activity and how this literacy starts building skills in a child's life which will have long term effects, the article proper is prefaced by a brief discussion of the importance of television literacy and its importance in the promotion of young children's mental health in terms of cognition. In order to make clear this importance the article then proceeds with the results obtained from the present study and the discussions about the relation of children's viewing skills to their reading and listening skills. The article then concludes with 3 guide-lines for teachers, parents and TV producers in handling the children's television dilemma.

Television and literacy

The discussion about television literacy begins with the level and value of understanding and the ability to communicate with this medium. This needs a special education which contrasts with our conventional perception of verbal and mathematical literacy.

In the current literature of television studies, a real concern about the utilisation of television by children is that they are unable to decode the flow of the messages which emerge from this one-way medium. This arises not only because this medium is new to them or because it delivers a lot of information; but also because television lacks the necessary literacy for decoding its technical messages (e.g. formal features like zooms, fades, cuts, travellings, cromakees, etc.). This lack of knowledge in young children, according to many pioneers of television studies, damages their mental health.

Therefore, according to this viewpoint, television viewing causes quietness, silence and passivity in the audience, particularly in young children (Emery & Emery, 1974, 1976; Halpern, 1975; Krugman, 1971; Lesser, 1977; Mandler, 1978; Moody, 1980; Postman, 1979; Schorr, 1983; Singer, J., 1980; Singer & Singer, 1983; Swerdlow, 1981; Winn, 1985, 1987).

According to researchers, television viewing without enough knowledge of its literacy leads to low-level cognitive processing, and it needs less mental effort compared with other media utilization (Featherman et al., 1979; Krugman, 1971; Moody, 1980; Morgan & Gross, 1982; Postman, 1979; 1982; Solomon, 1979, 1981a, 1981b, 1983; Singer, J., 1980; Singer & Singer, 1983; Weinstein et al., 1980; Winn, 1985).

This argument concerning the low cognitive level involved in young children's television viewing was first initiated by Krugman (1971) and mainly activated by Salomon (1979) and it soon began to gain some support from others. But later Roberts et al. (1984) and Beentjes (1989) provided some evidence which challenged the above claim. The claim that less mental effort is involved in television viewing, has been denied by other theorists (e.g. Anderson & Lorch, 1983; Anderson et al., 1981a; Huston and Wright, 1983; Wright and Huston, 1983; Wright et al., 1984), who only blamed the lack of television literacy for this inferior understanding.

In terms of the social psychological point of view, throughout history, any new communication medium that has been introduced has been accompanied by its own literacy (or package-of-rules) which had to be learned. Reviewing the details of the history of human communication, suggests that literacy rules have been delivered before or along with the acquisition of each medium by the inventor(s) or the creator(s) of the message. In the case of television, following its antecedents of cinema and radio, it has had no literacy rules or directions accompanying its introduction.

Perhaps this arose because these facilities were created following widespread industrialization and the necessity for mass production of uniform messages. During human civilization, there has never been a time man has experienced so many changes in sign and symbol systems as he has after the two world wars. On the other hand, no time can be found in human history during which man has invented so many different communication channels in such a short period of time. The time man learned to communicate with the print medium (written language) occurred centuries after he learned how to use oracy and painting for his communication. But the time he became a television user took approximately less than a decade after radio.

According to McLuhan (1964), the appearance of each new medium of communication throughout history has changed the whole pattern of civilization, the entire life patterns of people, and consequently, man's perception of the world and his behaviour. With each new medium literacy, educational systems were tremendously affected. But what about television literacy?

While television did not bring its own package of literacy along with its introduction, people spent a large amount of time in front of this medium. And, this massive use of television made parents and educators concerned about the potential effects of television on children's educational achievements.

Sensitivity to television's impact on schooling arose mainly because the fundamentals of education, from its very origin, have been rooted in the acquisition of verbal skills and the skills of computation. Television is blamed for reducing these skills, or for the willingness to downgrade them. These theorists were concerned about the social and psychological impacts of television on the time children spent on cognitive activities. They regarded this as an indirect effect of television on children's cognitive and mental growth from the aspect of health. They raised concerns on the part of social observers: policy makers, educators, and particularly parents.

They said if children spend so much time on watching television without thoroughly understanding it, what would be displaced? This major argument assumes that the time spent on television viewing activity is taken from other cognitive activities. Therefore, television viewing displaces activities such as:

- play
- homework and serious studies
- leisure reading (mainly comics)
- other leisure activities (e.g. cinema & theatre going, radio listening)
- social gatherings with friends and going out
- and causes children to go to bed late and miss their early school class topics.

(Belson, 1960; Coffin, 1955; Cramond, 1976; Fiske, 1978; Furu, 1971, 1977; Gadberry, 1977, 1980; Harrison & Williams, 1986; Himmelweit et al., 1958; Lu & Tweenten, 1973; Morgan & Gross; 1982; Murray & Kippax, 1978: Paschal, Weinstein & Walberg, 1984; Riley, Cantwell, & Ruttinger, 1949; Robinson, 1969; 1972a; Rubinstein & Perkins, 1976; Schramm, Lyle & Parker, 1961; Scott, 1956; Slater, 1963; Starkey & Swinford, 1974; Timmer, Eccles, & O'Brien, 1985; Walberg, 1984, Walberg & Tsai, 1985; Werner,

1975; Williams & Handford, 1986; Witty, 1967; Wolfe, Mandes & Factor, 1984).

Considering the power of literacy, it is assumed that literate people not only use different patterns of mental effort in their problem solving; they also use higher mental capabilities (Scribner & Cole 1978, 1981). Nevertheless, perhaps no experiment can yet demonstrate whether in fact a wholly literate or wholly illiterate society would be possible at all.

On the other hand, however, considering many other cognitive aspects of literacy, it cannot be accepted that the mere sum of verbal skills per se, without sensible developments in our imagination and creative reasoning, can be regarded as a general literacy.

It has been argued that if the basis of education and literacy is to teach children how to think properly and accurately, then perhaps television is furnishing this goal in accordance with new world requirements and in its own way (e.g. Rice et al., 1983; Wright and Huston, (in press)). Perhaps, as Illich (1969) puts it, television would be only suitable for post-literacy environments.

In processing television, the viewer engages in activities that are comparable to other cognitive activities that are usually taught at schools. If learning and literacy is regarded as the development of connected circuits in the brain (Thompson, 1985) (in terms of knowledge schemata), then these connections presumably may occur as a result of viewing conditions and a form of cognition will take place which will result from television literacy (Abelman and Courtright, 1983).

Television viewing as a cognitive activity

In television literacy, practices like 'selective attention', 'reading formal features of television', drawing inferences (focusing on important information and discarding the rest)', 'applying one's existing knowledge to what is presented on television', and 'decoding the main ideas' provide examples (Abelman and Courtright, 1983).

In the limited existing literature which has concerned this matter, it has been argued that if any increases in the viewer's interpretation ability take place, they would reside in the learning of formal features. Anderson and Lorch (1983) in their comprehensive review on this matter, have reported that this ability to interpret formal features is learned because it does not take place in young children under two and a half years of age.

According to them, children appear to learn television viewing strategies as they grow up with television. They become television literate people and use their know-how to better handle and manipulate television information. It has been suggested that children learn these strategies through their selective attention (Anderson and Lorch, 1983; Anderson and Collins, 1988).

Television literacy and attentional strategies are, therefore, geared with each other. Studies have so far found that there is a strong relationship between the comprehension of a television programme and maintaining attention (e.g. Abelman and Courtright, 1983; Afzalnia, 1992; Anderson et al., 1981; Burns & Anderson, 1990; Hornik, 1981; Salomon, 1979; Wright & Huston, 1983).

The more recent information on televiewing skills provides a base for speculating that television viewing is an activity which might develop into a skill by itself (Abelman & Courtright, 1983; Masterman, 1983a, 1983b, 1989). This skill could develop in children at about their tenth year, when the integration of audio and visual modalities is extensively experienced and exercised in a particular way. This decoding of integrated information might open a domain which has never been exercised to this extent before (Pezdek, 1987).

Salomon (1979) indicated that mastering the symbol systems which are emphasized by a particular medium eases decoding and learning from that medium. The long-run processing of television's formal feature and syntax of cinematic messages will provide a sort of expertise which eventually might lead to automation of this action. Just as one learns in reading: 'Symbols can stand for thoughts and ideas' (Hornik, 1981; P.229).

So, television is a vehicle for different symbol systems (verbal language, colour, space, depth, motion, positions, gestures, visual effects, sound effects, etc.). The unique pattern of combination of these various symbol systems in the form of television messages requires a particular kind of processing that other formats in print or aural communication might not need (Olson & Bruner, 1974).

In other words, the essential difference between a verbal statement, a visual medium like a poster a map, or a television presentation lies not necessarily in the content which is conveyed, but in the form of symbol systems which are used in order to convey a message. According to Salomon (1979), different codes or formats affect different clusters of mental skills which differentially mediate the acquisition of knowledge. Therefore, learning the formats typical of a particular medium enhances certain skills which are unique to that format alone. Learning to decode these symbols, by itself, can indeed improve the mastery of relevant skills (Hornik, 1981; Pezdek and Stevens, 1984; Rice, 1983, 1984; Salomon, 1979).

In the case of television, Rice (1983), (1984) and Rice and Haight (1986) suggest that learning of television language is achieved by mastering the ability to decode ikonic and linguistic information. These codes, according to research findings, require different kinds of viewer's knowledge.

Anderson and Collins' (1988) review of research on the impact of television on children's cognition proposes that children watching television usually 'deploy attentional strategies and engage in rich inferential activities much as they do during other receptive cognitive activities, such as listening, or reading' (p.16). Learning these attentional strategies, along with other viewing skills, will enhance cognitive skills and promotes children's mental health (Hornik, 1981).

In fact viewing skill consists of both verbal and visual abilities integrated into a single skill (Pezdek and Stevens, 1984). It is the ability to select a programme and interpret what is seen and heard. In order to get to this stage one needs a good knowledge of visual literacy and television syntax which applies to television literacy. In other words, **teaching television literacy to young children enhances their viewing skills that consists of abilities which are essential to decode the television message** (Abelman & Courtright, 1983; Greenfield, 1984; Masterman, 1983a; 1989; Salomon, 1979; Wober, 1988).

In order to investigate the linear relationship between children's viewing comprehension and their reading and listening skills as two aspects of their general cognition, and mental growth the present study has searched for the examination of the following hypothesis.

Hypothesis

children's viewing comprehension can significantly be related to their reading, listening and IQ achievements.

Subjects and the sample size

Since the intention of this study was to try to obtain a reasonably representative sample of British 9-10 year old children, 78 pupils from three parallel classes in the same junior school, ranging from 9.3 to 9.11 years old were chosen as a sample.

From a socioeconomic point of view, the sample was restricted to middle-class English children. In terms of the sample homogeneity, these groups of students were said by the school to be consistent groups. The results from various test scores obtained in this study also confirmed that this claim was indeed true.

Measurements

Measuring the variables considered in this study, different instruments were needed which are discussed below:

Teachers' questionnaire

This questionnaire was designed to explore the participants' academic performance in the school. In it, I asked the three form teachers in the school to report on each child's ability in skills related to all of the children's verbal communication skills including speaking, listening, reading, and writing. Also they were asked to report children's reading scores obtained in their reading test.

Reliability

Each of the teachers was asked to repeat the questionnaire for several pupils in their class chosen at random. The percentage agreement between first and second version was nearly 90%. The internal consistency of groups of related questions provided further supportive evidence of reliability. For example, in a group of three questions asking about children's reading abilities the teachers provided answers which were highly correlated [r **questions related to reading ability were = 0.95, 0.90, 0.88; all Ps were < 0.001**].

In another group of four listening questions the teachers responded such that they were highly consistent with each other [r **questions related to listening ability were = 0.98, 0.78, 0.92, 0.80, all Ps < 0.001**]. In the three question group related to speaking ability the results were similar [r = **0.88, 0.87, 0.90, all Ps < 0.001**]. Also, in a four questions group related to children's writing ability they again provided answers which were highly consistent [r = **0.78, 0.67. 0.78, 0.64, all the Ps were < 0.001**].

Validity

The close relationships between the teachers' reports on their children's reading and listening with the scores obtained on nationally standardised reading test results provided support for the validity of this questionnaire.

School based tests of reading and IQ

There were two groups of tests which were used in this study: In the first group, two ready-made tests were chosen in order to assess children's reading skills and IQ level. The Suffolk Reading test and AH1 perceptual reasoning test (taken as non-verbal IQ test) were obtained from NFER to perform the required measurements. In the second group, two listening tests and one viewing comprehension test were developed by the investigator (Afzalnia, 1992).

The listening test

According to the literature, one of the difficulties in studying relation-ships between reading and listening in the past has been the lack of suitable instruments to measure listening ability. Researchers have suggested that listening to a story requires the ability to concentrate and decode the entire idea through a meaningful discourse analysis (Afzalnia, 1992; Beery, 1954).

However, the ability to detect and identify sounds from background noise or in particular positions is another aspect of listening skill. It has been suggested that these two basic skills together form the essential parts of the whole that make up listening ability (Afzalnia, 1992; Barbe & Roberts, 1954). Therefore, for the purpose of this study, two listening tests were needed. One to measure children's listening comprehension and the other to measure their listening accuracy.

After two pilot versions, a 20-question test that measured listening comprehension of a story and a 30-question test that measured children's ability in detecting different sounds and noises was created. The corre-lation between these two tests [$r = 0.40, P < 0.001$] and their reliability and validity measures were quite acceptable for the purpose of this study (Afzalnia, 1992).

The viewing comprehension test

A viewing comprehension test was created based upon a ten minute cartoon programme. After two pilot studies of this test, I was able to select 30 questions for the final version. In order to test different aspects of comprehension, I organised the items in the following way: There were **six** questions which asked about information related to **sequences of events** (questions 11, 12, 13, 16, 18, and 23).

There were **six** questions which asked about information related to **central themes**; of which **three** were related to **pictures** and **three** were related to **sound/sound-effects** (questions 2, 8, 14, 17, 21, and 25).

There were **six** questions which asked about information related to **incidental events**; of which **three** were related to **pictures** and **three** were related to **sound/sound-effects** (questions 6, 3, 5, 10, 29, and 30).

There were **six** questions which asked about information related to the child's **inferences**; of which **three** were related to **pictures** and **three** were related to **sound/sound-effects** (questions 7, 9, 15, 19, 20, and 24).

There were **sic** questions which asked about information related to **details**; of which **three** were related to **more obvious** ones and **three** were related to **less obvious** ones (questions 1, 4, 22, 26, 27, and 28).

Thus, the **aim** of this viewing test was, therefore, **to assess the children's** understanding of the television cartoon programme that was used in this study.

Reliability

In the analysis of results, the internal consistency values for the 'viewing comprehension' test were derived from the **Kuder-Richardson** (Guildford, 1982), formula 21 and indicated that the R_{xx} for the 'viewing comprehension' test was significant [**r = 0.87, P < 0.001**]. This shows that the viewing comprehension test was highly reliable in its measurement.

Validity

When this test was piloted the distribution of the test results (both times) fell within a normal curve. Furthermore, in terms of **criterion validity**, the test's high correlations with children's major abilities supports its validity [**r Suffolk = 0.73 r listening scores = 0.63, r IQ = 0.53**]. Therefore, the test is appropriate for its uses to be reported. Having these measures, it was found that this measurement tool was significantly reliable and valid for the purpose of this study (Afzalnia, 1992). Thus the children completed these five tests, and the teachers their questionnaire. The results were as follows.

Results and discussion

A calculation of linear correlation between the test results indicated that the test outcomes were significantly and highly related to each other. Table 1 shows the results.

Table 1
Cross-relationships between tests' results

Correlations	B	C	D	E
A	.70***	.71***	.73***	.63***
B		.63***	.63***	.57***
C			.58**	.47***
D				.53***

N = 78   1-tailed Signif: *.05   **.01   ***.001

A = Suffolk Reading Test Scores
B = Sum of both Listening Test Scores
C = Teachers' Reading Test Scores
D = Viewing Comprehension Test Scores
E = Perceptual Reasoning Test Scores (IQ)

As can be seen, all of these test results are reasonably and significantly correlated with IQ with the highest correlation between the Suffolk reading test results and IQ [r = 0.63, P< 0.001]. Also it is shown that the viewing comprehension test scores have the highest relationship with Suffolk reading test results [r = 0.73, P < 0.001].

Table 2 shows that the correlations between children's viewing comprehension and their verbal receptive skills, obtained from the teachers' reports are also high, positive, and significant at P< 0.001.

Table 2
The relationships between children's IQ and viewing comprehension test scores with the teachers' estimates of their verbal communication skills

	IQ	Television Comprehension
using active vocabulary	0.55**	0.52**
speaking long sentences	0.59**	0.53**
making speech clear	0.48**	0.52**
reading accuracy	0.48**	0.54**
reading speed	0.51**	0.53**
reading comprehension	0.53**	0.56**
spelling speed	0.50**	0.50**
spelling accuracy	0.54**	0.52**
writing composition	0.48**	0.61**
writing - letter formation	0.44**	0.56**
listening accuracy	0.46**	0.51**
listening comprehension	0.43**	0.49**
listening attentiveness	0.46**	0.49**
listening speed	0.49**	0.58**
N = 78 1-tailed signif:	**0.001	

As can be seen, all the correlations are highly significant. The above data support the information presented in the previous table regarding the high correlation between children's IQ and viewing comprehension test scores with their reading and listening test scores.

As the data in Table 2 revealed, the relationship between children's 'general listening' and 'reading' skills with their 'viewing comprehension' was highly significant. These relationships are found to be [$r = 0.73$, 0.58, and 0.63, $P< 0.001$] respectively. This finding suggests that **children's IQ, reading, and general listening scores can be predictive of their comprehension of television, and vice versa.**

These results are consistent with that of Alvarez et al. (1988) and with Brooks (1984) who also found a close relationship between children's viewing comprehension and IQ with children's reading skills. Also, the high correlations between television viewing, and children's reading and listening obtained in this study is consistent with those of Neuman (1988) and Furu (1977) who also reported similar results.

Summary and conclusion

The hypothesis, which predicted that children's viewing comprehension can be predictive of their reading, listening and IQ achievements, is strongly confirmed in this study. This shows that children who had a lower score in viewing comprehension skills had also lower grades in their IQ, reading and listening skills.

Therefore, it can be inferred that if as the results of the present study show, the correlations between IQ, reading and listening ability with television comprehension are significantly high, and as the results of several other studies (e.g. Sticht et al., 1974) have indicated that the correlations between all four verbal communication skills are also high, then it is likely that viewing comprehension skill will also be correlated with other verbal skills (e.g. speaking and writing) to a high degree as well. This assumption adds to the importance of television literacy for children at a young age.

Sticht et al., (1974) having had a comprehensive study on the relationships between verbal communication skills have suggested that promotion of one verbal skill (e.g. listening), through effective instructions, will lead to the promotion of the others. Having the above results shows that this might be the case for the viewing comprehension skill as well. Therefore, it can be implied that having television literacy for children may help them to promote their general cognitive abilities.

Summing up the above discussions, the present study has yielded some implications and insights for parents and for policy makers and educational psychologists involved in making decisions concerning television education, and reading and listening curricula. Therefore, there are three major guide-lines which could be drawn up: One for education officials, one for parents, and one for tv producers.

Guide-line One

It is important for practitioners to remember that, in order to develop viewing skills, consideration needs to be made of formal education for teaching viewing skills. Some schemes, which are already running on a small scale, (e.g. Kelley et al., 1985, 1987) could be implemented more widely.

Guide-line Two

Parents need to recognize the importance of television viewing skills as an important element in their children's education. Instead of constantly blaming television they need to recognize the development of viewing skill which deserves careful attention. Parents, also, need to be informed about the importance of the quality of viewing and about the benefits of the television viewing skills for their children's cognitive growth.

Parents should reward their children when they are selective in their viewing activity and watch programmes that include more than pure entertainment programmes. In other words they should feel responsible in directing and orienting their children's viewing activities and not merely critical of their amount of viewing.

Guide-line Three

Television makers need to produce particular programmes which teach appropriate strategies to parents concerning how best they can handle their children's viewing activity along with their formal schooling. Such programmes should help parents to decide more positively on how to organise their children's viewing time. Also, the priority in the production of television programmes which teaches photographic, cinematic and television language should lie in simple explanation. Other related teaching materials and guides should be added to this in order to make a package which can provide a comprehensive tele-literacy delivery for nursery and primary school teachers.

References

Abelman, R. & Courtright,J.(1983).Television literacy: Amplifying the cognitive level effects of television's prosocial fare through curriculum intervention. *Journal of Research and Development in Education*, **17**, (1), 46-57.

Afzalnia, M.R. (1992). *Reading, listening and television viewing: A study of children's cognition.* Doctoral thesis submitted to Keele University, England.

Alvarez, M.M., Huston, A.C., Wright, J.C., & Kerkman, D.D. (1988). Gender differences in visual attention to television form and content. *Journal of Applied Developmental Psychology*, **9**, 459-475

Anderson, D.R., & Collins, P.A. (1988). *The impact on children's education: Television's influence on cognitive development.* Washington, DC: U.S. Department of Education

Anderson, D. & Lorch, E. (1983). Looking at television: Action or reaction? In J. Bryant & D.R. Anderson (Eds.), *Children's understanding of television: Research on attention and comprehension* (pp. 1-34). New York: Academic Press.

Anderson, D.R., Lorch, E.P., Field, D.E. & Sanders, J. (1981). The effects of TV program comprehensibility on pre-school children's visual attention to television. *Child Development,* **52**, 151-157.

Bandura, A. (1967). Behavioural psychotherapy. *Scientific American*, **216**, 3, 78-86.

Barbe, W.B. & Robert M.M. (1955). Developing listening ability in children. *Elementary English*, **54**, 82-84.

Beentjes, J.W. (1989). Television and young people's reading behaviour: A review of research. *European Journal of Communication.*

Beery, A. (1954). Interrelationships between listening and other language arts area. *Elementary English*, **3**, 164-172.

Belson, W.A. (1960). The effects of television upon family life. *Discovery*, **21**, (10) 1-5.

Burns, J. & Anderson, D. (1989). Cognition and watching television. In D. Tupper and K. Cicerone (Eds.) *Neuropsychology of everyday life.* Boston: K9iwer.

Choat, G.H. (1986). Young children, television and learning: Part II. Comparison of the effects of reading and story telling by the teacher and television story viewing. *Journal of Educational Television*, **12**, 2, 91-103.

Coffin, T.E. (1955). Television's impact on society. *American Psychologist*, **10**, 630-641.

Cramond, J. (1976). The introduction of television and its effects upon children's daily lives. In R. Brown (Ed.), *Children and television*. Beverly Hills, CA: Sage.

Emery F.F. & Emery M. (1974). Participation design: Work and community life, CCE., A.N.U.

Emery, F. & Emery, M. (1976). *A choice of futures*. Leiden: Martinus Nijhoff Social Sciences Division.

Featherman, Friesen, Greenspun, Harris, Schramm, & Grawn (1979).

Fiske, E.P. (1978). *Illiteracy in the U.S.: Why Johny can't cope*. New York Times.

Furu, T. (1971). *Function of television for children and adolescents*. Tokyo: Sophia University.

Furu, T. (1977). *Cognitive study and television viewing patterns of children* (Research Report). International Christian University, Department of Audio Visual Education.

Gadberry, S. (1977). *Television viewing and school grades: A cross-lagged longitudinal study*. Paper presented at the Biennial Meeting of the Society for Research in Child Development, N. Orleans, March, 17-20. (Eric Document Reproduction Service Number Ed140973).

Gadberry, S. (1980). Effects of restricting first graders' TV viewing on leisure time use, IQ change and cognitive style. *Journal of Applied Developmental Psychology*, **1**, 45-57.

Gibson, E.J. & Spelke E.S. (1983). The development of perception. In J.H. Flavel & E.M. Markman (Eds.) *Handbook of Child Psychology, Vol. 3, Cognitive Development* (pp.1-76) NY: John Wiley.

Gibson, E.J. & Walk, R.D. (1960). The visual cliff. *Scientific American*, **202**, (4), 64-71.

Greenfield, P. (1984). *Mind and media: The effects of television, video games, and computers*. Cambridge, MA: Harvard University Press.

Guilford, J.P. & Fruchter, B. (1982). *Fundamental statistics in psychology and education*. Auckland: McGrahill.

Halpern, W. (1975). Tuned-on toddlers. *Journal of Communication*, **25** (4), 66-70.

Harrison, L. & Williams, T. (1986). Television and cognitive development. In T.M. Williams (Ed.), *The impact of television: A natural experiment in three communities* (pp. 87-142). New York: Academic Press.

Himmelweit, H.T., Oppenheim, A.N. & Vince, P. (1958). *Television and the child*. London: Oxford University Press.

Hornik, R. (1981). Out-of-school television and schooling: Hypothesis and methods. *Review of Educational Research*, **51**, 199-214.

Huston, A. & Wright, J.C. (1983). Children's processing of television: The informative functions of formal features. In J. Bryant & D.R. Anderson (Eds.), *Children's understanding of television: Research on attention and comprehension* (pp. 35-68). New York: Academic Press.

Illich, I. (1974). *After de-schooling, what?* Writers' and Readers' Publishing Cooperation.

Kelly, P., & Gunter, B., Kelley, C. (1985). Teaching television in the classroom: Results of a preliminary study. *Journal of Educational Television*, **11**, 1, 57-63.

Krugman, H. (1971). Brain wave measures of media involvement. *Journal of Advertising*.

Lesser, H. (1977). *Television and the pre-school child*. New York: Academic Pres.

Lu, Y. & Tweeten, L. (1973). The impact of busing on students' achievement. *Growth and Change*. **4**, 4, 44-46.

Mandler, J.M. (1978). *Four arguments for the elimination of television*. New York: William Morrow.

Masterman, L. (1983a). Media Education in the 1980s. *Journal of Educational Television*, **9, 1**, 7-20.

Masterman, L. (1983b). Media education: Theoretical issue and practical possibilities. *Prospect*, **46**, XIII, 2, 103-191.

Masterman, L. (1989). *Media education*. London: Routledge

McLuhan, M. (1964). *Understanding media: The extensions of man*. New York: McGraw-Hill.

Moody, K. (1980). *Growing up on television: The TV effect*. New York: Times Books.

Morgan, M. & Cross, L. (1982). Television and educational achievement and aspiration. In D. Pearl, L. Bouthilet & J. Laser (Eds.), Television and behaviour (Vol. 2) Technical reviews (pp. 78-90). Washington, DC: Department of Health and Human Services.

Murray, J. & Kippax, S. (1978). Children's social behaviour in three towns with differing television experience. *Journal of Communication*, **28**, 19-29.

Neuman, S.B. (1988). The displacement effect: Assessing the relation between television viewing and reading performance. *Reading Research Quarterly*, **23** (4), 414-440.

Olson, D.R. & Bruner, J. (1974). Learning through experience and learning through media. In D.R. Olson (Ed.). *Media and symbol: The forms of expression, communication and education*. (pp. 125-150). Chicago: University of Chicago Press.

Paschal, R., Weinstein, T. & Walberg, H. (1984). Effects of homework on learning: A quantitative synthesis. *Journal of Educational Research*, **78**, 97-104.

Pezdek, K. (1987). Television comprehension as an example of applied research in cognitive psychology. In E.B.K. Dale Pezdek & W.P. Banks (Eds.). *Applications of cognitive psychology: Problem solving, education and computing*. Hillsdale: L. Erlbaum Associates.

Pezdek, K. & Stevens, E. 1984). Children's memory for auditory and visual information on television. *Developmental Psychology*, **20**, 212-218.

Postman, N. (1979). First curriculum: Comparing school and television. Phi Delta Kappan, **61**, 163-168.

Postman, N. (1982). *The disappearance of childhood*. New York: Dell.

Resnick, L., Levine, J. & Teasley, S. (1991). *Socially shared cognition*. Hyattsville: APA.

Rice, M.L. (1983). The role of television in language acquisition. *Developmental Review*, **3**, 211-224.

Rice, M.L. (1984). The words of children's television. *Journal of Broadcasting*, **28**, 445-481.

9   Mental health – A primary care perspective

E. Armstrong

Introduction

To most people - and that includes most health professionals - the two words 'Mental Health' mean Mental Illness. Even the Services we call Mental Health Services aren't - for the most part they offer treatment and support to those who are mentally ill.

This is certainly not to denigrate the excellent work that is often being done by those who work in the specialist services. Those who suffer from mental illness need care - in the same way that a person with cancer needs care. Their carers need help and support too.

But in primary health care, the focus is somewhat different. It is in the primary health care sector that prevention and the promotion of health can really come into their own - though, even there, we must not forget that GPs are involved in treatment too.

I'm not intending to offer any kind of definition of mental health - I leave that to the philosophers. What I am trying to do is suggest some practical ways of coping with the mental health problems that arrive every day on the doorstep of those who work in the primary health care sector - the GP, the practice nurse, the receptionist in the surgery, and the health visitor and district nurse too.

You'll notice I haven't mentioned the Community Psychiatric Nurse - for a very good reason. Because what all those other people have in common is that they are non-specialists. They have no specific qualification which will equip them to care for people who are mentally ill.

And yet, over 90% of people with psychiatric disorder are cared for within the primary care sector, and are never referred to the specialist services! (Jenkins and Shepherd 1983).

Going to see your family doctor when you're ill or in distress is a perfectly socially acceptable thing to do. Going to see a psychiatrist - or any other person with 'psych -' in their title, is much less acceptable.

This even though it is well known that up to a half of the mental illness that presents to the GP is not recognised - and therefore presumably, not treated.

In 1981, the Royal College of General Practitioners produced a report called 'Prevention of Psychiatric Disorders in General Practice'. It talked about the desirability of early detection and preventive interventions at times of life change. It may have had some effect (Newton, 1989) - but it had nowhere near the impact of another report produced in the same year.

This was the major report on the 'Prevention of Cardio-vascular Disease in General Practice' (RCGP 1981). Much more exciting, heart disease. Its dramatic to die of a heart attack. Prevent that and you'd really be doing some good! What the report suggested was that every adult should have his/her blood pressure measured at least once every five years, that GPs should ask their patients about their smoking habits and that weight should be monitored. Believe it or not, in 1981, that was revolutionary!

The major statement of the Report was that, 'A half of all strokes and a quarter of deaths from coronary heart disease in people under 70 are probably preventable by the application of existing knowledge'.

This challenge, to apply existing knowledge, was very quickly taken up by a team in Oxford. Facilitator, Elaine Fullard, and her colleagues - Godfrey Fowler, a GP and Muir Grey, a public health physician, devised a practical way of implementing the report's recommendations in every-day primary care situations (Fullard et al., 1984).

In the introduction to her new book on 'Preventing Mental Illness in Practice', Jennifer Newton suggests that 'current knowledge (about mental illness) is sufficiently impressive that we can at least begin to think about prevention, and about how existing services might be influenced by current research'. As before, the challenge is to put knowledge into practice.

Elaine Fullard was not the first to use the facilitator idea in general practice. The credit for that usually goes to an Islington GP, Dr Arnold Elliott, who showed that personal contact and help from a trusted colleague could be more effective in achieving change than any number of directives which frequently remain unread. (Allsop, 1990).

What Fullard did was take the idea and develop it to the point where there are now more than 250 primary care facilitators in post nationwide.

She was awarded the MBE for her work with the Oxford Prevention of Heart Attack and Stroke Project, and the project celebrates its 10th anniversary this year.

What, then, do facilitators do that has earned their pioneer such an accolade, and, in our present context, what do they have to offer the cause of the promotion of mental health?

What do facilitators do?

The British primary care system is based on general practice, that is, on our network of family doctors offering a consultation service to those who perceive themselves as ill. Over the last ten years, this illness-led model has gradually changed. The doctor still offers the consultation service, but in addition a variety of other services have been added, which are designed to encourage the maintenance of healthier lifestyles and to detect illness at an early, and more easily treatable stage.

Facilitators, who have been described as agents of change (Allsop, 1990), have been very active in enabling this to happen. There are four main areas of concern in their work.

1. The early detection and prompt treatment of illness - The classic example in which facilitators have been involved is the detection of previously untreated hypertension - an important risk factor leading to strokes.
2. The prevention of disease - for instance immunisation.
3. The management of chronic ill-health - for example clinics for people with asthma or diabetes.
4. The promotion of good health - helping people give up smoking, and providing information about healthy living.

From the beginnings of the Oxford Project, facilitators have been working to introduce into the primary care system this more health-oriented approach to care. For the most part they are not directly involved in giving care. What they do is help others, notably practice nurses, acquire the skills necessary to enable them to develop this different approach to practice.

Sometimes, facilitators are involved in providing training themselves. However, there is now an increasing variety of courses available for practice nurses - for instance, the excellent course run by Greta Barnes, herself a practice nurse, at the Asthma Training Centre in Stratford upon Avon. Facilitators help practice nurses identify their training needs and gain access to the courses to meet those needs.

In this paper I am suggesting that methods which have been used by facilitators in physical health are transferable to the mental health field. I propose to describe some of those methods, with examples from my own experience.

The KCW FHSA Mental Health Facilitator Project

For nearly two years now, I have been working on a Department of Health funded research project which is designed to evaluate the facilitator role in primary care in two important areas:

1. The early detection and prompt treatment of people with depression and anxiety.
2. The identification and support of people at risk of these conditions.

I came to this project as an experienced community nurse and facilitator. I am a health visitor, have also worked as a district nurse - and I was about the 18th primary care facilitator to be appointed in the country, following the initial success of Elaine Fullard's work. Like most of the people I work with - the GPs, practice nurses administrators and managers - I am not a specialist in mental illness - but I am a specialist in health.

The methods I use to achieve change are not vastly different from those I've used before, nor are they very different from those used by other facilitators, though the words we use may not always be the same.

1. Audit

Before initiating any kind of change, it is of course necessary to know where you are starting from!

Results from previous research help, but it's very easy for people to say that research findings apply to the others, not to us. Or to criticise the methodology. Or to say the research is old, was done in a different area - or any number of other excuses to avoid having to face up to the implications. Life in general practice is incredibly pressured. Change implies making an effort. If you already feel stretched to the limit, you need a pretty good reason why you should stop and think about changing the way you work. Audit can provide that reason.

Some people see audit as threatening. In this context it simply means asking one very basic question:

How are we doing?

In our audit, we wanted to be able to show GPs and their staff how they were doing in relation to the care of people with mental health problems. It would be specific to their practice and their patients, and it would be confidential. In other words, the result wouldn't go outside the practice without the express permission of the GPs involved. Confidentiality means that the facilitator can discuss the results of the audit freely with the GPs in an atmosphere of trust.

The audit provides a starting point for discussion with the practice about the care they are offering. It helps to identify areas of change which are needed. Most importantly, it raises awareness and provides motivation, which can be very difficult to achieve by other means.

There are other ways of identifying possible starting points for change. One such would be to 'sit in' with each member of the practice during their working day - GPs, nurses and reception staff. This is a good way of getting to know the personalities and the dynamics of the practice, and is a generally acceptable approach. It can be used as the basis of a report to the practice with recommendations for change.

However, such a report lacks the force of audit figures and is easier to ignore. Simply being in the practice conducting an audit is an equally useful way to getting to know it.

Audit seems to me to underpin much of the facilitator's work. Basing other interventions on audit results will help to ensure that they are relevant to individual practitioners.

2. Training

Most change involves the need for some kind of training. The facilitator's job here is to identify the particular needs of individual practice team members for extra training, and to see that it is made available to them. This may mean providing information abut outside courses, but where these are either inaccessible, too expensive or not appropriate, it might mean arranging 'in house' sessions.

Much educational work done by facilitators is informal and arises directly from audit or other observations. In discussing audit results with practice members, the facilitator will be suggesting ways in which care could be improved. He/she might also provide copies of suggested protocols or guidelines as well as relevant research reports.

There is currently a lack of suitable courses on mental health issues for primary health care workers, particularly practice nurses, though a number of different organisations are beginning to address the problem.

3. Employment advice

Traditionally, an important part of the facilitator's work was encouraging and supporting the employment of practice nurses. Much of this has now been taken over by practice nurse advisers and other FHSA managers, but in the present project, it is apparent that without a considerable increase in clinical expertise in general practice, the scope for improving primary mental health care is strictly limited. To some extent this means more training, but it also means more people - and not necessarily more doctors.

Nurses have a lot to offer, and their role in general practice is often circumscribed by the need to achieve such things as cervical cytology targets which bring in remuneration. Their skills are thus under used. It has been demonstrated that, with appropriate extra training, non-specialist nurses can assess people for depression, and can monitor those taking anti-depressants personal communication. I have also devised a systematic method of identifying people at risk of developing mental health problem, especially depression, which is being piloted by a number of practice nurses and has proved acceptable in use to both nurse and patient.

There is, it seems to me, potential to develop this tool further. Newton's work strongly reinforces the idea that targeting support -perhaps in the form of problem-solving skills - at vulnerable people may be a valuable way of preventing more serious mental health problems.

Such tools as are presently available are often time-consuming to use - and in general practice time is at a premium. Tools therefore need to be easy and quick to use. Questionnaires for self-completion by patients are especially popular, particularly where they can be used to measure change over time.

But without a considerable increase in practice nurse numbers, these interventions are unlikely to be widely taken up.

There is also, it seems to me, a need for many more counsellors in the primary care sector. Counselling is a preferred method of treatment for depression in polls of consumer attitudes (Mori 1992), but their employment raises a number of difficult issues, not least of which is 'What is a Counsellor?' GPs need someone to whom they can turn for advice on these matters. The well-informed facilitator could fulfil that function.

4. Bridge-building/networking

Although my main area of work is not the care of the long-term mentally ill, this is a group about whom GPs worry a great deal. They can cause problems out of all proportion to their numbers. Even more worrying has been the lack of support some GPs and practice nurses experience from the specialist services. It is not unusual to find that these non-specialist nurses are regularly providing depot injections to patients with chronic schizophrenia without knowing to whom they should turn if a crisis arises. The patients too, frequently seem to have no contact with the specialist services, which means that they could be losing out on the essential social care and support which they need to prevent relapse (Jenkins et al., 1992). I do not think that this phenomenon is confined to central London!

Part of the solution is undoubtedly better training for practice nurses. But there is clearly a need for much better liaison between specialists and primary care. Perhaps what should happen is for some form of shared care to evolve. It has happened in diabetes care, and in the maternity services. Why not in mental illness?

Conclusion

I have tried in this paper to suggest some of the ways in which I think workers in the primary health care sector could contribute to better mental health care, to the prevention of mental illness and the promotion of mental health.

An overall aim would be to have mental health seen as part of health, and not as something separate, to be talked of in hushed tones, if at all. Mental health care audit typically finds more than 2/3 of patients attending surgery have mental health problems. Yet our approach is always to look for physical symptoms first.

Is this logical? We certainly haven't yet really begun to look at the whole person.

It might cause some raised eyebrows to suggest that doctors and nurses should assess the mental state of their patients first - but it's surely not unrealistic to make attention to mental health and well being an integral part of every consultation.

References

Allen, P., et al., Nurse Depression Study (personal communication).

Alsop J. (1990). Changing primary care: The role of facilitators, Kings Fund Centre: London.

Davies, T.M. (1992). Schizophrenia: Issues for General Practice in the primary care of schizophrenia. R. Jenkins, V. Field & R. Young, (Eds.), HMSO:London.

Fullard, E.M., Fowler, G.H., & Gray, J.A.M. (1984). Facilitating prevention in primary care, *BMJ*, **298**, 1582-1587.

Jenkins, R. & Shepherd, M. (1983). *Mental illness and general practice in mental illness: Changes and trends*. In P. Bean (Ed.). London: John Wiley and sons Ltd.

Mori poll for Defeat Depression Campaign, (1992). RCGP/RCPsych, London.

Newton, J. (1989). *Preventing mental illness*. London: Routledge.

Newton, J. (1992). *Preventing mental illness in practice*, London:Routledge.

Prevention of Arterial Disease in General Practice (1981). Report from General Practice 19, RCGP, London.

Prevention of Psychiatric Disorders in General Practice (1981), Report from General Practice 20, RCGP, London.

10 Community mental health care: Promoting a better quality of life for long-term clients

M. Barry

Abstract

The increasing emphasis on quality of life issues in the mental health literature signals a shift to a more holistic model of care. Improved quality of life has become an explicit priority of the community alternatives to hospital-based care. This paper considers the role of quality of life issues in the provision of community care for people with long-term mental health needs. Research findings from an ongoing study concerned with the impact of community care on the quality of life of long-stay patients discharged from psychiatric hospital are presented. This paper concentrates on the initial impact of resettlement on residents' quality of life at six months following the move to the community. Information concerning residents' self-assessed judgements of quality of life is presented and a comparison is made with the quality of life experienced by the same individuals in hospital prior to their discharge. The paper also relates the impact of changes in care environments and care practices following the move to the community care schemes on the reported changes in quality of life.

Introduction

The extent to which community-based residential care programmes succeed in improving the quality of life of their clients is an important test of the feasibility of the new community care policy. The importance of quality of life as a desired outcome for care programmes for the chronically mentally ill has been highlighted by a number of practitioners and researchers in this area (Anthony, 1980; Bachrach, 1980; Baker & Intagliata, 1982; Bigelow et al., 1982; Lehman, 1988; Wilde & Svanberg, 1990). The objective of maximising quality of life is of particular relevance to clients who are in need of long-term residential care. The assumption is that the quality of life of such clients will be enhanced through the provision of noninstitutional care. However, as pointed out by Shadish, Orwin, Silber and Bootzin (1985), this assumption needs to be tested by investigating the extent to which community residential programmes are a) providing noninstitutional care and b) are enhancing the quality of life of their residents. Determining which elements of the care process are critical to ensuring a high quality of life for residential care clients is an important research goal in this area.

This paper reports on the quality of life of the residents of specially established community care schemes for patients being resettled from the North Wales Hospital. The paper examines residents' perceptions of their quality of life experienced by the same residents on the hospital wards prior to discharge. In addition to residents' self-reports of their quality of life, the paper also considers the broader impact of changes in residential setting and care process on the quality of life of residents of the care schemes.

Methodological issues surrounding the conceptualisation and measurement of quality of life of long-term clients have been addressed in an earlier paper by Barry and Crosby (1992). Research work to date does suggest that a multi-dimensional construct such as quality of life provides a useful evaluative framework against which to assess the outcome of care and is also a useful source of information concerning the subjective perceptions and life situation of individual clients. Barry, Crosby and Mitchell (1992) reported on the standard of quality of life offered by conventional hospital care to a group of long-stay psychiatric residents at the North Wales Hospital. The present study follows up the first research cohort of 62 clients, 34 of whom have been discharged into community settings. The baseline phase of the study was carried out on the rehabilitation wards of the North Wales Hospital and a quality of life interview was administered to each of the 62 clients on the wards. The study reported that the quality of life of the residents as objectively measured was quite low, yet the majority of the residents evaluated their subjective quality of life in a positive manner. Despite poor living conditions, restricted social lives and limited leisure, financial and employment opportunities, residents reported high levels of satisfaction across a number of different life areas. Difficulties surrounding the interpretation of the data, in particular the lack of correlation between the objective and subjective indicators, were highlighted. The influence of such factors as positive response bias, standards of social comparison and the effects of institutionalisation and psychopathology on self-assessed judgements of quality of life were also documented. Global quality of life ratings were found to be correlated with levels of depression and thought disorder and with overall levels of dependency. The importance of relating the data derived from the quality of life schedule to the other indicators of client welfare being used in the study was therefore highlighted by the baseline results. The influence of residential care settings and care practices was also noted as a potentially important determinant of the quality of life of clients receiving long-term residential care. The present paper will therefore attempt to relate the information derived from the quality of life schedule to a range of client outcome and care process variables in order to assess residents' quality of life from a number of different perspectives using a range of data sources.

The present study

The original group of 62 residents were followed-up as they were discharged from hospital and the present paper reports on the impact of community care on the lives of 30 of the 34 discharged clients six months after their move from hospital. The study evaluates the effects of resettlement in the initial period following hospital discharge. The following dimensions of client welfare are addressed:
- individual adjustment to living in supported accommodation in the community following lengthy periods of hospitalisation
- the impact of community care on clients' self-assessed judgements of their quality of life
- the effects of the move from hospital on clients' level of psychiatric symptomatology and levels of social and behavioural functioning
- the impact of changes in care environments and care practices on residents' quality of life

Method

Measures

Data presented in this paper are drawn from research instruments adapted or developed by the Health Service Research Unit (HSRU) team and include;
- A quality of life interview specifically designed for use with a sample of long-stay patients. The redesigned schedule is adapted from Lehman's (1982) quality of life interview, covering objective and subjective indices of quality of life in nine life areas together with indices of general well-being. A fuller description of the

115

development of the schedule and its psychometric properties may be found in Barry, Crosby and Bogg (1992).

- A standardised psychiatric interview was also developed for use in the study. The schedule contains 45 items and allows for ratings to be carried out on scales such as the Brief Psychiatric Rating Scale (BPRS) of Overall and Gorham, 1962 and the Krawiecka Rating Scale (KRS) of Krawiecka, Goldberg and Vaughan, 1977, (for details of the interview see Mitchell, 1990).

-Levels of behavioural and social functioning were rated on the REHAB scale (Baker and Hall, 1983) which was completed by care staff trained in its use.

- Assessment of the care regime was carried out by members of the research team in conjunction with staff and managers of the care schemes using the Hostel and Hospices Practices Profile (HHPP) adapted from Wing and Brown (1970), and Staff Attitudes and Management Practices Schedule (SAMPS) adapted from Garety and Morris (1984).

The settings

Hospital reprovision consists of four main types of residential settings; a supported housing scheme consisting of 5 houses with 24-hour staffing, a registered care home managed by a voluntary agency, private homes for the mentally ill in the local area, and a small number of clients (4) in independent living situations. The care processes in the housing scheme and the group home were examined for the purpose of assessing the impact of changing care environments and care practices.

The housing scheme, which is managed by the local health authority consists of five houses in pleasant residential areas in a North Wales town and nearby village. Each house in the scheme provides attractive, well-furnished residential accommodation and has three or four bedrooms. The physical environments are completely domestic. The registered care home consists of a large town house providing residential care for people in six flats. The scheme, which is managed by a voluntary agency, offerers twenty-four hour support. Each flat has its own kitchen, bathroom, living room area, and individual bedrooms. The physical environments are predominantly domestic, but there are some institutional features such as a communal lounge and staff office accommodation. The majority (83%) of the residential care staff of the two schemes had previous care related experience and had previous contact with people who experienced mental health difficulties, but only 19% had qualifications related to psychiatric nursing per se.

The care environments of the new community schemes contrast sharply

116

with those of the hospital wards from which the residents were discharged. The four wards selected were those from which patients were prepared for their move into the community care schemes. The quality of the physical environment in these wards was generally poor, affording little opportunity for privacy, personalisation, independence and access to community facilities (see Crosby, 1990). Two wards housed old long-stay patients and these had the poorer environments in terms of access to facilities, such as shops and cafes, degree of privacy for residents (dormitory sleeping arrangements) and the maintenance of cleaning, decoration, and repairs. The two rehabilitation wards for the new long-stay patients were generally better maintained and, in one case, offered better accommodation including single bedrooms.

Profile of discharged group

Of the 34 clients who have been discharged from hospital to date, the majority are male, have a primary clinical diagnosis of some form of schizophrenia (79%), range in age from 27 to 77 years (mean age of 56 years) and have spent from .7 to 46 years of their lives in a psychiatric hospital (Mean number of years hospitalised = 23). The sample of discharged residents includes both the 'old' and 'new' long-stay patients. During the course of the six months following discharge, three of the residents died due to natural causes and one was re-admitted to hospital, leaving a total sample of 30 residents. Clients currently residing in the housing scheme and in private care homes may be characterised as old-long-stay psychiatric patients, with a mean age of 66 years, having spent most of their adult lives in hospital (mean number of years hospitalised = 33 years). On the basis of their psychiatric assessments this group presently exhibits relatively few active or florid psychiatric symptoms. In comparison, the clients selected for the care home scheme and/or living independently are comprised of relatively younger individuals (mean age = 48 years), who have had more frequent and shorter periods of hospitalisation and exhibit more florid symptomatology.

Of the original cohort, 28 are currently residing in NWH awaiting resettlement. Three of this group also died due to natural causes and one was transferred to another hospital. The baseline characteristics of the research cohort were examined in order to identify any differences between the group of leavers and those who have remained in hospital. No significant differences were found between the sample of leavers and stayers in relation to demographic and clinical characteristics, attitude to discharge, overall level of dependency or in the level of active psychiatric symptomatology. The only significant difference to emerge between the

117

leavers and stayers was in relation to the level of deviant behaviour as measured on the REHAB scale ($F=18.50$, $p<.001$). Those clients who have remained in hospital show a higher incidence of occurrence of such problem behaviours as incontinence, violence, verbal aggression and talking/laughing to self, making their discharge to the community potentially more problematic. In essence the clients who have remained in hospital consist of either EMI patients or those younger clients with challenging behaviour.

Design of the study

The study employs a longitudinal repeated-measures design which permits the collection of data at a number of points prior to and following discharge from hospital. Three baseline assessments are carried out on the hospital wards prior to discharge and three repeat assessments following discharge from hospital are also carried out, at six weeks, six months and twelve months post-discharge . The design permits a comparison of clients' quality of life while in hospital with that experienced by the same clients following their move to the community. The paper concentrates on the initial findings from the six months followup in the community.

Results

Adjustment to life in the community care settings

Six months after the move from hospital, residents express very positive attitudes about the community settings. 93% describe their lives in the community residences as either much better (80%) or somewhat better (13%) than in hospital. Despite an initial unwillingness to leave the hospital, particularly for the older clients, many now describe their lives as having improved following the move to the community settings. Roughly one third of the discharged group reported not having wanted to leave the hospital, but six months on, they report feeling much better for having made the move; **'I didn't want to move, but its much better here'**. None of the clients express a desire to return to hospital.

When questioned about which areas of their lives were most affected by resettlement, the majority of the responses (48%) refer to the greater freedom and independence experienced in the community settings; **'They were too strict in hospital, your life wasn't your own, there's real freedom here'**, **'I'm more independent, I can handle my own food and money, I can go shopping, self-medicate....'**. Of the discharged group, 57% express a desire to remain in their present accommodation which they describe as being comfortable (93%), providing an opportunity to do things when they want to (78%), and an opportunity to plan their own activities (50%). With regard to the clients who feel they would be better off if they were moved (23%), the majority express a desire to live with family, even when this is no longer feasible or a realistic option. Despite this preference for family life, 73% of the resettled group feel that they belong in their new homes.

Changes in clients' perceived quality of life

At six months post-discharge the residents report very favourable comments about their life in the community. As shown in Figure 1, residents express generally higher levels of satisfaction with their lives in the community compared to hospital. Reported levels of satisfaction in each of the life domains ranged from 60-93%, with the highest levels of satisfaction being expressed in relation to living situation (93%) and social relations (90%). High levels of satisfaction were reported in relation to the accommodation (80%), food (90%), privacy (93%), bedroom (100%) and the freedom (97%) provided by the community settings. The majority of residents express high levels of satisfaction with their relationship with other residents (87%) and with the care staff 90%) and 47% report having friends within the house/home. Satisfaction with the treatment received in the community settings was also high, with 73% expressing satisfaction with the medical treatment and 80% satisfied with their opportunity to consult staff. Safety issues do not present as a problem, with 90% of residents reporting satisfaction with personal safety in the community homes and 80% satisfied with safety in the neighbourhood.

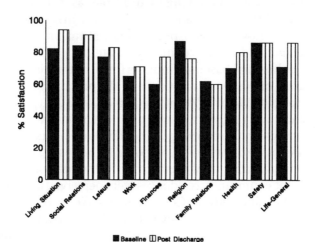

■ Baseline □ Post Discharge

Figure 1 Quality of Life: satisfaction ratings at hospital baseline and six months post-discharge in the community(N=30)

The life areas that elicited the highest levels of dissatisfaction were frequency of family contact (27% dissatisfied), lack of employment (25%) and finances (20%). Residents expressed a desire to see their families more often with many wanting to live with family, even when this is not a feasible option. Levels of contact with family did not change appreciably following the move to the community, with 43% of community residents receiving family visits on at least a monthly basis compared to 39% of the hospital baseline sample. The majority however, were content with the frequency of contact with family (57%), and with how they got on with family (63%). Dissatisfaction with not having a job was voiced mainly by the younger clients, many of whom had been attending the hospital's industrial therapy unit. This service has not been replaced for residents in this group since the move from hospital and it would appear that some form of occupational or training activities would be of benefit to the younger clients. With regard to finance, residents reported receiving on average £26.67 per week which was managed by residents with help from staff as appropriate.

The drop in levels of satisfaction with religion in the community may be explained by the fact that some of the clients were regular attenders at the hospital chapel which was located in the grounds of the hospital. The percentage of weekly church goers has dropped since the move to the community. With regard to life in general, residents expressed higher rates of satisfaction with their life overall in the community (87%) compared to that expressed when in hospital (71%). Many describe their life as having improved following the move from the hospital **'I'm much happier here.... my life has changed and I feel as if it's a new life'.**

In order to assess the significance of the changes in residents' quality of life following the move from hospital, statistical analysis was carried out on the subjective and objective quality of life indices in each life area, comparing the hospital baseline findings for 30 of the discharged clients with the quality of life reported at six months post discharge. Repeated measures analysis (MANOVA) of the subjective quality of life indices revealed a statistically significant improvement in satisfaction with living situation, with residents reporting higher levels of satisfaction with their new residences in the community compared to the hospital wards ($F=6.20$, $p<.05$). Nonparametric analyses of the individual objective indices revealed that the community residences were perceived as more comfortable than the hospital setting (Cochran's $Q=4.00$, $p<.05$), and residents were more likely to report that they belonged in the community settings (Cochran's $Q=4.00$, $p<.05$), and that they had greater opportunity to plan their own activities (Cochran's $Q=5.00$, $P<.05$). A number of other

120

individual indices were also found to show significant improvements; residents reported feeling less lonely in the community compared to hospital (Friedman's x2 = 4.32, p=.04), and were also more likely to perceive their medication as being helpful (Friedman's x2= 5.14,p<,05).

Analysis of the objective quality of life indices revealed increased levels of social interaction in the community residences (F=18.62,p<.001). Higher levels of interaction were reported by residents, both within (F=14.74,p<.001) and outside (F=10.41, p<.01) the facility. The main improvements to date appear to be in relation to higher levels of contact among the residents and the care staff. The low rates of interaction between the residents in the hospital setting was commented on in an earlier report (Crosby et al., 1990) and it would appear that the smaller, more domestic, units in the community schemes have successfully facilitated higher levels of interaction among the residents and staff. The changes in levels of interaction are reflected in residents' reports of feeling less lonely in the community settings. The increased level of social interaction outside the facility is mainly attributable to contact with other clients, resident in either another house in the resettlement scheme or still resident in hospital.

(see Table 1)

Due to the small number engaged in employment, the work scale was not included in the analysis.

(*p<0.05, **p<.01, ***p<.001)

A significant increase was also found in relation to leisure activities (F=4.68,p<.05) with residents participating in more activities such as day trips, outings and making greater use of local community facilities such as shops and cafes.

Residents were also found to be more likely to express greater satisfaction with their life overall in the community settings than they were while in hospital (F=6.53,p<.05).

Changes in the care environments and care process

Two of the newly established community schemes were examined in order to assess the effects of changing care environments and care management practices on residents' quality of life. Assessment of the care regime using research instruments such as the Hostel and Hospices Practices Profile (HHPP), and the Staff Attitudes and Management Practices Schedule (SAMPS), indicated that the move from hospital to the community has resulted in a substantial reduction in restrictive care practices. The HHPP, which provides a means of assessing the extent to which care regimes and environments are resident orientated or institu-

Table 1

Life domain composite indices at baseline and six months post-discharge for long-stay patients resettled in the community(N = 30)

Life Domain	Hospital Baseline Mean	(S.D.)	6 months post discharge Mean	(S.D.)	MANOVA F-Ratio
Subject Indices					
Living Situation	13.14	(2.58)	14.43	(.92)	6.20*
Social Relations	8.40	(1.44)	8.92	(.28)	2.99
Family Relations	4.84	(1.39)	4.95	(1.27)	.06
Leisure	5.21	(1.13)	5.64	(.91)	2.63
Finances	2.29	(.98)	2.54	(.84)	2.03
Religion	2.89	(.43)	2.65	(.80)	2.37
Health	13.48	(1.69)	13.56	(2.06)	.07
Personal Safety	5.46	(1.07)	5.57	(.92)	.17
Objective Indices					
Living Situation	7.80	(1.48)	8.90	(.99)	3.77
Frequency of Social Contacts	17.67	(5.31)	21.29	(4.67)	18.62***
Within the facility	8.62	(3.62)	11.31	(3.03)	14.74***
Outside the facility	4.89	(2.69)	6.12	(2.63)	10.41**
Frequency of Family Contact	5.46	(2.62)	5.71	(2.48)	.71
Leisure Activities	19.52	(2.69)	20.48	(2.31)	4.68*
Weekly Spending Money	13.70	(9.08)	26.67	(21.90)	8.77
Physical Illness in Past year	3.75	(.65)	3.86	(.45)	1.00
Frequency of Religious Practice	2.41	(1.50)	1.91	(1.27)	2.01
Victim of Robbery/Attack	1.43	(.50)	1.75	(.65)	3.53
Global Quality of Life	2.36	(.99)	2.82	(.55)	6.53*

tionally orientated (Wykes, 1982), found that the care regime in the community care schemes is some 20% less restrictive for residents than was the hospital care regimes. This greater autonomy and the increase in freedom achieved by the new care regimes has registered with users as the major difference they note between hospital and community care. Analysis of the HHPP data identified five areas which are the main components of client-orientated care management; a high degree of independence for clients, satisfactory privacy for clients, the extent to which the living environment is 'personalised', for example by the users' own possessions, the extent to which the environment and care management symbolise liberal care regimes and a high degree of community accessibility available to users. In each of these areas there have been substantial gains for residents following the move from hospital to the community care schemes (Crosby, Barry, Cater and Bogg, 1992).

Examination of the care practices also revealed a greater involvement of clients in decision-making and taking responsibility for making choices in their lives. Increased personal responsibility for clients was seen as an important part of the care process by 61% of community care staff, together with developing increased self-confidence and mixing in the community. There was also evidence of increased working with individual clients on a one to one basis, made possible by higher client - staff ratios compared to hospital. Interaction with clients was perceived by 86% of the staff as the most rewarding aspect of their work. Staff morale was high, with the majority expressing high levels of satisfaction with their work in the new schemes; 97% of the staff reported being pleased with their move to the community schemes and 89% felt that the resettlement process was successful to date (Carter, Bogg, Crosby and Barry, 1992).

Changes in level of functioning

The level of clients' psychiatric symptomatology at six months post-discharge shows no significant changes from that measured at hospital baseline (see Table 2). The findings from the psychiatric rating scales indicate that to date the move from hospital has not resulted in a significant deterioration of clients' level of psychiatric functioning. The initial differences in psychiatric state at baseline between the clients discharged to the housing scheme and the group home are still evident at six months post-discharge. The younger clients in the group home continue to exhibit higher levels of symptoms such as delusions and hallucinations than the older clients in the supported housing scheme.

Levels of social and behavioural functioning show marked improvements following the move from hospital. A comparison of ratings on the REHAB scale at baseline and six months post discharge show significant improvements in relation to clients' social activity, level of self-care, community skills and speech skills (see Table 3). The overall level of dependency, as measured by the total general behaviour score on the scale, also shows significant improvements ($F=27.55, p<.001$). Retrospective analysis of the REHAB ratings at baseline shows the older clients in

Table 2
Psychiatric ratings: hospital baseline and six months post-discharge

	Hospital Baseline Mean	(S.D.)	6 months post discharge Mean	(S.D.)	F-Ratio
KRS Ratings					
Depression	.39	(.82)	.32	(.53)	.17
Anxiety	.80	(.96)	1.09	(.99)	1.70
Coherent Delusions	1.24	(1.70)	1.19	(1.61)	.03
Hallucination	.85	(1.56)	.57	(1.32)	1.06
Incoherence of Speech	.67	(1.08)	.68	(1.20)	.01
Poverty of Speech	.69	(1.15)	.71	(1.17)	.01
Flattened Incongruous Affect	.64	(.95)	.62	(.93)	.01
Psychomotor Retardation	.47	(.77)	.38	(.76)	.46
BPRS - Factor Scores					
Anxiety - Depression	.72	(1.03)	.75	(.77)	.03
Anergia	.62	(1.11)	.33	(.68)	2.71
Thought Disorder	1.19	(1.43)	1.10	(1.48)	.27
Activation	.68	(.71)	.91	(.81)	2.77
Hostility - Suspiciousness	.50	(.75)	.67	(.81)	1.66

the supported housing scheme to have higher overall dependency scores (i.e. total general behaviour scores) than the younger clients in the group home. The differences were found to have significantly diminished at six months after the move from hospital.

These improvements may be interpreted as reflecting the more liberal and client-oriented care regimes in the community care settings, which give residents greater opportunities for carrying out basic self-care functions and utilising basic social and community skills. As outlined, the community schemes have an explicit policy of encouraging client independence and self-reliance wherever possible.

Discussion

From the results it may be seen that the movement to the community has produced positive outcomes for clients, reflected in significant improvements in quality of life and levels of behavioural and social functioning

Table 3
REHAB: Hospital baseline and six months post-discharge
scores for additive scales

	Hospital Baseline Mean	(S.D.)	6 months post discharge Mean	(S.D.)	F-Ratio
Deviant Behaviour	1.36	(1.12)	1.61	(1.59)	.75
Factor Scores					
Social Activity	25.58	(13.58)	16.89	(12.29)	20.04***
Speech Skills	6.72	(5.19)	4.69	(4.33)	8.47**
Disturbed Speech	4.70	(4.07)	4.03	(3.71)	1.49
Self-care	15.48	(11.40)	11.66	(9.73)	5.74*
Community Skills	9.88	(5.94)	7.11	(4.94)	14.91***
Total General Behaviour	60.02	(29.89)	43.95	(26.40)	25.88***

*p<.05, **p<.01, ***p<.001

compared to that found in the hospital setting. Overall, clients have reacted well to the changes in their care settings and care regime. The move to the community has resulted in improved objective standards of living for the resettled group, i.e. more comfortable living conditions, higher levels of contact within and outside of the facility, and greater freedom and independence, all of which are reflected in residents' comments concerning their quality of life. The majority appear to be adapting well to their life in the community. This is worthy of comment given the relatively lengthy periods this group had spent in hospital and the relatively short time they have spent living in the community. As expected, the most significant changes in quality of life at this early stage have been in relation to the immediate living situation, with residents reporting significant improvements in their general well-being. As may be seen from the results, significant changes were not found in all life areas e.g. family contact, unemployment and finance remain common sources of dissatisfaction. It is to be expected, however, that changes in the more long-term patterns of behaviour will take longer than six months to be attained.

It would appear from the results to date that the reduction in restrictive and institutional care practices in the community schemes has had a positive impact on clients who are responding well to the increased opportunities for greater self-reliance and a more independent life style. The reported increase in social interaction within the community facilities, together with the improved Rehab ratings on social activity, is consistent with the findings from other studies of people moved from large institutions to smaller domestic units (Gibbons and Butler, 1989; Garety and Morris, 1984). The location and lay-out of the care settings, i.e. smaller domestic units located in residential areas, has facilitated higher rates of social interaction within the care facilities and greater take-up of local community facilities.

What emerges clearly from clients' comments about the differences between hospital and community living is the greater independence and freedom afforded by the community settings. Although lack of freedom per se did not emerge in residents' accounts of life in the hospital, it would appear that independence and being able to do things for oneself, once experienced, is an important consideration for clients with long-term needs. As such, clients' comments suggest that the objectives of the community schemes in encouraging independence and self-reliance are thus far being achieved. The increased levels of expressed satisfaction in the community are notable given the high baseline levels expressed by clients in the hospital setting. It will be interesting to observe whether the standards of comparison employed by the community residents in their judgements of life quality will change as a result of increasing levels of independence and greater exposure to the standards of living in the local community.

Generally, the findings suggest that the outcome measures used in the evaluation study, such as the Rehab and the quality of life measures, are sensitive to change and can discriminate life areas which have been affected by a change in care setting and the style and delivery of care. Although implied in some of the quality of life indices, the addition of items specifically tapping independence and freedom may be an important outcome indicator and may increase the content validity of quality of life scales for long-term psychiatric clients. The lack of change in the levels of psychiatric functioning is consistent with that reported by other studies and may be attributed to the stabilising effects of medication on levels of symptomatology.

The findings from the repeated measures carried out while in hospital allow greater confidence to be placed in the findings of the present study. Both the quality of life and Rehab measures produced stable hospital baseline measures against which to assess the significance of the changes following the move to the community. The comparison of each individual client's level of functioning and quality of life under both the hospital and community settings also strengthens confidence in the outcomes of the study, providing a truer assessment of the impact of resettlement. The convergence of information derived from different sources, i.e. clients and staff, allows greater confidence to be placed in the validity of the study's findings.

The results indicate a number of areas on which rehabilitation strategies might focus in order to maximise the quality of life of their clients. The observed improvements in social and behavioural functioning most likely reflect increased opportunity to practice previously existing skills in the new community settings rather than the acquisition of new skills since leaving hospital. However, the acquisition of new skills e.g. domestic, educational and social skills and the fostering of greater independence, self-determination and control over one's life should continue to be encouraged and, where possible, developed in a structured manner. The need for structured day time activities and in particular recreational and occupational/training activities for younger residents clearly emerges from the quality of life data. At this stage it is difficult to judge the actual level of community integration and acceptance as no systematic investigation has been undertaken. However, the social networks of the resettled groups would still appear to be restricted to contact with other clients and support workers in the scheme. In this respect, encouraging outside contact with other agencies and services, particularly day centres or evening classes, may be desirable in order to broaden the opportunities available to residents for wider social contacts. Sustaining the high level of staff commitment and enthusiasm in the care schemes over time is also an important consideration in relation to residents' quality of life. Developing relevant training opportunities for care staff and providing the necessary support to enable them to meet the needs of residents is vital to the overall success of the new schemes.

It is important to stress that the findings from the study remain tentative at this stage owing to the relatively short period of time spent by residents in the community settings. It will be necessary to await later results to ascertain if initial outcome patterns are maintained over a longer period of time. However, if these positive outcomes are maintained they will provide support for the claim that it is possible to maintain even the more dependent, chronic psychiatric clients in the community and enhance their quality of life through the provision of carefully designed, and adequately supported, community residential schemes. Small scale, carefully designed studies such as the present one help to provide useful empirical information on the impact of community care on the lives of individual clients and provide feedback on the positive elements of the care processes which facilitate improved quality of life for residents. As well as identifying elements of good practice, the study also points to areas where further improvements may be made. Further analysis of the study's findings will seek to determine the strength of the relationship between the care process and client outcome variables in order to determine which variables are most critical for ensuring effective outcomes and a high quality of life for clients receiving long-term care in the community.

Acknowledgements

The work reported in this paper forms part of a longitudinal study commissioned by the Welsh Office, The Department of Health, Clwyd and Gwynedd Health Authorities, and Clwyd and Gwynedd Social Services Departments. The cooperation and assistance of residents and staff at the community care schemes in Clwyd is gratefully acknowledged. The views expressed in this paper represent those of the authors and do not necessarily reflect those of the sponsors.

References

Anthony, W.A. (1980). *The principles of psychiatric rehabilitation*. Baltimore: University Park Press.

Bachrach, L.L. (1980). Is the least restrictive environment always the best? Sociological and semantic implications. *Hospital and Community Psychiatry*, **31**, 97-103.

Baker, R. & Hall, J. (1983). *User's manual for rehabilitation evaluation: Hall and Baker*. Aberdeen: Vine Publishing Ltd.

Baker, F. & Intagliata, J. (1980). Quality of life in the evaluation of community support systems. *Evaluation and Programme Planning*, **5**, 69-79.

Barry, M.M., Crosby, C. & Mitchell, D.A., (1992). Quality of life issues in the evaluation of mental health services. In D.R. Trent (Ed.), *Promotion of mental health* (Vol.1), (pp.152-163). Aldershot: Avebury.

Barry M.M. & Crosby, C. (1992). Quality of life and mental health: Evaluating the impact of long-term care. In I. Markova & R.M. Farr (Eds.), *Representations of health, illness and handicap*. Harwood (in press).

Bigelow, D.A., Brodsky, G., Stewart, L. et al. (1982). The concept and measurement of quality of life as a dependent variable in evaluation of mental health services. In G.J. Tash and W.R. Tash (Eds.), *Innovative approaches to mental health evaluation*. New York: Academic Press.

Carter, M.F., Bogg, J., Crosby, C., & Barry, M.M. (1992). *Evaluation of resettlement from North Wales Hospital: Report on staff attitudes and management practices in two community residential care schemes and North*

Wales Hospital, Denbigh. Health Services Research Unit, Department of Psychology, University College of North Wales: Unpublished Manuscript.

Crosby, C., Barry, M.M., Carter, M.F. & Bogg, J. (1992). *Evaluation of resettlement from North Wales Hospital: Brief report on the care process in two community care schemes*. Health Services Research Unit, Department of Psychology, University College of North Wales: Unpublished Manuscript.

Crosby, C., Barry M.M., D.A., Horrocks, F.A. & Littlejohns, C.S. (1990). *Evaluation of the Clwyd mental health community service: An interim report*. Health Services Research Unit, Department of Psychology, University College of North Wales: Unpublished Manuscript.

Garety, P.A. & Morris, I. (1984). A new unit for long-stay psychiatric patients: Organisation, attitudes and quality of life. *Psychological Medicine*, **14**, 183-192.

Gibbons, J.S. & Butler, J.P. (1987). Quality of life for 'new' long-stay psychiatric in-patients: The effects of moving to a hostel. *British Journal of Psychiatry*, **157**, 347-354.

Krawiecka, M., Goldberg, D. & Vaughan, M. (1977). A standardised psychiatric assessment scale for rating chronic psychotic patients. *Acta Psychiattrica Scandinavica*, **55**, 299-308.

Lehman, A.F., Ward, N.C. & Lynn, L.S. (1982). Chronic Mental patients: The quality of life issue. *American Journal of Psychiatry*, **139** (10), 1271-1276.

Lehman, A.F. (1988). A quality of life interview for the chronically mentally ill. *Evaluation and Programme Planning*, **11**, 51-62.

Mitchell, D.A. (1990). Cohort description: Demographic, psychiatric and behavioural characteristics. Paper 2 in Crosby, C., Barry, M.M. Mitchell, D.A., Horrocks, F.A., & Littlejohns, C.S. *Evaluation of the Clwyd mental health community service: An interim report*. Health Service Research Unit, Department of Psychology, University College of North Wales: Unpublished Manuscript.

Overall, J. & Gorham, D. (1962). The Brief Psychiatric Rating Scale. *Psychological Reports*, **10**, 799-812.

Shadish, W.R., Orwin, R.G., Silber, B.G. & Bootzin, R.R. (1985). The subjective well-being of mental patients in nursing homes. *Evaluation and Programme Planning*, **8**, 239-250.

Wilde, E.D. and Svanber, P.O. (1990). Never mind the width - measure the quality. *Clinical psychology Forum*, 2-5.

Wykes, T. (1982). A hostel ward for 'new' long-stay patients: An evaluative study of 'a ward in a house'. In J.K. Wing (Ed.), Long-term Community Care: Experience in a London Borough. *Psychological Medicine Monograph Supplement 2* (pp.57-97). Cambridge University Press.

11 Bereavement care as a preventative health measure in older adults

R. Barry

The focus of this conference is on 'preventing mental illness' and 'promoting mental health'. Although the text books provide us with neat definitions of these terms (see Dr Trent's paper), many health professionals remain confused as to where the barriers are between health and illness. This is because there are no clear cut-off points, as research into the (un) reliability of psychiatric diagnosis shows us. It can be difficult to determine exactly at which point someone becomes 'ill'.

An alternative view, however, is of a society which comprises a continuum of people who experience a continuum of situations, problems, psychological distress, resources and coping abilities. Whether a particular individual at any given time crosses the boundary from health to illness depends largely on social factors. These include the individual's own perception of their emotional state as normal or abnormal; society's perception of their emotional state as healthy or sick and, on a practical level, whether there is any help available to that distressed individual at that time, other than a visit to their G.P.

The very painful experience of grief is an example of a natural process which often becomes medicalised due to lack of understanding and, if mis-managed or ignored, often leads to health problems.

Bereavement, above any other life situation, has been associated with the onset of physical and emotional health problems (Stroebe and Stroebe 1987) and this is especially true for those in the older age groups. The Samaritans' (1990) regular statistical review of suicide rates shows that those aged 65 plus and 75 plus consistently show higher suicide rates than younger age groups. Since only 10.7% of *known* suicides are by means of

131

poisoning by gases, it is highly unlikely that the introduction of the catalytic converter in cars will achieve the desired goal of a 15% reduction in suicide rates proposed by the new Government White Paper on Health.

Given the high rates of depression in older people (Fielden 1992) and the strong link between depression and suicide, the aim should be to alleviate the sources of depression, rather than the means of suicide, as a way of both preventing ill health and promoting good health.

A model of health care

Dr Albee refers to a model of mental health promotion which suggests the need to be proactive in offering help to those in 'at risk' groups. This is exactly what I am going to suggest that we do for bereaved elders.

Research into bereavement care can now indicate both the best means to facilitate transition through the grieving process and can help us to identify the factors which would indicate that a person might be at risk of suffering a particularly difficult reaction.

How effective is bereavement counselling?

Whether or not bereavement counselling works is dependent on several factors. Questions such as who are the counsellors, who receives counselling and when and for how long counselling is done, must be considered. Parkes (1980) has reviewed several studies which have attempted to evaluate counselling services. These include professional services by trained doctors, nurses, social workers and psychologists, services provided by trained volunteers supported by professionals and self-help groups, most of which had similar aims and approaches to counselling. Parkes concluded that 'professional services and professionally supported voluntary and self-help services are capable of reducing the risk of psychiatric and psychosomatic disorders resulting from bereavement. Services are most beneficial among bereaved people who perceive their families as unsupportive or who, for other reasons are thought to be at special risk' Worden (1982) states that his own clinical experience supports this conclusion.

Probably the most convincing evidence for the effectiveness of professional bereavement counselling comes from a study by Raphael (1977). In this study a group of widows assessed as being at 'low risk' were compared with two groups of 'high risk' widows who had been randomly assigned to intervention and control groups. Counselling was provided by Raphael herself, an experienced psychiatrist and bereavement counsellor. Clients had an average of four sessions (the range was from one to nine) which took place within their own homes between six and twelve weeks after bereavement. Assessment of general health was made thirteen months after the death. This indicated a poor outcome for approximately twenty percent of both the low risk group and the high risk group who received counselling compared with almost sixty percent in the high risk control group.

Parkes (1979, cited in Parkes, 1980) conducted a similar study to that of Raphael in order to evaluate a bereavement counselling service provided by selected and trained volunteers. Measures of change in health in the four years following bereavement were made. No differences between groups were found in the first year but thereafter significant differences favouring the supported group were found on two out of the three measures of change in health. As in Raphael's study the effect of counselling was to reduce the risk in the high risk group to about that of the low risk group. A further study of the volunteer service by Cameron and Parkes (1983) confirms these positive findings.

There appear to be very few empirical studies which investigate the impact of self-help intervention on bereavement outcome. However a controlled study by Vachon et al (1980) indicated beneficial effects of a combination of individual and group support provided by people who had themselves lost a spouse. Intervention was particularly effective for high risk widows (defined as those with high pre-intervention scores on a general health questionnaire). The counsellors in this study had received training from a professional nurse counsellor and a psychiatrist and, as such, may not be typical of those who generally work in self-help programmes. Parkes (1980) concludes that self-help groups that lack this type of professional backing are unlikely to provide so effective a service.

Early intervention is generally preferable but should be offered at least a week or so after the funeral (Worden, 1982). A counsellor who has been in contact with family members prior to the bereavement may be more able to offer help at an early stage. Both Worden and Parkes (1980) suggest that the home is likely to be the most suitable setting for counselling. Although most therapists (and some counsellors) require the formality of a professional setting, I would suggest that the very nature of bereavement counselling necessitates that the client feels as secure and comfortable as possible in his or her surroundings. For elderly people and others who may have difficulties travelling there is also the practical consideration of getting to the office.

What else helps?

Studies into what helps people to cope with a bereavement have generally found similar factors rated as most important.

133

Lehman et al (1986) and Janice Harris-Lord (1989) both report that what bereaved individuals rate as most helpful are contact with similar others, someone just being there, listening to them and letting them talk. Early on in the process practical help is valued e.g. helping organise the funeral and providing meals, etc. What is viewed as least helpful is people offering platitudes which minimise the loss e.g. 'he was 82, he'd had a good innings' or 'well, he is better off out of it now'. Even though people often come to think that themselves, they generally find it very upsetting to hear it from others and it is similarly unhelpful to tell people that "I know how you feel", when, in fact, no matter how similar the loss, no-one can know exactly how another person feels. Some people may find it helpful to discuss religion and their own philosophical perspectives but most people do not wish to have other people's thrust at them, you really have to take your cue from them..

Overall, the most helpful service would seem to be contact with other bereaved people, who it is felt, have experienced a similar loss, but with the training in counselling skills necessary to know how to listen and support without saying the wrong thing or being too directive.

Risk factors

Table 1
Assessing complicated grief risk factors

1. **Circumstances of the loss.**
   After long illness - dependency
   Sudden. Unexpected. Untimely. Uncertain e.g. missing.
2. **Social Factors.**
   No-one to listen or support. Relatives/friends acting as if nothing has happened.
   Not allowed to grieve in their own way.
3. **Relationship with the deceased.**
   Ambivalent/Dependent
4. **Bereaved person's history.**
   History of depression. Past complicated grief reactions. Bereavement/loss as a child.

Studies by Raphael (1977) and Parkes (1980) highlight the benefits of counselling for those who are at high risk of poor outcome. Later physical and psychological problems can be prevented if counselling is offered early to those identified as being at highest risk of poor outcome. A comprehensive review of studies is provided by Stroebe and Stroebe

(1987). The most important factors include the following:

(1) Circumstances of the death

These have been shown to have the highest relationship to outcome. If the loss is sudden, unexpected or untimely (as a child dying before a parent) then the bereaved is likely to need support. If a carer has been heavily involved in the care of a relative who died, the sheer physical impact, coupled with the frequent loss of a role upon the death, can lead to problems.

(2) Relationship with the deceased

When a relationship has been highly dependent and a widow(er) is left unable to fulfil certain needs, for which they have always depended upon their spouse, or at the other extreme, highly ambivalent, - for example where there had been a violent relationship - the grief process is likely to be complicated by guilt, rather than the death being a source of relief, as might be expected.

(3) Social factors

These have been shown to be very important not only in enabling people to cope with grief but also as a mediating factor in depression in older people (Murphy 1985).

It is very important that a person is allowed to grieve in their own way and there may be problems if friends and relatives put pressure on them to behave in a certain way, for example, to go out or not to go out. Most important is the bereaved persons perception of their level of support from others. When assessing risk factors it is important to look not only at the numbers of family and friends available to support the bereaved but also at whether they are perceived as helpful by the bereaved. Lack of social support or just someone to talk to have been identified as risk factors.

(4) Bereaved person's history

If the person has a history of depression or has had past losses which they either did not grieve or had difficulty with, this is likely to contribute to difficult reactions to a current loss. Also if they suffered a close loss as a child this may be a risk factor (e.g. Brown and Harris, 1980).

The relevance of bereavement counselling for older adults

A quick glance at the above list highlights the particular problems associated with bereaved elders. They are most likely to suffer loss after a long (more dependent) relationship, to suffer multiple losses, yet to lack the social support so necessary to help them through. Added to this there

135

is a small body of findings relating specifically to older people.

Table 2
Grief in older adults
variations

Raphel (84)	Many do not show grief directly but through impairment in physical health
Stern (51)	Minimal conscious guilt, tendency to self isolation, hostility towards members of family and friends
Samaritans(1990)	Highest suicide rate in 65+ and especially for 75+
Shulman (78)	Role of bereavement in this
Sanders (81)	18-20 months after death, older adults showed exacerbated grief reactions compared to younger adults
Gerber (75)	Physical health of elderly bereaved, worse for those whose spouse died following a lengthy illness than a short illness
Raphel (84)	Older more inclined to deny reality of loss, defense reaction
Sanders (81)	Deceased person may be idealised, resistance to relinquishing the spouse

An early study by Stern et al. (1951; cited in Diamond 1981) investigated grief reactions in a small sample of elderly people and found that these people showed minimal conscious guilt, a tendency to replace emotional reactions with somatic complaints, and a tendency to self-isolation and hostility toward members of the family and friends. It may be useful for the counsellor to bear in mind these factors when offering bereavement counselling to the older adult. One of the most profound losses, the death of a spouse, is more likely to occur in later life. In addition, many of the older bereaved may not show their grief directly, but rather through an impairment in their physical health (Raphael, 1984). Information from the Samaritans (1990) shows that in 1988 the suicide rate for elderly people was fifty percent higher than the overall rate for adults. The rate is particularly high for those aged over seventy five. The role of recent bereavement in increasing this risk is highlighted by Shulman (1978).

Elderly people are more likely to have experienced previous health problems and it may be expected that this would increase their risk of a poor bereavement outcome. Studies focusing on older age groups have highlighted the effects on both mental and physical health (Gallagher et al., 1983; Thompson et al., 1984). A longitudinal study by Sanders (1981 cited in Stroebe and Stroebe, 1987) found that shortly after widowhood, younger spouses seemed to suffer the most severe consequences but appeared to be able to adjust over time. Eighteen to twenty four months later, it was the older bereaved who showed exacerbated grief reactions. Contrary to general evidence regarding the greater impact of expected death, Gerber et al. (1975a) found the physical health of the elderly bereaved to be worse for those whose spouse had died after a lengthy (as opposed to a shorter) chronic illness. This finding was attributed to the strain of being a care-giver throughout a long illness, along with possible neglect of personal health and the vulnerability to ill health in old age. The findings of Lundin (1984) support this interpretation.

A counsellor attempting to help an elderly person adjust to the loss of a spouse needs an understanding of the social and environmental context in which the bereavement process occurs. As mentioned earlier, a perception of poor social support is a risk factor in bereavement outcome. An elderly person has usually spent a long time with his or her marital partner. This person may well have been the only really close relationship left and the last remaining source of physical affection. Following the loss of a partner many elderly people may feel particularly isolated and helpless. Financial hardship may limit the extent to which older people can build up supportive social networks and few of the elderly bereaved remarry (Moss and Moss 1979; cited in Raphael, 1984). Cultural and social attitudes towards the elderly are likely to be important factors in the availability of support. In many Western societies older people tend not to be valued and often lack status and resources. For these reasons counselling may be particularly appropriate for the older bereaved person.

It is not only spouses who are likely to die in later life but also other relatives and friends. As Diamond (1981) points out, the older person may not have time to finish the 'grief work' associated with one loss before another loss occurs. In addition to the death of close friends and family, older people are likely to experience numerous other kinds of loss. Retirement, the loss of a home and neighbourhood and physical deterioration such as the loss of mobility, sight or hearing are all losses associated with ageing. Diamond suggests that since the probability of 'bereavement overload' of this kind is high for the elderly, they are likely to experience a different kind of grieving process to younger people.

Older people may be more inclined to deny the reality of their loss and, in so doing, may not complete the grieving process (Raphael, 1984). It is particularly important for the bereavement counsellor to be aware of this. The older the bereaved person, the less of a future he or she perceives and so the less the motivation to fully accept the death and adjust to a new life.

Sanders (1981) suggests that initially denial acts as a defense mechanism which offers older people some protection against an adverse grief reaction. The deceased person may be idealized and, particularly in the very old, there may be a great resistance to relinquishing the spouse. There may be times when this has to be accepted by the counsellor and when it might seem almost unethical to encourage a reluctant elderly person to experience the pain of grief.

Table 3
Why do older adults need bereavement counselling?

1. Same reasons younger adults do.
2. Lack of perceived social supports - isolation.
3. Bereavement overload - multiple losses.
4. Older people do not acknowledge the need for counselling - then go to a GP with physical symptoms.
5. Different culture - not used to seeking help for emotional problems.
6. More likely to appear to cope well initially and then suffer exacerbated reaction.
7. A sense and awareness of their own mortality.
8. High rates of depression and suicide in older adults.
9. Lack of mobility, and cash, to seek social supports

In what appears to be one of the few controlled evaluations of bereavement interventions for elderly people, Gerber et al. (1975) considered the effect of a brief crisis intervention offered by trained psychiatric workers to elderly people who had lost a spouse. This consisted of emotional support, companionship and practical help. The findings indicated that the intervention was generally effective; those with therapeutic support received fewer prescriptions, consulted their doctor less frequently and reported feeling ill less often than those in the control group. The positive effects of the service began to be apparent approximately three months after the start of the intervention. Findings were linked to gender and cultural differences. There appears to be a lack of adequate research into the effectiveness of bereavement counselling with the elderly. In view of the possibility that the effects of bereavement in the elderly may be delayed initially, there is a particular need for longitudinal research in this area.

Table 4
Possible further developments in bereavement care for older adults

1. Counselling to be offered early to everyone.
2. Widow-to-Widow, Peer support.
3. Development of voluntary services, e.g. CRUSE, who provide social support groups for older age groups.
4. Development of social support for Sundays.
5. Preparation for death - how many never think about it?
6. Support and practical help to elderly caring for a dying spouse to lessen the impact of exhaustion and poor self-care.
7. Use of touch. Pets, Children.
8. Management of death in hospitals.
9. Manner of breaking the news. Explanations.

Not all older people either need or want help in coming to terms with their loss. However, in terms of preventing problems I believe that there are certain developments which could be beneficial (see Table 4). Counselling could be offered early (within three months of a death) to everyone identified as being at risk. Possibly this could be done via a widow to widow scheme as in the U.S.A (given that support from' similar others' is perceived as most helpful). I firmly support the role of voluntary agencies in providing this type of help, but believe that they need more help in terms of finance and professional support in training, supervision and as a resource to take over where they feel out of their depth with an individual. Closer links between voluntary agencies and professionals would facilitate early and smooth transition to a more professional service where this is necessary but save professional time being spent with individuals who do not need it. At the moment who you see for counselling is a lottery.

More support groups based in the community are needed, especially for difficult days like Sundays.

Preparation for death in terms of lifting the taboos so that the topic becomes more openly discussed and people prepare in advance for the reality of being alone (see Plenary Report, Barry).

The management of death in hospitals or at home and the manner of telling people could be improved. A lot of pressure is put on people to die in hospital rather than to provide sufficient support to care for them and allow them to die in dignity at home.

People are often told at the time of the death what is the cause of the death, which, due to the numbness characteristic of the first stage of grief, they usually forget. They should have a routine follow up visit by a G.P. or nurse to go through it with them later when they are more able to take it in. This could also be a way of monitoring how well they are dealing with their grief.

Conclusion

Bereavement is strongly implicated as a factor in both physical and psychological health problems in older people. In terms of preventing the development of these problems I believe there is a lot we can do. We should develop pro-active services, largely based on well-financed and supported voluntary agencies, backed by professional time, aimed initially, primarily, at those who can be identified as being at risk for the development of problems, so that people are contacted and offered support before they have to identify themselves as 'sick' and go to the services looking for it.

References

Cameron, J. & Parkes, C.M. (1983). Terminal Care: Evaluation of effects on surviving family of care before and after bereavement. *Postgraduate Medical Journal.* **59**,73-78.

Diamond, M. (1981). Bereavement and the elderly: A critical review with implications for nursing practice and research. *Journal of Advanced Nursing.* **6**, 461-470.

Fielden, M. (1992). Depression in older adults: Psychological and psychosocial approaches. Br.J.Social Wk, **22**.

Gerber, I., Wiener, A., Battin, D. & Arkin, A.M. (1975). Brief therapy to the aged bereaved. In B.Schoenberg, A.C.Carr, A.H.Kutscher, D.Peretz & I.Goldberg (Eds.), *Bereavement: Its psychosocial aspects.* New York: Columbia University Press.

Harris-Lord, J. (1988). *Beyond sympathy: What to say and do for someone suffering an injury, illness or loss.* Ventura: Pathfinder Publishing.

Lehman, D.R., Ellard, J.E., & Wordman, C.B. (1986). Social support for the bereaved: recipients and providers perspectives on what is helpful. *J.Couns & Clin. Psychol.* **54** (4) 438-446.

Lundin, T. (1984). Morbidity following sudden and unexpected bereavement. *British Journal of Psychiatry.* **144**, 84-88.

Murphy, E. (1985). The impact of depression in old age on close social relationships. *Am.J.Psychiatry,* **142**, 323-7.

Parkes, C.M. (1980). Bereavement counselling: Does it work? *British Medical Journal*, **281**, 3-6.

Raphael, B. (1977). Preventive intervention with the recently bereaved. *Archives of General Psychiatry*, **34**, 1450-1454.

Raphael, B. (1984). *The anatomy of bereavement*. London: Hutchinson.

The Samaritans, (May 1990). Information Sheet.

Sanders, C.M.(1983). Effects of sudden versus chronic illness death on bereavement outcome. *Omega*, **13**(3), 227-241.

Shulman, K. (1978). Suicide and parasuicide in old age: A review. *Age and Aging*. **7**, 201-209.

Stroebe, W. & Stroebe, M. (1987). *Bereavement and health; The psychological and physical consequences of partner loss*. Cambridge: C.U.P.

Thompson, L.W., Breckenridge, J.N., Gallagher, D. & Peterson, J. (1984). Effects of bereavement on self-perceptions of physical health in elderly widows and widowers. *Journal of Gerontology*. **39**(3), 309-314.

Worden, J.W. (1982). *Grief counselling and grief therapy*. London: Tavistock.

12 Experiences of collaborative community research and action in Nottingham

J. Bostock

Abstract

The principal tenet of this paper is that mental health promotion is best achieved via social interventions that allow people to have control over their circumstances. I begin with a critical examination of the meaning of 'mental health promotion' and argue for an ecological approach. I then discuss the research and community development activities of a group of residents and professional workers in Nottingham.

What is mental health promotion?

Trent (1991) has described five senses that are required for positive mental health: a sense of trust; a sense of challenge or curiosity; a sense of confidence, power and control; a sense of accomplishment; and a sense of humour. He has pointed out that mental health may be viewed as an entirely different construct to mental illness. Indeed mental health promotion is usually defined as improving the strengths and well-being of people (particularly vulnerable groups) at an individual or systems level (Ketterer, Bader and Levy, 1980) rather than treating so-called mental illness.

Mental health promotion is a term that carries medical connotations and therefore there is an erroneous tendency to think of mental health as a potentially normative condition, akin to physical fitness, to which we may all aspire. This assumes that our social and material worlds are organised in a way which is functional for most individuals. Even the mental health promotion rhetoric of preventing distress in 'vulnerable' groups may avoid the issue of eradicating the reasons for them being so defined (such as racism or unemployment).

We all live with a constellation of negative and positive feelings, strengths, weaknesses and resources that are inextricably linked with our actual experiences and situations. So, for instance, our senses of trust, challenge, control, accomplishment, and humour are not personality attributes which can inform us about how healthy we are. They are part of a complex web of personal resources which are inseparable from our past and present experiences and opportunities for actual control and agency.

Adding the term 'promotion' to 'mental health' further encourages a view of people's subjective experiences as individual possessions or commodities that can be improved like merchandise. This again is in danger of negating an environmental perspective. There is a vital need for research and theoretical developments that are more sensitive to social, cultural and ideological issues (Edwards, 1989; Smail, 1991; Orford, 1992). Although contemporary psychological models of stress purport to represent a transactional relationship between individuals and their environments, (Cox, 1978), in actuality the main thrust of empirical and practical work is with individuals.

There is some evidence to suggest that lay people are less likely to use a narrow individualistic definition of health than professional workers (Dun, 1989). The Edinburgh Research Unit in Health and Behavioural Change (1989) has reported on a study of a community development approach to health issues that indicates that health professionals are more concerned with changing individual behaviours than members of the public, who are more inclined to relate their health to such things as the prescription of tranquillisers or poor housing.

What is an ecological perspective and why is it relevant to mental health promotion?

An ecological approach recognises the reciprocal relationship between individuals' resources (e.g. education, problem solving strategies) and environmental influences (e.g. opportunities at school). Psychological distress is viewed as arising from a discordant 'fit' between persons and their social and physical environments rather than because of intrapsychic causes. (Rappaport, 1977)

Epidemiological data support such an explicit recognition of social as well as individual factors influencing psychological functioning. For instance, unemployed people are found to report higher levels of distress than employed people (Francis, Rajan, and Turner, 1989; Warr, Jackson and Banks, 1988); and Platt and Kreitman (1984) report high correlations between rates of unemployment and parasuicide among men in Edinburgh over a fourteen year period - the incidence of parasuicide among the unemployed was nearly ten times that in the employed group. Recent figures about suicide rates in young men aged between 20 and 24 years indicate a rise of 71% between 1980 and 1989 (HMSO, 1992) - a fact that cannot be separated from diminishing employment opportunities and increased poverty.

An ecological perspective is also supported by evidence that physical environments may adversely affect people although this is not a straightforward deterministic relationship. Chavis and Wandersman (1990) cite evidence that such things as litter and abandoned cars can engender fear of crime, lower property values and social withdrawal. Traffic level, community facilities, and residential designs can all affect social interaction and mental health (Rohe, 1985).

The American community psychology literature has done much to promote interventions consistent with an ecological perspective and to change social conditions in preference to offering individual treatment or therapy (Albee, 1988; Wolff, 1987). Such activity is located within a radical frame of reference concerned with structural social and economic change to foster a more equitable distribution of resources in society. This is a very different priority from much of the usual work undertaken by psychologists and mental health professionals, which tends to be reactive, and unquestioning of the economic and social reasons underlying many of the referrals of people to mental health services (Holland, 1988). Albee (1988) advocates diverse preventive practices such as laws to ensure equal opportunity, public education, and changes in the way the mass media portray certain groups. He also recommends empowering individuals or groups in order to strengthen their psychological resources to overcome adverse circumstances. The usual activity of mental health professionals can be represented within functionalist or interpretive paradigms, whereas Albee's exhortations suggest more radical activity - according to an analysis based on Whittington and Holland's work (1985).

The Sneinton and Bakersfield survey reported here illustrates how research or survey work can be a vital tool in understanding the needs of a community in order to respond to these, and can become a helpful intervention in itself. The way that research is carried out and the results disseminated can facilitate or undermine people's control or empowerment. Collaborative and interdisciplinary social action research tends to be associated with an ecological approach to mental health promotion and a commitment to public participation and empowerment (Rappaport,

1992). The survey discussed here involved many different people in its implementation, the discussion of the results and what to do with them. A community development worker and myself worked particularly closely together in ensuring that the project did not lose momentum. This was a good illustration of Florin and Wandersman's point (1990) that community development workers offer community psychologists an excellent opportunity to work collaboratively on citizen orientated research. The survey was not an academic exercise or an end in itself but aimed to be a catalyst for generating social change.

The Sneinton and Bakersfield community survey

The area this survey relates to is situated approximately two miles from the city centre of Nottingham and covers a population of approximately 35,000 people. There is a mixture of housing that includes three council estates, three tower blocks of flats, suburban semi-detached houses, and many Victorian Terraces which are Council/Housing Association/privately rented or owner-occupied. There is an active environmental group in the area which takes pride in some historical features and in preserving and restoring these, so there are definitely positive aspects to the area. However, there are signs of extreme poverty and deprivation in that the average rate of unemployment is 22%, and up to 25% of the population are single parents in some areas.

The Sneinton and Bakersfield Community Forum set up the survey. Their diverse membership includes a Tenants' Association Representative, community development workers, a GP, a community psychologist, the warden of an elderly person's housing scheme, an employment development worker, clergymen, representatives from community centres, a policeman, a City Councillor. They originally met in order to exchange local information (for example about summer playschemes) and to respond to local issues. The survey was initiated because of concern that the Forum was predominantly made up of professional workers and there was insufficient participation of local residents. It aimed to (1) gain systematic knowledge about living in the area and what people thought affected their physical and psychological health; (2) engage with people proactively; and (3) encourage residents' participation in addressing the issues identified as important (reproduced from Bostock and Beck, in press).

Undertaking the survey meant Forum members working together to decide on what we wanted to know and how we would gather the information. It began with semi-structured group interviews and the final interview schedules were based on twenty three pilot interviews that drew on the group interviews and on a survey done in West Lambeth (Dun, 1989). The questions asked and the results obtained have been written about in more detail by Bostock and Beck (in press). The interview included open and closed questions that asked about what people liked and disliked about living in the area, what they thought affected people's health and what adversely affected their own health or caused them stress.

Interviews were conducted by fifteen interviewers. Most of the hundred and twenty three interviews took place with people they met through their work or voluntary activities. This method of recruitment was used after much discussion in preference to a random population sampling technique because Forum members were keen to work with networks of people they came across fairly naturally. Thus the second aim of the research was immediately met because the survey provided a means of engaging with people. For instance some people were met and interviewed because they were patients at the GP surgery, or as users of community centres.

The qualitative data were coded by two of the Forum members and their categories were checked for reliability by an independent assessor and found to be satisfactory (94% agreement). All the data were then discussed at length by the Forum before the summary of results was publicised. A short summary was sent in a letter to 79 of the people interviewed who had expressed an interest in receiving them along with an invitation to a public meeting to discuss the findings in more depth. The results of the survey and the public meeting were also publicised via posters and a press release to the local radio and press.

Results

Most of the people interviewed were positive about the Sneinton and Bakersfield area for reasons such as being close to the city centre, having a sense of community and friendliness, good shopping facilities and proximity to parks and open spaces. Common aspects of the area that were disliked were dirty streets and litter, petty crime and vandalism, dog dirt, and traffic and busy roads.

Similar themes were mentioned with regard to problems people identified as affecting their health which were mainly environmental rather than personal such as, air and traffic pollution, dogs, and litter/dirt. More personal issues such as diet and exercise were raised by the question asking about what contributes toward a healthy life. Smoking was the most frequently cited harmful aspect of daily life.

Dog mess was most often mentioned in response to a question which asked people to say which of twenty two factors they thought affected their health or caused them stress. The ten responses most commonly identified were: dog's mess on pavement or play areas; dangerous traffic; rubbish on the streets; dirt and pollution; fear of crime; feeling it is not safe to go out; having to manage on a low income; lack of places for young people to go; lack of places for children to play; and noise.

The non random nature of the sample means that these results cannot be said to represent the views of a cross-section of the Sneinton/Bakersfield population. The results were used by the Forum members as a starting point for further engagement with the community that was fairly systematically based. They decided upon the following broad themes as starting points for discussion at the first public meeting: the environment, crime and safety, youth provision and child and play provision.

In order to avoid an intimidating traditional public meeting format, it was planned that four groups would discuss each of these themes and then report back to pool their ideas. These small groups were led in a way that encouraged the discussion of possible solutions rather than generating further concerns.

Since then there have been further bi-monthly public meetings and a new structure for public participation has emerged. A steering group coordinates the publicity and communication between the different groups of people now involved in the Forum. 'Working groups' have developed in conjunction with the broad themes discussed - an area improvement group, a childcare and play provision group, a crime and safety group and a youth provision group. They have differed in the extent of their activity but have become involved in such things as consulting with young people about youth clubs; setting up a parent and toddler group; developing a patch of derelict land into a children's play area; developing communication between neighbourhood watch groups; lobbying for better leisure facilities and setting up support groups in a community centre.

This structure has also provided a means for some representation of local people in Nottingham's City Challenge initiatives, for example in defining the job description of a play development worker. The scope of my community and preventive work as a community psychologist has been enhanced as I am able to have easier contact with people to offer advice and support outside a formal referral system.

Using collaborative research and action for the promotion of mental health: some reflections

Research: a catalyst for community development

The Sneinton and Bakersfield community survey did not purport to promote the mental health of the local community but has done so by providing a means of understanding and changing adverse aspects of the social and physical environment. The actual results of the survey have become less important than the network of activity that has been generated. The survey provided a way of involving people on the basis of some systematically derived evidence - albeit methodologically flawed because of the unknown effects of interviewer bias and the unrepresentative sample. The survey was more successful in encouraging people's participation than previous efforts at inviting people to the Forum meetings via displays in the library and press releases. Over a hundred people have been involved in various meetings over the past year.

It seems likely that the process of doing the research and sharing the results helped to galvanised local action. The publicising of the first public meetings coincided with Nottingham winning City Challenge status and this has fired people's interest. Some people attending the meetings were hoping to secure funds for particular projects and this is likely to have been a motivating factor in engaging popular support.

Mental health promotion at an ecological level

One can argue that the groups' activities have taken a collective, radical humanist approach to tackling sources of psychological and physical suffering (Whittington and Holland, 1988). The groups are helping people to gain more from an existing social structure. They are concerned with improving conditions at a local and proximal level rather than challenging macro economic structures.

Acknowledgement of limitations

A realistic awareness of the limitations of this project needs to be maintained. The community psychology and mental health promotion literature tackles the issue of empowering vulnerable groups without questioning whether this is a realistic long-term strategy for fundamental social change. Empowerment needs to be concerned with more than giving people an opportunity to voice their opinions, but with effecting real opportunities for power, influence and control. There is often an optimistic assumption of a benign social context while in practice this may not be true. For instance, one of the Sneinton and Bakersfield groups is interested

149

in setting up a community nursery and training facility but, realistically, unemployment is still likely to be an extremely difficult hurdle to overcome. While an energetic and sustained commitment to such endeavour is essential, an apolitical, evangelical enthusiasm for collective action is in danger of underestimating the odds that are against changing the status quo.

Methodology

Another issue that this survey highlights is the difficulty of obtaining valid and reliable data in a way that involves people in the data gathering and dissemination. A good deal of time, organisation and mutual cooperation and compromise was entailed. Those of us educated in a positivist tradition as psychologists are wary of research designs with unrepresentative samples or a likelihood of interviewer bias. However, I suggest that we generated rich data that people found interesting and relevant. The methodological limitations mean that generalising the findings is not possible, but that was not our aim.

The need for evaluation

A further question that needs addressing is the understanding of the groups' participants and activities in order to consider whether they are involving people who are actually already well-resourced and empowered. The extent to which the groups are involving people who most need the social support and empowerment has yet to be established.

The Forum's actual achievements and disappointments need continuous monitoring, bearing in mind that there is a high failure rate for community groups (Florin and Wandersman, 1990). There has been a differing rate of activity for the Sneinton and Bakersfield groups and it would appear that the involvement of active professional workers has been an important influence. There is considerable scope for the development of further lobbying and supportive structures in this community.

Professional's involvement

The sneinton and Bakersfield Forum has always involved a diverse range of people and the survey was a shared enterprise that involved considerable cooperation and mutual learning. People with different experiences and strengths were able to share these. For example, administrative and research skills, and familiarity with community development. Flexibility has also been demanded in undertaking tasks that may not traditionally be seen as part of one's professional role, like making tea and addressing envelopes!

Professionals sharing resources with each other and with local residents, is a delicate issue because of the propensity for professionals to be patronising, over-controlling and therefore disempowering. Using jargon and a glib familiarity with a perplexing bureaucracy can be very alienating for people. The nature and duration of the professional workers' involvement remains a difficult question to resolve and needs negotiating with the groups' participants. It has to be said that most health professionals and psychologists are still very concerned with a treatment mode of working and are largely inexperienced in relating to people outside a health care setting. This puts people in a situation without familiar ways of operating or 'rules' which can be very challenging and potentially threatening for all concerned.

The Sneinton and Bakersfield Community Forum is not a mental health forum but an organisation committed to improving social and physical conditions in the area. The groups that have been set up are building social structures that foster public representation and participation in overcoming harmful circumstances - mental health promotion attained via pragmatic and collective action.

References

Albee, G.W., (1988). Prevention is the answer. *Open Mind*, 35,14-16.

Bostock, J., & Beck. D., (1992). The Sneinton and Bakersfield Community Survey: A collaborative approach to community action and research. *Journal of Community and Applied Social Psychology.* In press.

Chavis, D.M., & Wandersman, A., (1990). Sense of community in the urban environment: A catalyst for participation and community development. *American Journal of Community Psychology*, 18 (1), 55-82.

Cox, T., (1978). *Stress.* London: Macmillan

Dun, R., (1989). *Pictures of Health? A Report of a Community Health Survey carried out in Clapham, South London.* West Lambeth Health Authority Community Unit.

Edwards,G., (1989,April). Finding that Broad Street pump. *Changes,*(pp.61-64)

Florin, P., & Wandersman, A., (1990). An introduction to citizen participation, voluntary organisations and community development: Insights for empowerment through research. *American Journal of Community Psychology*, 18 (1), 41-54.

Francis, W.M., Rajan, P., & Turner, N., (1990). British community norms for the Brief Symptom Inventory. *British Journal of Clinical Psychology*, 29,115-116.

Holland, S., (1988) Defining and experimenting with prevention. In S. Ramon & M.G. Giannichedda (Eds.), *Psychiatry in transition: The British and Italian experiences*. London: Pluto Press.

H.M.S.O. (1992). *The Health of the Nation*.

Ketterer, R.P., Bader, D.C., & Levy, M.R. (1980). Strategies and skills for promoting mental health. In R.H.Price, R.F.Ketterer, B.C.Bader, & J.Monahan (Eds.), *Prevention in mental health. Research, policy and practice*. Beverley Hills: Sage.

Orford, J., (1992). *Community psychology: Theory and practice*. Chichester: Wiley.

Platt, S., & Kreitman, N., (1984). Trends in parasuicide and unemployment in men in Edinburgh. *British Medical Journal*, 289,1029-1032.

Rappaport, J., (1992). The dilemma of primary prevention in mental health services: Rationalise the status quo or bite the hand that feeds you. *Journal of Community & Applied Social Psychology*, 2,95-99.

Research Unit in Health and Behavioural Change, University of Edinburgh. (1989). *Changing the public health*. Chichester: Wiley.

Rohe, W.M., (1985). Urban planning and mental health. In A.Wandersman & R.Hess (Eds.), *Beyond the individual: Environmentalist approaches and prevention*. US: Hawarth Press Incorporated.

Smail, D. J., (1991). Towards a radical environmentalist psychology of help. *The Psychologist*, **4** (2), 61-64.

Trent, D., (1992). Breaking the single continuum. In D.Trent. (Ed.), *Promotion of mental health, (Volume 1)*. UK: Avebury.

Warr, P., Jackson, P., & Banks, M., (1988). Unemployment and mental health: Some British Studies. *Journal of Social Issues*, **44**, 47-68.

Whittington, C., & Holland, R., (1985). A framework for theory in social work. *Issues in Social Work Education*, **5** (1),25-50.

Wolff, T., (1987). Community psychology and empowerment: An activist's insights. *American Journal of Community Psychology*, **15** (2), 149-165.

13 A follow-up study of people with mental health problems attending an office technology training scheme

D. Buglass, M. Coutts and J. Tate

Introduction

The Scottish Association for Mental Health started training in office technology in Edinburgh in 1987. Training was targeted at people who had mental health problems. The scheme was originally funded under the MSC Community Programme and has since been variously funded by the European Social Fund, Employment Training, Local Enterprise Board and the local authority. Financial support has been varied and uncertain and the number of places has fluctuated accordingly, rising from an initial 10 places to 30 at present.

This paper presents the experience of those trainees who entered the programme from its start in December 1987 and who had left by November 30 1990. It considers their training experience and their work history after they left. The building in which training is located is called Atlantic House and 'Atlantic Text' was adopted as the name for the programme as a whole. The usual expected length of stay is one year.

Trainees were selected by interview, much as if they were applying for a job. Motivation to tackle the training and to find work were factors which favoured acceptance. The number of suitable applicants soon exceeded the number of places and a waiting list was established. Applicants were reconsidered from the waiting list as places became available.

Method

All trainees who enrolled and actually attended the project were listed and basic information about them was culled from the project notes and from the recollections of the two workers who had long association with the project. A questionnaire was then sent to the last known address of each individual. The questionnaire asked about subsequent employment, education, current health and recollections of their time at Atlantic Text. Respondents were asked to return the questionnaire by the end of April 1991. A reminder was sent out in May encouraging the return of outstanding questionnaires.

April 30th 1991 was taken as the cut-off date for calculating the period of follow-up. This meant that the time since leaving the project ranged for individuals from 5 months to two and a half years.

The statistical significance of some comparisons has been tested (Chi-squared test); results are deemed significant if the probability of the difference occurring by chance is less than 1 in 20 (P<.05).

Results

1. Characteristics of the total group

By November 1990, 63 persons had left the project after spending time at Atlantic Text. Their characteristics are summarised in Table A

Age and sex

Thirty six (57%) were men and 27 (43%) women. The group had an average age of 31 years. The youngest was 18 at the start of the programme, the oldest 57. Most trainees were in their twenties (44%) and thirties (40%). Only one person was over 50 years.

Education prior to the programme

The educational level of the trainees was high. 79% had at least one CSE or 'O' level; 11 (17%) had a degree or professional qualification, for example in nursing, teaching or accountancy, and a further 17 (27%) had at least one year at college or university.

Previous work

A third had less than a year's experience of paid work; a third between one and 5 years experience and a third over 5 years. 32% had previous experience of a SAMH training scheme (in the main SPROUT, a market garden training scheme).

Source of referral

The psychiatric hospital was the single greatest referral agent (42%); 23% of trainees approached the project direct.

Previous health problems

Only minimal information was kept on previous illness because the philosophy of the project was to accept people as they were and to assist them in planning for the future rather than dwelling on past difficulties. Nevertheless it was ascertained either from records or from the recollections of the workers that at least 34 (59%) persons had been psychiatric in-patients during the 12 months prior to commencement of the project. At the time of starting the programme, 25% were living in supported accommodation and one person was still in hospital. Although diagnostic labels were not recorded, it was clear that the majority of trainees had had serious and long-term problems.

Length of stay, completion of programme and position on leaving

22 trainees completed the full programme. The mean and median length of stay was 7 months. Some left early because they had found work.

22 left for open (10) or sheltered employment and 2 transferred to another Employment Training Scheme.

13 were too sick to continue and a further one was readmitted to hospital.

The follow-up questionnaires

The follow-up questionnaires achieved 68% response rate (or 74% if death and addresses not known are excluded).

Table 1
Number of respondents who returned followup questionnaires

Questionnaire:	Number	Percent
Completed	43	68.3
Refused	1	1.6
Not returned	14	22.2
Returned by PO, address N/K	4	6.3
Died	1	1.6
TOTAL	63	100

155

Typicality of people who returned the questionnaire

In any survey it is useful to know whether the people who responded were markedly different from those who did not. In this study we found that people who returned the questionnaire were more likely to have finished the programme provided by Atlantic Text and were more likely to have employment when they left. In addition there was a trend - just below the level of statistical significance - for people over 35 years to be more likely to return their questionnaires. In other respects the characteristics of those who returned the questionnaires were similar to those who did not. These differences are summarised in Table A (Appendix). The remainder of this paper describes the results for the 43 respondents who returned the follow-up questionnaire.

2. Respondents and work

Employment after the programme

One expectation of an employment programme is that it leads to a job. 44% of the respondents (19 persons) left Atlantic Text for work, either open or sheltered. 49% (21 persons) were in work at the time of the survey; two more were doing further training on Employment Training schemes. 28% had been continuously employed since leaving and 47% had worked for about half the available time. Four ex-trainees had been in full time further education and 4 in part-time. Ten (23%) had done some voluntary work since the end of the programme.

Table 2 shows the relationship between leaving the programme for a job, the proportion of time in work and being in work at the time of the survey. It is clear that these three items are highly related. People who left Atlantic Test for a job were very likely to be in work now and to have worked for at least half the time available since leaving. Those who did not have a job to go to when they left Atlantic Text have rarely worked since that time. Being in current work can, therefore, be considered a fair indication of a good employment record after Atlantic Text; likewise not being currently in work was generally indicative of little or no work since the programme. In subsequent analysis current work is used as a key variable against which all other aspects of the respondents' life experience are reviewed.

Predictors of subsequent employment

Does any of the information available about trainees while they are on the programme indicate whether they will subsequently have a good work record? Table 3 shows current work status in relation to respondents' characteristics at the start and finish of the programme. None of the initial

156

Table 2
Current work and other measures of employment

| | Current Employment Status | | Total |
	Employed	Not employed	
Total	21 100%	22 100%	43 100%
Position on Leaving: Employed Other	 17 81% 4 19%	 2 9% 20 91%	 19 44% 24 56%
Proportion Time Employed: Half or more Less than half	 18 86% 3 14%	 2 9% 20 91%	 20 47% 23 53%
Months Employed: None <12m 12m+	 0 0% 9 43% 12 57%	 20 91% 2 9% 0 0%	 20 47% 11 26% 12 28%

characteristics are related to subsequent employment. Gender was not significantly related to being in work but women were a little more likely to be working. Age - being under or over 35 years - was quite unrelated to being in work. Level of previous education, length of time previously in work, whether SAMH training (usually market gardening) had been undertaken previously, source of referral, type of accommodation and whether an in-patient in a psychiatric hospital during the year preceding the programme were all unrelated to being in work.

The predictors of a good work record are staying on the programme for 12 months, completing the programme and (as noted above) having a job to go to at the time of leaving. Those people whose health, motivation and persistence enabled them to see the programme through and who left for work were much more likely than their fellows to be in work at follow-up.

Work histories

What sort of work did trainees find? Did they make use of their training? At the time of follow-up 14 people were in open employment, 7 in sheltered employment and 2 in further employment training. Since leaving the programme, 12 had been in work for 12 months or more (4 of

Table 3
Characteristics of respondents and current work

	Current Employment Status			Total	
	Employed		Not employed		
Total	21	100%	22	100%	43	100%
Sex						
Male	10	48%	15	68%	25	58%
Female	11	52%	7	32%	18	42%
Age						
Under 35	11	52%	11	50%	22	51%
35 and over	10	48%	11	50%	21	49%
Previous Education						
Minimum to A level	9	43%	14	64%	23	53%
At least 1 yr coll	12	57%	8	36%	20	47%
Previous Work						
<5yr	15	71%	10	45%	25	58%
5yr+	6	29%	12	55%	18	42%
Previous SAMH Training						
Yes	8	38%	7	32%	15	35%
No	13	62%	15	68%	28	65%
Source of Referral						
Self	4	20%	4	18%	8	19%
Psych Hosp	10	50%	6	27%	16	38%
Other	6	30%	12	55%	18	43%
Accommodation at Start						
Supp Accom	6	29%	6	27%	12	28%
Other	15	71%	16	73%	31	72%
In-pt in Previous Year						
Yes	10	53%	11	55%	21	54%
No	9	47%	9	45%	18	46%
Length of Stay*						
Under 12 mths	9	43%	17	77%	26	60%
12 mths +	12	57%	5	23%	17	40%
Completed Programme*						
Yes	13	62%	6	27%	19	44%
No	8	38%	16	73%	24	56%
* Difference statistically significant						

these for over 2 years); seven had been in work for 6 - 12 months. People were asked whether they had used the skills learned at Atlantic

Text and those in work were much more likely to have done so, (Table 4). In particular they had used their computer, keyboard, wordprocessing and general office skills. Spreadsheet and database skills were not often

Table 4
Skills used since leaving Atlantic Text

	Current Employment Status				Total	
	Employed		Not employed			
Used skills since AT*	19	90%	9	41%	28	65%
Computer skills*	14	67%	7	32%	21	49%
Keyboard skills*	15	71%	7	32%	22	51%
Word processing*	15	71%	7	32%	22	51%
General office skills*	17	81%	5	23%	22	51%
Spreadsheets	4	19%	2	9%	6	14%
Databases	9	43%	5	23%	14	33%
How to prepare a CV	8	38%	6	27%	14	33%
Total respondents	21	100%	22	100%	43	100%
* Difference statistically significant						

required in their work. People not in work had used the training in preparation of a curriculum vitae almost as often as those who were working.

The type of work obtained by trainees was mainly clerical and secretarial. There were two exceptions - a woman who was back in Employment Training after working in a factory and as a cleaner and a man who had been employed as a laboratory assistant then as a lifeguard. The remainder - both open and sheltered - were clerical assistants, secretaries, technical clerks, accounts assistant or book-keeper. One person worked as an office manager, another, after a spell as a clerk, obtained open employment in a voluntary organisation. In all, 4 people moved, or were about to move, from sheltered to open employment; another, after a year's open employment, had her secretarial job redesignated as sheltered.

The respondents were not fickle in their work. Since the follow-up period for individuals was very variable - 5 months to 31 months - the average length of time employed is not a relevant measure. However, respondents who obtained work tended to remain there. Changes of job were not frequent. Sometimes people consolidated their work position, for example by moving from a temporary to a permanent post within the same organisation.

Comparison of Year 1 and Year 2

Certain features distinguished the people who started the programme in the first year, Dec 1987 - Nov 1988 from those in Year 2, Dec 1988 - Nov 1989. (The eight people in the study who started the programme in Year 3 are excluded from this comparison because they are all early leavers. The cut off date for the study was November 1990; anyone starting the programme in Year 3 who had left by then had not had time to complete the programme - though some left for work).

Two of the 13 people starting in Year 1 went to open employment and eight to sheltered employment. Only 3 did not have work when they left. Of the 22 people starting in Year 2, 5 went to open employment, 1 to sheltered employment and 16 to neither of these. Respondents from Year 1 were significantly more likely to be in work at the time of follow-up than

Table 5
Employment and starting date

	Year Programme Started			
	Year 1		Year 2	
Total	13	100%	22	100%
Position on Leaving				
Open employment	2	15%	5	23%
Sheltered employment	8	62%	1	5%
Unemployed	1	8%	10	45%
Further education	0	0%	2	9%
Sick	1	8%	3	14%
ET	1	8%	0	0%
Other	0	0%	1	5%
Current Employment Status				
Open employment	6	46%	7	32%
Sheltered employment	5	38%	1	5%
ET	0	0%	2	9%
Not in work	2	15%	12	55%

160

were people from Year 2. More respondents from Year 2 (59%) had not worked at all since leaving compared with Year 1 (15%). The difference was accounted for by the greater proportion of Year 1 who found sheltered work, (Table 5).

Health

Over half the respondents reported that their health was 'good' at the time of the survey; 20 said it was fair or poor. Respondents in work were much more likely than those not employed to say that their health was good (71% compared with 36%). People in work were also significantly less likely to say that their health had prevented them from obtaining work (Table 6).

Table 6
Health and current work status

	Current Employment Status		Total	
	Employed	Not employed		
Total	21 100%	22 100%	43	100%
Present Health*				
Good	15 71%	8 36%	23	53%
Fair to poor	6 29%	14 64%	20	47%
Health Prevented work*				
Yes	6 29%	15 68%	21	49%
No	15 71%	7 32%	22	51%

3. Activities after the programme ended

What happened to the trainees after they left Atlantic Text apart from work? Did they go for further education or voluntary work? Had their health problems been resolved? Did their experience vary greatly according to whether they had work? Trainees' responses are summarised in Table 7.

Further education

Four people had experience of full time education, four of part-time. Two trainees who left Atlantic Text for further education were unable to continue in it. One gave up a computing course after a month; another abandoned a post-graduate diploma because of the difficulty in settling

161

Table 7
Activities after the programme and current work

	Current Employment Status			
	Employed	Not employed		
Total	21 100%	22 100%	43	100%
Further Education				
Yes	5 24%	3 14%	8	19%
No	16 76%	19 86%	35	81%
Voluntary Work				
Yes	4 19%	6 27%	10	23%
No	17 81%	16 73%	33	77%
Day Time Activities				
Yes	4 19%	11 52%	15	36%
No	17 81%	10 48%	27	64%

in lodgings in a strange town. Only one of the four who entered full time study is now in work (as a clerical assistant). Those people who were able to integrate further studies with their work, perhaps on a day release basis, were more successful. One is currently doing a printing course, another accounting and two others took courses in other aspects of computing. All those doing part time courses are currently in work.

Voluntary work

Ten - 4 now in work, 6 not employed - respondents said they had done some voluntary work since the programme. This included being a befriender of people with mental health problems; helping in a charity shop; typing a student's thesis and tutoring people with learning disabilities in word processing and databases.

Day activities

A higher proportion of people not employed (not quite statistically significant) said that they participated in some form of structured day activity - for example attended a day centre or a day hospital or a job club. (11 of the not employed compared with 4 of the employed). One employed person combined a job with spending the lunch hour at a day centre; another in sheltered employment attended a day hospital four times a week as well. Others said that when not in work they occupied themselves with the tasks of everyday living.

Some of their comments illustrate their daily routine:

- 'Going shopping (window shopping); visiting friends; looking for a job'. (employed 3/4 of available time since leaving).
- 'I am in contact with a Resettlement Officer from Lothian Region Social Work Department who helps me find work. I go to the Job Centre and buy newspapers for job vacancies. I socialise with friends who have been made unemployed'. (no employment).
- 'Attended job club (Executive Club) at end of 1989 and from March-September 1990' (employed 1/2 available time).
- 'Mainly in looking for work; I find it difficult to make good use of time when I don't have anything in particular'. (employed 3/4 available time).
- 'NSF Centre. I am a very regular attender. Meeting, talking to people at the Centre; reading, watching TV, going out with friends, writing poems, visiting my mother.' (no employment).

Readiness to leave

Two thirds of respondents said they were ready to leave the programme at the time of departure, but 12 said their departure came too soon. Those who were not ready were rather less likely to be in employment now (just below the level of statistical significance).

Continuing contact

Respondents were asked whether they remained in touch with staff and fellow trainees. Sixteen said they remained in touch with Atlantic Text staff and 19 were in contact with other trainees. Those in employment were rather more likely to keep in touch with Atlantic Text staff but those who kept contact with fellow trainees were equally likely to be unemployed.

4. Looking back

Recollections of the Atlantic Text programme

The programme devised for Atlantic Text trainees is intended to be responsive to their individual needs. The trainees learn about all aspects of office technology and office practice; they are shown how to prepare a curriculum vitae and try out interview techniques. They learn specific computer packages for word processing and for database and spreadsheet skills. Some of their courses take place in local colleges, some in Atlantic Text premises. Efforts are made to find placements which give them experience of the working world and complement their training. Placements are tailored to individual need and may, for example, be a block placement of two or three weeks or a half-day a week over a period of months. In addition the programme seeks to provide a positive and supportive experience to people whose lives have mostly been seriously disrupted by illness. At the time of follow-up, therefore, respondents were asked about their recollections of the course and whether it had helped them develop attitudes which would assist them in work and also which would improve their general well-being. Table 8 summarises their responses.

Table 8
Views of the programme

	Employed		Not Employed		Total	
Total	21	100%	22	100%	43	100%
Having a work routine helped me with my timekeeping	14	67%	11	50%	25	58%
The support of people with similar problems was helpful	17	81%	14	64%	31	72%
I felt I was part of a team wiht similar aims	15	71%	10	45%	25	58%
The demands of a work routine were difficult to cope with	0	0%	7	32%	7	16%
I gained confidence in interview technigues	12	57%	5	23%	17	40%
Difficult to be with people with mental health problems	3	14%	3	14%	6	14%
I developed my ability to take responsibility for work *	16	76%	8	36%	24	56%
My expectations of getting work were raised too much	2	10%	6	27%	8	19%
I became more aware of current office practices	19	90%	15	68%	34	79%
I enjoyed the challenge of working with other people	17	81%	10	45%	27	63%
I felt the course was too demanding	0	0%	5	23%	5	12%
I became more confident in my dealings with other people*	18	86%	11	50%	29	67%
Working alongside other people was difficult to cope with	1	5%	5	23%	6	14%
I felt more confident about myself	15	71%	14	64%	29	67%
I didn't learn anything very much	2	10%	1	5%	3	7%
* difference statistically significant						

More than half the respondents said that the programme had provided a situation in which they found:
- a work routine which helped timekeeping
- the support of people with similar problems which was helpful
- they were part of a team with similar aims
- they developed ability to take responsibility for work
- they were more aware of current office practices
- they enjoyed the challenge of working with others
- they were more confident in their dealing with other people
- they were more confident about themselves.

Two of the items - the ability to take responsibility for work and confidence in dealing with others - were endorsed significantly more often by people now in work. In addition, seven people who are not in work said they had found the work routines at Atlantic Text difficult; none of the employed said this. Similarly 5 of the unemployed felt the course too demanding but none of the employed endorsed this item. In general, the other items fell in the expected direction - people in work expressed a more positive view and felt they had gained more from the course than those not working.

Two items, however, are of interest because they did **not** discriminate between the employed and the unemployed. Fifteen of the employed and 14 of the unemployed said that the course helped them to feel more confident abut themselves. Six people in all - 3 employed and 3 unemployed - said that they 'found it difficult to be on a course with people who had mental health problems'. Only three people said that they didn't learn anything very much; two of these are now in employment.

Attitudes to college training

The programme provided by Atlantic Text has varied over time. In the early days, particularly in the first two years, part of the training was provided at a local further education college. This was partly for practical reasons and partly because it was thought to be beneficial for trainees to attend a mainstream resource. This issue has at times been controversial for both staff and trainees. Some trainees disliked going to college. Some trainees also followed courses at another FE college as 'open-learning students'. Trainees were given the opportunity to comment on the mix and location of training. They were also presented with eight statements describing possible reactions to College attendance and asked to say which applied to them. Table 9 shows their responses. Seventeen respondents said that success in gaining modules increased their confidence; 12 said it was difficult to study in a large institution. Nine said they

Table 9
Statements about college training

	Current Employment Status				Total	
	Employed		Not employed			
Total	20	100%	16	100%	36	100%
Gaining modules increased my confidence	10	50%	7	44%	17	47%
I found it difficult to study in a large institution	6	30%	6	38%	12	33%
I became more able to tackle problems	7	35%	3	19%	10	28%
I discovered I was capable of more than I thought	4	20%	6	38%	10	28%
I found studying for a module created stress	3	15%	4	25%	7	19%
I found lecturers supportive	5	25%	4	25%	9	25%
More possibilities in education than I realised	5	25%	2	13%	7	19%
I felt lecturers didn't understand my problems	3	15%	4	25%	7	19%

found lecturers supportive; 7 that lecturers did not understand their problems.

Thirty-one trainees offered some comment on the location and mix of training and/or on their reactions at the end of College training. Of these only three were firmly positive and nearly half were unequivocally negative; the remainder were mixed or neutral. One person wrote:

'In my circumstances College did me a lot of good and I acquired new skills. [When I left] I felt more confident and felt a lot of achievement'.

Another said: 'The mix of training was about right'.

Several gave thoughtful and balanced assessments of the pros and cons of their experience.

- 'College was a little daunting at first but it gave me a great sense of achievement'.
- 'On site training is very good for general office and computing; College work is more suitable for trainees who would like special-ist subjects not given at Atlantic Text'.

For others College proved a stressful and painful experience:

- 'Had difficulty coping with other students. Felt awkward and nervous'.
- 'I found College very intimidating, unsupportive to individuals and almost a total waste of time'.

Other reasons for not liking College were its geographical location on the edge of the city, which meant a long and inconvenient journey for some trainees; one respondent complained that it was not sufficiently demanding:

Trainees were asked to complete the sentence: By the end of my course at college I felt .... Their responses reflected the same division between people who were satisfied to have achieved some skill or academic success (e.g. 'satisfied that I had something on paper to show for it') and those who were simply distressed by the experience, for example:
- 'Thank God! I don't need to go back!'
- 'That I never wanted to return to College for any reason'.

Employment placement

Nineteen respondents had experience of an employment placement. People who had had a placement were more likely to be in current work. However, this is likely to be a reflection of the fact that placements mostly took place in the later stages of the programme and those who stayed the course were both more likely to have a placement and to find work.

Fifteen of the 19 said they found their placement helpful; 4 did not. Most people (17) said they received enough support while they were on their placement.

Support during and after the programme

Most respondents (85%) also said they received enough support while they were on the programme, this was not the case after they left. Only 16 (40%) said they received enough support afterwards.

5. An alternative outcome measure: confidence in self

The results so far have used employment as a criterion of good outcome. It is arguable that employment is not the only suitable measure of outcome. In the present economic situation with high unemployment some people will have difficulty in finding work even if their health and motivation are good. People with long experience of mental health problems may have been notably helped if they feel better about themselves, despite the fact they are not in work. Therefore the item 'I felt more confident about myself' was examined in more detail and the 29 people who answered 'yes' were compared with the 13 who did not. (One did not reply). It was noted earlier that this item was not related to being in current work. Present health was also unrelated to increased confidence at the time of finishing the course. Table 10 shows the items most highly associated with increased confidence.

Table 10
Items related to increased confidence in self

	Yes		No		Total	
Total	29	100%	13	100%	42	100%
Used computer skills	19	66%	2	15%	21	50%
Used keyboard skills	20	69%	2	15%	22	52%
Used general office skills	19	66%	3	23%	22	52%
Work routine helped timekeeping	21	72%	4	31%	25	60%
Developed ability to take responsibility for work	21	72%	3	23%	24	57%
Kept in touch with trainees	17	59%	2	15%	19	45%

The most striking relationship with increased confidence in self was having made use of the skills learned since leaving the programme. Those with increased confidence in themselves also said they had developed the ability to take responsibility for pieces of work and that the work routine had helped their time-keeping. Failure to improve self-confidence was reflected in negative views of the course. The numbers were often too small for a formal test of significance but, for example, 4 of the 5 who thought the course too demanding and the three people who said they 'didn't learn anything very much' also said their confidence had not improved. This negativity was reflected in continuing contact and people whose confidence did not improve were also less likely to keep in touch with Atlantic Text staff and significantly less likely to keep in touch with fellow trainees.

6. Improvements

Could the training or the programme have been improved?

Fifteen respondents thought the programme could be improved. The suggestions for improvement in specific aspects of the training reflected personal interests, for example:

- 'More accounting work for those who want it. Too much emphasis on keyboard skills. Felt I was forced into doing this.'
- 'Without being sexist I feel that it is too much geared to skills which

168

employers expect (being sexist) from women. Men need a different emphasis'.

Someone asked for more time to develop interview skills; another said:
- 'Yes, improvements can always be made in any training programme. It should not have been so rigid. Flexibility should have been allowed where appropriate'.

The one person who viewed the programme very negatively said:
- 'Yes. They could have given trainees more encouragement, tried to understand their problems and what's more, they didn't help me find a job. I did it on my own'.

Two people had problems with work experience, either because it was not available or because it should have been selected more carefully. One or two experienced some difficulty in transferring from an earlier training programme in information work to one in secretarial and office studies. One would have liked a talk on stress management; another would have liked more male staff; another thought that trainees should be able to stay two years rather than be restricted to one.

A few respondents recognised that they were unable to benefit from the programme for reasons of their mental health problems.

Another concluded:
- 'So when taking all facts into consideration I can't see that the programme could have been improved on except in the manner which I've described - through experience and flexibility'.

When discussing the programme in more general terms, some trainees thought the programme could have been more flexible and that discipline was too strict. There was also considerable empathy with the staff and recognition that a new project has to find its way:
- 'As this was a comparatively new venture for both trainees and staff, I felt that it was a well-balanced and very instructive course and any misgivings and/or deficiencies in respect of the course were quickly identified and this enabled action or a suggestive approach to be pursued as the time progressed and as staff and trainees gained mutual respect and confidence'.

7. Looking back, do you feel that Atlantic Text was helpful to you?

Most of the respondents (35-83%) said that Atlantic Text had been helpful to them. Two said it had not; the remainder were uncertain or did not answer. Respondents had the opportunity to expand on their reply and most took this up. The most negative respondent said:
- 'I learnt how to use my computer but there was no interest given by the

169

staff e.g. they never helped me find a placement without me having an argument with them'.

Another commented:

- 'I was not ready. I did not like computers'.

The majority, however commented very positively. The themes most frequently encountered were improved confidence and the opportunity to gain skills and qualifications, followed by greater ability to obtain work and the personal and social benefits of having a structured activity. These views are illustrated in the respondents own words:

Confidence

- 'After prolonged illness the Text gave me the support, confidence and qualifications I needed to obtain my aim, full time employment'.

- 'It gave me a purpose, something to get up for every morning. I achieved more than I thought I could at that particular time. I gained confidence by working and socialising with people'.

- 'It provided a way of getting out of a vicious circle of unemployment and depression at a time when I probably couldn't have coped with most other schemes'.

Obtaining skills

- 'Learning new skills such as typing and word-processing'.

- 'At the moment I have still to find employment but the skills I learnt at Atlantic Text will be helpful either in employment or voluntary work'.

Work:

- 'Yes, if it hadn't been for Atlantic Text, I wouldn't be in a job today'.

- 'It made me very confident in the possibility of getting work. It gave an excellent and comprehensive training for the type of work I wished to do. It raised my self-confidence. I had a lot of support when I was in difficulties with the work and also when I was unwell'.

Personal help

- 'It was helpful in providing a structure so that I could leave hospital with something concrete to do'.

- 'It kept me occupied and gave me a direction for so long'.

- 'Yes it was useful though not for the fact that I was doing office training (as yet) but in the general aspect of working life'.

Discussion

The lack of suitable occupation for people after they leave hospital has often been noted, e.g. McCreadie, (1984). A desire for employment is also

170

frequently expressed by people who have had severe mental health problems, many of whom attend day facilities because there are no appropriate job opportunities. Hatfield et al. (1992), for example, found that almost a half of service users interviewed in the Northern Town study said they needed help in finding a job; only 8% were in full or part time employment. The authors commented that 'a substantial level of expressed need for employment was elicited from the Northern Town sample of mental health users.' The training scheme described in the present study was set up to meet such needs.

The trainees on the Atlantic Text programme are already a highly selected group. Their previous educational level is generally high and they had been successful in the initial interview for admission to the course. This may explain the discrepancy between the present study and some reports in the literature (e.g. Vostanis, 1990), which suggest that youth and having long experience of previous employment are predictive of regaining employment after a mental illness. In the present study neither age nor length of time previously employed was related to a good employment record after the course.

Many aspects of the present study are very encouraging; half the respondents were in work at the time of follow-up; a quarter had been continuously employed since leaving the training scheme and a half had worked for about 50% of the time available. It is probable that the outcome for respondents was better than for non-respondents since people who left the programme for employment were more likely to reply; nevertheless the results show that at the very least a third (21 out of 63) of all trainees enrolled on the office technology course were working at follow-up. Most of those who obtained work stayed in work.

The contrast between the first and second years was also of interest. People starting the programme in Year 1 had a more favourable outcome in terms of employment because they had greater opportunity for sheltered work. Under the sheltered placement scheme employers of a limited number of people with long term disabilities can be given subsidies which offset the loss incurred to the employer through the worker's reduced capacity. The number of places for which subsidies are available is quite small. Since demand exceeds supply, and those who obtain posts tend to remain in them, capacity to provide for new applicants is soon exhausted. Sheltered work placements can provide an excellent opportunity for people to work in a range of employment situations at reduced pressure. The value of sheltered work in its various forms is well attested, for example by Harding (1991), who also emphasises the importance of preparation for work, careful introduction to a placement and good support after starting a job. Atlantic Text seemed to provide the initial preparation very well but many trainees would have liked more support afterwards. Midgely (1990) notes the need for rehabilitation agencies to have employment officers who help negotiate job opportunity for clients and assist them in the transition.

The respondents' views of the training scheme were strongly positive. The majority thought they were helped by the programme and they particularly mentioned its value in increasing confidence and providing skills; some thought they would have been unable to find work without it. About three quarters of all respondents felt more confident about themselves after the course. Increased self-confidence was not related to being in work but was related to having made use of the skills learned. Perhaps an extension of skills provides a source of self-esteem in its own right. This would accord with Vostanis' (1990) observation that work is of value in its own right and, indeed, can often be regarded as therapy.

Respondents' views of that part of their training which took place in a further education college was in strong contrast to their response to the programme in general. A few exceptions apart, they found the college experience difficult and distressing. The present study does not allow us to identify which aspects of the college experience were so disturbing. However, it raises questions about the assumption among some professionals that all 'segregated' activities are wrong. Vulnerable people need varying degrees of support. (More recently, Atlantic Text has modified its practice; college attendance is less integral to the course and can be better tailored to individual needs; in addition, trainees and their instructor from Atlantic Text go together to the College).

Most respondents said that the support of people with similar problems was helpful; a minority thought it was difficult to be on a course with people with mental health problems. The balance of opinion was that being with people who could understand their problems from the inside was a benefit not a hindrance to greater development.

Not all the respondents in this study experienced good employment outcomes. Some have protracted health problems and others are still seeking work. The difficulties experienced after a period of training has terminated have been noted elsewhere, (McCollam, 1988). When people are vulnerable, training should be regarded as making a contribution to the quality of life of which achieving employment is only one part. The findings of this study pose the question of whether training schemes are evaluated within too narrow a framework. One aim of such schemes is certainly to enable trainees to find work, and in this the present scheme was successful. However, the programme produced wider effects and work should not be the only criterion. In a time of high unemployment, it is inevitable that some people will not be readily absorbed into the labour market. For those who are not, a scheme should, and can, provide other benefits. Midgely (1990) has commented on the thinking underlying training for employment and suggested that it is dominated by an overly individualistic social philosophy. To use economic outcomes as the sole criterion is both short sighted and inhumane.

Conclusion

The office technology training scheme described in this paper was successful in getting people back to work; 49% of respondents were in work at the time of follow-up and 28% had been continuously employed since leaving training. The training had other benefits, especially in terms of increased self-confidence and the acquisition of skills. It is suggested that work should not be the only criterion of success of training schemes and that more personal, social and health related measures should be agreed as satisfactory outcomes. Sheltered placements in ordinary work environments are a great benefit to people returning to work and an increase in their number is much to be desired. Greater flexibility in the length of training would enable schemes to respond more fully to individual need. There is a definite need for continued support after training ends.

Acknowledgements

We should like to thank the former trainees of the Atlantic Text programme for their time spent in completing the questionnaires and their comments which made this paper possible. Out thanks also go to Anne Pearson and Cheryl Minto of the Scottish Association of Mental Health who generously gave of their time and knowledge of Atlantic Text.

References

Harding, A. (1991). Returning to work: A realistic aim? *Rehab Network*, Winter (pp.6-8).

Hatfield, B., Huxley, P., & Mohamad, H. (1992). Accommodation and employment: A survey into the circumstances and expressed needs of users of mental health services in a Northern Town. *British Journal of Social Work*, 22, 61-73.

McCollam, A. (1988). *Working at SPROUT: The evaluation of an employment project for people with experience of mental illness*. Scottish Association for Mental Health.

McCreadie, R. G., Robinson, A. D., & Wilson, A. O. A. (1984). The Scottish survey of chronic day-patients. *British Journal of Psychiatry*, **145**, 626-630.

Midgely, G. (1990). The social context of vocational rehabilitation for ex-psychiatric patients. *British Journal of Psychiatry*, **15**, 272-277.

Vostanis, P. (1990). The role of work in psychiatric rehabilitation: A review of the literature. *British Journal of Occupational Therapy*, **53**, 24-28.

Appendix A
Characteristics of trainees

	Questionnaire				Total	
	Completed		Not completed			
Total	43	100%	20	100%	63	100%
Sex						
Male	25	58%	11	55%	36	57%
Female	18	42%	9	45%	27	43%
Age						
Under 35	22	51%	16	80%	38	60%
35 or over	21	49%	4	20%	25	40%
Previous Education						
School	23	53%	12	60%	35	56%
College or Univ	20	47%	8	40%	28	44%
Previous Work						
<5 years	25	58%	15	75%	40	63%
5 years +	18	42%	5	25%	23	37%
Previous SAMH Training						
Previous ET at SAMH	15	35%	5	25%	20	32%
No previous SAMH training	28	65%	15	75%	43	68%
Source of Referral						
Self	8	19%	6	30%	14	23%
Psychiatric Hospital	16	38%	10	50%	26	42%
Other	18	43%	4	20%	22	35%
Accommodation at Start						
Supported	12	28%	5	25%	17	27%
Other	31	72%	15	75%	46	73%
In-pt in Previous Year						
Yes	21	54%	13	68%	34	59%
No	18	46%	6	32%	24	41%
Length of Stay						
<12 m.	26	60%	16	80%	42	67%
12m+	17	40%	4	20%	21	33%
Completed Programme*						
Yes	19	44%	3	15%	22	35%
No	24	56%	17	85%	41	65%
Position on Leaving*						
Employed	19	44%	3	15%	22	35%
Other	24	56%	17	85%	41	65%
*Difference statistically significant p < .05						

175

14 A community group for women who have or are at risk of having mental health problems

L. Collins

Introduction

This paper will discuss the Wimbledon Women's Group - this is a community group for women who have been identified as having had or being at risk of having mental health problems. The two group facilitators are employees of the London Borough of Merton - a Wimbledon District Office Social Worker and a Day Care Officer at Chapel Orchard Mental Health Project (the author of this paper). It is under the preventative brief of Chapel Orchard's Operational Policy that this group exists.

The paper will be presented under a number of headings - The nature and aims of the group, Background to the group. Who are the users of the group? How the group has changed over time and finally, Evaluation and discussion.

It would be stated from the outset that the facilitators are committed to the non pathologising of women and to preventing their further involvement with traditional mental health services where appropriate.

The nature and aims of the group

The Wimbledon Women's Group is an eight member group with two women facilitators. It meets weekly for two hours in a room attached to a sheltered housing block and has been in existence since March 1991. The group is for women who have been identified and referred by a Health Authority or Social Services professional as having or being at risk of having mental health problems.

It is an open group and the membership has changed over time, however there has been a core of the same five women for over a year at the time of writing. The facilitators have encouraged the women to decide how they use the two hours and the group has evolved into a talking group which covers a wide range of content - current affairs, members news, ventilation of problems, discussion of personal issues, advice seeking and nostalgic accounts. This is not a psychotherapy group but the women can use the space to discuss personal issues if they so wish and there is a group rule that everything that is said in the group is confidential.

The group is aimed at local women and the expectation is that they will transport themselves. Wimbledon is a mixed area both in cultural and socio-economic terms (it's not all tennis!).

The facilitators take responsibility for encouraging the women to 'take space' but very much seek to avoid 'sitting in the therapist's chair', and encourage a sharing of responsibility for group facilitation. They do however provide tea and biscuits, a resource box of advice and information, keep track of the group book loan scheme and do the initial home visits - these follow the referral and are aimed at sharing information about the group and inviting interested women to come along.

It is the aim of the facilitators that the group provides a weekly supportive space for isolated women, to talk and be listened to, a place where they can negotiate what the rules are and decide what the content of the group will be - that they will use the time to ventilate, solve problems or meet with others socially. It is encouraged that they bring their 'whole' selves and not just their psychiatric label. Purposefully, very little information is known about their previous encounters with mental health services except that which is self reported.

It is the overall aim to prevent a deterioration in the mental health of these women if possible, through the support of other women, and where appropriate, reduce future encounters with the psychiatric system and prevent the development of a 'psychiatric career'.

Background to the group

There is much research and writing on the subject of women and mental health or rather, how women are ill served by services for their difficulties that are socio-political in origin as opposed to biological.

It appears that depression and anxiety are twice as common in women as in men (Paykel 1991), and married women suffer the most. Women are far more likely to be diagnosed as having some kind of psychiatric condition, and double the number of prescriptions for psychotropic drugs are given to women compared with men, to help them deal with their mental health problems (Neustatter, 1989).

178

Phyllis Chesler's work in the early 70's was in part a reaction to the relative silence in professional practice about any link between women's psychological problems and their position in society. The Women's Movement raised people's awareness about the relationship between women's social roles and their mental health problems.

Brown and Harris in Social Origins of Depression (1978) summarise that the root cause of depression is a situation in which a woman 'cannot feel good about herself'. They stress the value of a close friend or confidant, ideally a partner, with whom a woman has developed a trusting, caring relationship - a support system which may affect or alleviate depression. They say 'a relationship that makes a woman feel positive about herself provides valuable support, and friendships between women are very important'.

(Paykel, 1991) explains that depression may cumulatively result from: the social effects of stress, social vulnerability factors (Brown and Harris 1978), the absence of support, and women's role in society. There is particular vulnerability to depression in married women aged 20-40 years with young children.

It is the White City Project in West London with its emphasis on empowerment, raising the awareness of women and preventative mental health care ethos that has actively moved forward ideas as to what constitutes real help for women with mental health problems. Sue Holland, initiator of the project at White City says, 'any venture in the field of preventative work in mental health must make its central task the transformation of passive receivers of mental health services into active participants in the understanding and solutions of their own and their neighbours' distress'.

The Wimbledon Women's Group evolved from the view that many women are treated by the psychiatric services when they simply need to make connections with others, have a place to be listened to, valued and understood. It also was based on the assumption that the position of women in society adds to, if not creates, the mental health difficulties that women seek treatment for.

This, coupled with an individual caseload at the Mental Health Project, of women telling similar stories, experiencing 'symptoms' of loneliness, feeling misunderstood and disconnected, having difficult family relationships and often no structure outside of their home, led to the creation of the Wimbledon Women's Group.

Over a period of six months and prior to the group starting the facilitators met for two hours a week. This was an essential time both for planning and for them to develop their co-working relationship. Much time was spent sharing views and ideas, developing the necessary paperwork, circulating publicity and liaising with professionals in Health and Social Services who were to become the referring agents to the group. Initial home visits began two months before the group started in March 1991.

Who are the users of the group?

The group is ongoing and there is a maximum of eight members at any one time. Since the group began there have been fourteen women who have come to the group. Seven have left the group four for positive reasons - either work or a training course and two have left because they could not use the group. All of the women have had contact with mental health services and this ranges from fortnightly ongoing contact with a community psychiatric nurse to just 'brushing sleeves' with the referring agent e.g. a one off, G.P. referred appointment with a psychiatrist. The referrals have come from a number of agencies: occupational therapists (5), social workers (4), outpatient psychiatry/psychology (3) and community psychiatric nurses (2).

The age range of the women who have used the group is 24 to 58 years and the mean age is 44 years (appendix 1). Although the age range clusters around the 40's and 50's and much of the subject matter of the group is age related as are the family circumstances, there is an understanding that each person needs space and it is often acknowledged that members have different but equally important issues regardless of age. At times there is a maternal feel to how the younger members are supported. It is thought to provide some balance that the facilitators are both in their late 20's.

The cultural background of the women is mixed (appendix 1) but the group is all white. This is disturbing given that the percentage of Black and Asian people in Wimbledon is between 12% and 22%. A fuller discussion will follow later but it is interesting, if alarming, to note that none of the thirty six referrals received since the group began have been on behalf of Black or Asian women. The group facilitators are white, one English, one Irish.

With regard to marital status, more than half of the women have been married although some are divorced or widowed. Five out of fourteen women have never been married/co-habited although two of these are in their early twenties and therefore have had less opportunity to be married (appendix 1). All of the women who are or have been married identify difficulties with their partnerships to a greater or lesser degree.

The group members have a mean number of 2 children and a range from 0 to 5 children (appendix 1). Two of the women who have no children are in their early twenties and may go on to have children at a later time. For many women their children are teenage and are discussed often in the group and at times are felt to be the source of much anguish. A lot of the women whether they have grown up or school age children talk about having particular child care responsibilities that are not/weren't shared by a partner, if there was one.

The self reported psychiatric diagnoses of the women who use the group is mixed (appendix 1) however for the people with psychotic diagnoses they perceive depression to be at the core of their difficulties - so it seems fair to say that depression is a common factor among these women.

Wimbledon most certainly isn't all tennis and a look at the financial status of these women will demonstrate this (appendix 1). While most women have very little and live on state benefits there are a few people who are materially very well off although it needs to be said that these women are dependent on their partner's income and they are aware and concerned that their choice about whether to stay or leave is grossly affected by this fact.

The women who come to the group, while sharing the experience of depression also, identify three main issues that affect their mental health and feel that, prior to joining the group and making links with each other, probably added to its deterioration. They talk about isolation, difficult family relationships, and lack of structure/network as important factors. These, together with for some people recent significant life events, brought these women to the attention of professionals.

The women who use the group are similar and different from each other as group members always are and they take on different roles at different times - there is however an unspoken rule that they all adhere to - that each woman has a right to her space, to be valued and to be respected.

How the group has changed over time

There have inevitably been changes during the life of the group, membership is one. There has been a core of five women who have been regular attenders and it is these women that have given the group its shape. The addition of new members has always been planned as a slow and gradual process and it has, if anything become slower over time, especially as the group now need time to adjust to older members moving on before being open to accommodating someone new.

The facilitators, in designing the group aimed at a maximum of ten women - at the request of the group this has been reduced to eight; it was felt that the group would be too large and feel less safe with ten people.

In terms of group processes: 'forming', 'storming', 'norming' and 'performing', the group is now in the later stages; however there was much 'storming' in the first few groups. This was often aimed at the facilitators and included, for example, demands for information, 'what is this group about anyway?' along with questions about what was going to be 'provided'. While this was an uneasy time it was necessary in order that discussions could take place about what would be the most helpful structure for the group. It was also a time when there was clear acknowledgement of the different roles of 'worker' and 'user'. This 'storming' allowed us to 'clear the air' and develop the agreed aim of developing a useful space. From there the group moved on to a much more interactive stage where they looked less to the facilitators to hold the continuity and began to share responsibility much more for the content of each group. Around the same time the women started to arrive up to half an hour early for the group and have a 'pre group' meeting where they make each other tea and catch up on news before the facilitators arrive.

Another significant change has been the communication of absences - members now phone the group room during the hours of the group if they cannot attend, as opposed to phoning the workplace of one of the facilitators, as happened in the earlier days.

On a few occasions the women have met without the facilitators and while it is not possible to comment on what took place, all of the members attended and things were said to have gone well, so well that they were late in finishing! Following the first of these groups there was an obvious change in the rules. Tea making, was once something the facilitators took as their task, in the knowledge that for a lot of these women it would be the only time in their week when someone would make them a drink, however following the first group that was held without the facilitators the women elected to have a drink as they arrive and now take it in turns to organise this; the facilitators still make the mid group drink. The rules on smoking, which the group spent much time discussing at the outset, have become completely relaxed and people seem to smoke when they feel like it - this appears to suit both smokers and non-smokers, indicating it was much more of an issue for the facilitators!

The content of the group has changed, people know each other well now and feel safe to bring issues of a more personal nature. They are also more likely to come to the group when they are depressed whereas in the past they may have stayed away. Inevitably there are times of conflict, when people disagree, get angry, become competitive - because the members know a lot about each other and there is a commitment to the group this can be tolerated and contained, although, of course, it is not always comfortable. When new members start the safety of the group dilutes and for a couple of weeks the content of the group will be less personal.

Over time the women have become more politicised and many hours are spent exploring ideas - about their roles as women, why they have developed mental health problems, how these are misunderstood by friends and family and how the psychiatric system hasn't always offered them what they now know they needed at times of distress - essentially, some way of reducing the isolation that comes as a result of the misery of depression.

Of late there has been a lot of advice sharing between the women about available services and the group now has a resource box of information and also a loan scheme for half a dozen self help type books.

During the life of the group the women have experienced their own individual changes. A number of members have had significant life events which they have brought to the group and have received support with these. Some people have added to their external network since being in the group, both socially and in terms of getting appropriate help with other aspects of their lives. With regard to traditional mental health services only one out of the current seven group members has continuing contact, the other six have diminished their contact over time. People have recounted that in the past they have felt desperate but didn't know what could help them or what was available, these women say that with hindsight they were aware of 'upping the stakes' in terms of how they presented themselves to services, and if they hadn't found the group they may well have taken overdoses in the same way some of them had before.

Initially, the facilitators asked for a named keyworker for each woman and this would often be the referrer. This was an idea inherited from another group that worked mainly with women who had recently been in a psychiatric hospital, with the aim of having someone to contact should something alarming come up during a group. This idea has now been abandoned and any concerns would be raised directly with the women themselves and if it was felt that some follow up in the week between groups was appropriate the facilitators would do this.

The facilitators have changed in their role over time. Although uncomfortable, it was very freeing to acknowledge from the outset that there were clear differences in role between 'worker' and 'user'. While this difference is obviously still there and affects what happens it has been refreshing to feel that the connection is one of 'people' as opposed to 'client' and 'worker'. The facilitators have become more relaxed about sharing personal information and while they acknowledge that they are not there to use the group for themselves, it has been a relief to be freed from the strict boundaries that they had digested during social work training, about the sharing of personal information. In the Wimbledon Women's Group it would be inappropriate not to share something of themselves but of course there are limits to this.

In general the facilitators have been honest about their political beliefs and their commitment to the task of 'helping women to redefine reality, expand their available choices and achieve the desired changes - to encourage change and coping rather than adjustment and adaptation.' (Pollack & West 1987)

Due to the fact that there is now a waiting list for the group prioritising is having to take place. Women with other services and structure to their week may not be considered and the aim is to include in the group, women who are very isolated.

Concluding this section on changes, it seems fair to say that the group has evolved in to a group with a definite core membership, a culture that is self defined and has a shared identity.

Evaluation and discussion

The feedback from the women in the group is very positive - they feel safe to talk, they are respected and valued, they have some structure to their week, the group has become important.

So why has it worked? The main aim which was made explicit from the outset of the group was that, women could come and be their 'whole' selves and they would not be treated according to their psychiatric label. This has been a very important experience for these women who are often seen as 'sick' or 'mad' in their families and who have been frustrated at times by services that have given them little more than a diagnosis.

The facilitators' insistence that the women should decide how to use the time, and their willingness to change 'the rules', for example to reduce the maximum number of group members, has been important to the amount of control and decision making the women feel that they have in the group. Also, the toleration of challenges and conflict has been important. A balancing act of facilitation which enables people to take space alongside 'just letting them be' seems to have been pitched appropriately. The atmosphere that has encouraged people to share what is important for them, be listened to and validated has been central.

Prior to the group beginning, having a good amount of planning time was very helpful in the development of the co-working relationship between facilitators. Publicity and liaison work at the outset enabled the facilitators to reach potential referrers. The initial home visit stage weeds out most of the inappropriate referrals from professionals who think a women's group would be 'good' for someone. Women have a choice and when advised that there is absolutely no obligation to come to the group a lot of these people who are the victims of a referrers 'good idea' elect not to come. They will be told of other services at this stage if this is appropriate.

There are restrictions on who can use the group and the facilitators are very aware that the group cannot be all things to all people. There are no child care facilities, no transport is provided, the group meets during the day, and there is a criterion that women must be able to share space. So, there will be women who cannot use the group or people who would not feel contained in this sort of setting, for example, someone who was actively psychotic at the time of referral.

Over the last two years, the London Borough of Merton has seen the start of the Women's Groups' Development Network. This is a meeting for interested professionals to identify gaps in services and it is a forum for developing new groups (the author is the co-ordinator of this network). One of the concerns of the Network and of this paper is the adequacy of services to Black and Asian women. The Wimbledon Women's Group have no Black or Asian members and none of the thirty six referrals received since the group began have been for women of these ethnic backgrounds, despite the fact that there are between 12% and 22% of people in Wimbledon who are Black or Asian. It may be that the group is perceived as a white resource however, this still doesn't explain the lack of referrals at the outset. It may be possible that women are being referred to services which are specifically designed to meet their cultural needs - the fear is however, that these women are being offered very little given that it is often white professionals who are assessing their needs and may be making decisions that are unhelpful, inaccurate and at worst, racist.

It is terribly hard to find women who are depressed and isolated and many of the group users have reported being depressed and without support for a very long time, many since they had young children and very little help. There is now a bottle neck in the Wimbledon Group and more groups are needed. One main area for further exploration and development is primary care, liaising with G.P.s would be central to finding these women earlier.

Where does the group go now? There is no expectation that it will go anywhere and the women are under no pressure to leave. The hope of the facilitators is that it will become self running eventually but only time will tell. Realistically, the facilitators won't be able to allocate their time to the group indefinitely when there is so much need for similar services.

'As long as women are over represented among mental patients and family caretakers and under represented among psychiatrists, administrators and politicians, their lives will continue to be unhappily affected by decisions in which they take no part.' (Showalter, 1987)

Despite all of the writing and research on the subject of women and mental health, their needs and the prevention of mental ill health, very little is done to assist the empowerment of women that will enable them to define their needs and shape their services.

'Only those who are at present victims of the prevailing destructive social conditions will have a true commitment to the struggle towards prevention. It is also they who will be the main recipients of the British welfare state's attempt to treat, administer, therapeutize, tranquilize and neutralize them out of their justifiable rage.' (Holland. 1991).

The Wimbledon Women's Group is based on a simple idea - bring women together and offer them a space, they have shown that they will use it in the way that is most helpful for them.

Conclusions

People need to make connections with others and when they don't it can be quite mad-making. This paper has described one project which has attempted and, in its own terms succeeded, in helping women to connect with each other and by their own reports reduced their escalating contact with psychiatry and provided them with a network, some structure to their week, and important relationships with other women.

By using a supportive space on a weekly basis in an ordinary room in Wimbledon, these women have come together to talk, be listened to, valued and respected for themselves, away from their families, their loneliness and their psychiatric label.

References

Brown, G.W., & Harris, T. (1978). *Social origins of depression; A study of psychiatric disorder in women*. London: Tavistock.

Chesler, P. (1972). *Women & madness*. New York: Doubleday

Clark, M. & Kilworth, A. (1990). Why a group for women only? (13). In R. Jozef Perelberg & A.C. Miller (Eds), *Gender and power in families*. Tavistock: Routledge.

Ernst, S. & Goodison, L. (1981). *In our own hands*. Women's Press.

Gomez, V. (1987). Running groups on depression (8), Chaplin, J. & Noack, A. (1987). Leadership and self help groups (13). In S. Krzowski & P. Lane (Eds), *In our experience; workshops at the women's therapy centre*. Women's Press.

Holland, S. (1991). Defining and experimenting with prevention (11). In S. Roman & M.G. Giannichedda (Eds), *Psychiatry in transition; the British and Italian experiences*. (2nd Ed.). Pluto Press.

Neustatter, A. (1989, October 26). Headcounting. *The Guardian*.

Paykel, E.S. (1991). Depression in women. *British Journal of Psychiatry*, 158, (suppl 10), 22-29.

Pollack, L. & West, E. (1987). Women and psychiatry today. *Senior Nurse*, 6, (6), 11-14.

Showalter, E. (1987). *The female malady: Women, madness and the English culture 1830 - 1980*. London.

Starr, I. (1985, August 26). The depressed sex. *Social Work Today*.

Subotsky, F. (1991). Issues for women in the development of mental health services. British *Journal of Psychiatry*, 158, (suppl 10), 17-21.

Appendix 1

AGE	21-30	31-40	41-50	51-60
NUMBER OF WOMEN	2	2	5	5

CULTURAL BACKGROUND - SELF-DEFINED	WHITE BRITISH	IRISH	LEBANESE	JEWISH
NUMBER OF WOMEN	10	1	1	2

MARITAL STATUS	MARRIED	NEVER BEEN MARRIED	SEPARATED OR DIVORCED	WIDOWED
NUMBER OF WOMEN	4	5	3	1

NUMBER OF CHILDREN	0	1-2	3-4	>5
NUMBER OF WOMEN	4	4	5	1

PSYCHIATRIC DIAGNOSIS - self-reported	DEPRESSION	MANIC DEPRESSION	SCHIZOPHRENIA	AGITATED DEPRESSION
NUMBER OF WOMEN	7	3	3	1

FINANCIAL STATUS	DEPENDENT ON STATE BENEFIT	DEPENDENT ON PARTNER'S INCOME	FINANCIALLY INDEPENDENT
NUMBER OF WOMEN	9	4	1

15 Psychological well-being and gay identity: Some suggestions for promoting mental health among gay men

A. Coyle and M. Daniels

Introduction

Many studies have been undertaken which examine the prevalence of psychopathology among gay men, mostly prompted by the adoption of a medical model of homosexuality. The results of these studies have been decidedly mixed. Some have reported that, compared with heterosexual men, gay men are lower in psychological well-being on such dimensions as neuroticism (Van den Aardweg, 1985), self-esteem (Jacobs & Tedford, 1980), hostility (Rizzo et al., 1981) and emotional vulnerability (Williams, 1981). Other studies that have examined factors such as general psychiatric disorder, depression, extraversion-introversion, ego development, sex guilt and - once again - neuroticism and self-esteem have found no significant differences between heterosexuals and homosexuals (Carlson & Baxter, 1984; Harry, 1983; Hooberman, 1979; Pillard, 1988; Weis & Dain, 1979). Others still have reported higher levels of psychological well-being among gay men than among heterosexual men (Skrapec & MacKenzie, 1981). In reviews of studies of psychological well-being among gay men, Gonsioreck (1991) and Hart et al. (1978) criticised them on conceptual and methodological grounds. They concluded that there is no empirical basis for the belief that homosexuals are inherently any less psychologically adjusted than heterosexuals.

The following examination of psychological well-being among gay men takes as its starting point a study which used a self-completion questionnaire to investigate the gay identity formation experiences of a non-clinical group of 140 gay men from the Greater London area (Coyle, 1991,

1992). The questionnaire addressed a broad range of experiences that - in a pilot study and in previous work on the topic - have been described as instrumental in the formation of a gay identity (Cass, 1979; Coleman, 1982; Hencken & O'Dowd, 1977; Hetrick & Martin, 1987; Lee, 1977; Minton & McDonald, 194; Plummer, 1975; Troiden, 1979, 1988; Weinberg, 1983). As part of this study, respondents' levels of psychological well-being were ascertained by having them complete the 30-item General Health Questionnaire (GHQ-30) (Goldberg, 1978). The scores obtained by the gay men were compared with the scores obtained in a study by Cox et al. (1987) which applied the GHQ-30 to men from the general population (Coyle, in press).

Bearing in mind that the lower the score a person obtains on the GHQ-30, the higher is their level of psychological well-being, the mean score obtained by the gay men who participated in the gay identity formation study was 4.56, while the mean score obtained by single men in Cox et al.'s study was 3.67. The difference between these scores was statistically significant (z=2.08, p<.05). This difference persisted when the married men in Cox et. al.'s study were considered. Their mean score was 3.35 and the difference between this score and the gay men's mean score was again statistically significant (z=2.56, p<.05). Divorced/separated men and widowed men in Cox et. al.'s study obtained mean scores of 4.61 and 5.19 respectively. The differences between these scores and the gay men's mean scores were not statistically significant. In terms of psychological well-being, the sample of gay men was comparable with groups of men from the general population who have undergone potentially traumatic emotional life events that may have undermined their psychological well-being.

Psychological well-being and gay identity formation

Studies of gay identity formation have described the sorts of potentially traumatic experiences that men may encounter when constructing a gay identity against a background of negative social representations of gay men/homosexuality and that may impact negatively upon their psychological well-being. An indication of the nature and content of these negative social representations was obtained in the gay identity formation study when respondents were asked to report what they first learned about homosexuality and to describe what they thought a stereotypical gay man was like at that time. In addition to learning about the meaning of the gay/homosexual social category, i.e. that there were men who were called 'gay' or 'homosexual' and who were sexually attracted to other men, respondents said they had also learned that being gay was something to be despised and ridiculed; that it was associated with being effeminate; and that it was sick or abnormal. Respondents reported that at that time they saw a stereotypical gay man as someone who was effeminate; who was sexually attracted to other men; who wanted to have sex with young boys; who was 'a dirty old man in a dirty raincoat'; who wanted to be a woman; and who dressed in women's clothes.

Through the process of what Malyon (1982) called 'biased socialization', most people internalise these negative social representations of homosexuality. The suspicion that one is or might be gay/homosexual and that the socially devalued gay/homosexual category has relevance for the self may therefore be a source of considerable distress. This self-suspicion process has been linked with physical and psychosocial dysfunction, including feelings of alienation, isolation, loneliness and guilt, a diminution of self-esteem and a tendency towards depression and self-blame (Malyon, 1982; Remafedi, 1987a, 1987b; Richardson, 1981). Respondents in the gay identity formation study frequently reported having experienced fear, worry and uncertainty at this point. The self-suspicion stage also had social implications, as respondents thought they would have to be very secretive, felt socially isolated and became very concerned about what other people thought of them. These reactions persisted, although to a lesser extent, even when respondents had decided that they were definitely gay. At this point, however, more positive reactions did emerge, with many respondents feeling glad that all the doubting and questioning was over, and believing that they had been courageous in facing up to their socially stigmatised sexuality.

The process of disguising their homosexuality or of 'passing' as heterosexual (Goffman, 1963) appeared to exert particular strain on respondents. At the time of the study, over half the respondents disguised their homosexuality from at least one person or one group of people, most commonly from friends, family members, and work colleagues. However, some disguised their homosexuality from everyone in their non-gay social world. When asked to describe their feelings when they now passed as heterosexual, many said they felt that those from whom they disguised their homosexuality did not really know them and they wished they had the courage to tell them. They felt they were not being true to themselves, that they were 'letting the side down' and being hypocritical. Such feelings of guilt, dishonesty and estrangement from others and from oneself may prove highly detrimental to psychological well-being.

The fact that these feelings were *currently* reported by respondents demonstrates that the identity demands an individual faces in constructing a gay identity many continue, albeit in an attenuated form, in the maintenance of that identity. A further example of this is provided by Lee (1977), who noted that the disclosure of sexual identity is not a once-and-for-all task but rather involves continually risking the loss of different aspects of one's social world as these become new audiences for disclosure.

Two findings that emerged from multiple regression analyses of the gay identity formation data (see Coyle, 1991, 1992) and that concerned psychological well-being are of particular interest. Respondents' levels of psychological well-being were found to be significantly related to the extent to which they perceived being gay as holding salient personal advantages for them and to their degree of involvement in the gay subculture. Neither of these results were particularly surprising. If a person perceives being gay as personally advantageous, they are less likely to experience anxiety, stress or depression - the principal dimensions measured by the GHQ-30 - as a result of holding a gay identity. They may be said to feel positively about their gay identity and by extension about themselves. Nor was it surprising that a high degree of involvement in the gay subculture should be associated with a high level of psychological well-being. Through conversations with other gay men in the gay subculture, those who are engaged in identity construction can discover strategies for coping with the interpersonal problems that a gay identity may cause. They may be able to hear and internalise legitimating accounts of what it means to be gay and to normalise through mixing with similar others what society at large would regard as an aberrant sexual identity. They can key into what Golan (1981) termed the 'mutual help system' of the gay subculture and can obtain social support, new reference groups, and a social context in which a positively-evaluated gay identity can develop. In this way, a high degree of subcultural involvement can decrease the potential for gay men to experience anxiety, stress and depression as a result of their sexual identity.

The advent of HIV/AIDS constitutes a further factor that may depress the psychological well-being of gay men. Media constructions of the HIV/AIDS pandemic have variously represented it as a 'gay plague', transmitted through the unnatural sexual practices of irresponsible, immoral, promiscuous gay men (Armstrong, 1985; Watney, 1987). With the advent of HIV/AIDS, already negative social representations of gay men have become suffused with notions of physical disease, divine damnation and death. Although it has been contended that HIV/AIDS is no longer represented in this way in the media (Berridge, 1992), the extent to which the original media constructions of HIV/AIDS continue to inform public ideas about the condition is uncertain. It could be that the social representation of HIV/AIDS as a 'gay plague' has proven durable and retains a capacity to render the construction of the positive gay identity even more difficult and to undermine the self-worth of gay men (Feldman, 1988). Those gay men who have HIV/AIDS may have to cope with a range of issues that may exert extremely adverse effects upon their psychological well-being. These include multiple losses (for example, losses of finance, relationships, self-image, future, sexuality, and control over one's life), which may include multiple bereavement if many members of the person's social network have died from AIDS-related conditions; issues of dependency; the disguising and disclosure of HIV status; coming to terms with one's own mortality and coping with terminal illness; trying to obtain and co-ordinate services from diverse service providers; and coping with the social stigma associated with HIV/AIDS (Coyle and Craig, 1992; Martin, 1988; Morin and Batchelor, 1984; Morin et al., 1984; Sherr, 1989). The epidemic has also been found to have detrimentally affected the psychological well-being of gay men who do not themselves have HIV/AIDS (Hirsch and Enlow, 1984; Noh et al., 1990; Stulberg & Smith, 1988). In view of these considerations, it is apparent that the promotion of psychological well-being among gay men in the light of HIV/AIDS constitutes a separate topic in its own right. When examining how the mental health of gay men could be promoted, the topic of HIV/AIDS will therefore be dealt with only in terms of its most basic negative effects upon gay identity.

Neither will the promotion of mental health among lesbian women be explicitly addressed. Political differences between gay men and lesbian women and differences in the ways in which male and female sexuality are socially constructed mean that the issues faced by gay men and lesbian women in the establishment and maintenance of their sexual identities are not equivalent (Kitzinger, 1987). On account of this, the study of gay identity formation which informs the following discussion of mental health promotion strategies was not broadened to include the experiences of lesbian women. That is not to deny that there exists a considerable degree of cross-gender experiential convergence. In constructing positive sexual identities, both gay men and lesbian women face similar problems of disclosure, passing, overcoming the heterosexual socialisation process and coping with negative social representations of their sexual identity. Many of the mental health promotion strategies to be outlined could therefore be usefully adapted and applied to lesbian women.

Strategies for promoting mental health among gay men

The foregoing presentation of findings from the gay identity formation study may be regarded as a form of mental health needs assessment for gay men. The research offers empirical evidence that, in constructing and maintaining their sexual identities, gay men must negotiate tasks that may exert a detrimental effect on their psychological well-being. It affords insights into the nature of these tasks and allows the identification of factors that may mitigate their deleterious effects. The findings from the gay identity formation study provide an empirical framework within which to locate suggestions for interventions that would promote mental health among gay men.

When planning health promotion interventions, it is important to be aware of the variety of health promotion approaches available and to select those approaches that are most suited to the aims of the interventions. Most of the interventions that follow may be viewed as loosely residing within the community development and educational approaches to health promotion. The community development approach operates when 'a group or groups of like-minded people, who recognise themselves as having common experiences in health matters, come together to discuss and review their concerns, to take stock of their situations, to identify mutual problems and to share in the process of clarifying options, working out appropriate joint action and setting about the process of trying to change their circumstances' (Beattie, 1991, p.176). The educational approach involves presenting people with information and ensuring that they understand it so that they can make informed decisions about health-related behaviours (Tones, 1981). It is, however, difficult to fit health promotion interventions into mutually exclusive theoretical categories and it is often possible to discern characteristics of different approaches within the same intervention.

For health promotion workers who wish to become involved in promoting the mental health of gay men, gay social or political groups or gay contacts within the local community constitute a valuable resource. For example, one such group is Friend, an organisation with branches in many parts of the country which provides information, advice and social activities for gay men and lesbian women. Using a form of co-operative inquiry within a community development model (Daniels & Coyle, 1992), members of these groups may be consulted to help identify the most pressing mental health needs of those with whom they come into contact. At this stage, the findings from the research on gay identity formation may constitute a useful source of ideas. Group members may then be co-opted as voluntary workers in the establishment and maintenance of mental health promotion projects. Their roles could involve publicising the projects and recruiting men to participate in them; co-facilitating projects

194

with health promotion workers; and, after projects have been initiated, assuming the role of project facilitators themselves.

The precise nature of any mental health promotion interventions that are undertaken will depend upon the issues that they seek to address. This in turn will be determined largely by the developmental stage of the gay men at whom the interventions are targeted, i.e., whether the gay men are in their teenage years, young adulthood, middle adulthood, or older adulthood. At each stage of the life course, gay men must deal with issues additional to those faced by heterosexuals (Herdt, 1992). For example, although the multiple, simultaneous transitions of adolescence have been described as potentially stressful for all adolescents (Simmons et. al., 1979), gay adolescents must additionally negotiate the meaning, management and expression of their socially-devalued sexuality (Boxer & Cohler, 1989). As part of this process, they may experience grief and may require time, space and a context in which to mourn the loss of what Herdt and Boxer (1992) have termed 'previously internalized heterosocial life goals' such as marriage and heterosexual parenthood, and to construct new life goals.

Discussion groups

One very simple strategy that could constitute a mental health promotion intervention for gay men or that could act as a point of departure for such an intervention would be the establishment of discussion groups. These could be aimed at certain groups of gay men - such as young men, retired men or men who are actively constructing their gay identities - who would be responsible for setting their own agenda of topics for discussion. Alternatively, the groups could address predetermined issues, such as the management of sexual and emotional relationships. The benefits of simply discussing shared problematic concerns and exchanging shared experiences within a group context should not be underestimated.

Within a non-threatening context, the discussion of gay identity formation experiences that may have been traumatic can prove cathartic and can divest these experiences of their negative affective charge. During discussions, the men may find that their gay identity - related experiences overlap with the experiences of other gay men, which may serve to validate and legitimise these experiences. They may come to realise that, although they may have felt socially isolated when they first thought they might be gay, other men experienced similar reactions and felt similarly isolated. By openly sharing these feelings, the men can retrospectively receive the legitimation and social support they lacked at the time. If some men are experiencing difficulties with certain developmental tasks in gay identity formation, their range of coping strategies may be broadened by listening to the experiences of other men who have already negotiated these tasks. Moreover, they may feel reassured that others have trodden their path before and have survived. Finally, as Coyle (1991, 1992) has noted, through verbalising and sharing their experiences in a group context, gay men are given the opportunity of creating meaningful, cohesive and self-esteem-enhancing identity narratives. These functions are also partly fulfilled by the gay subculture but gay men may welcome the chance to meet others specifically to air and deal with the psychosocial difficulties of assuming and maintaining a gay identity within a society that devalues that identity. Thus conceived, such discussion groups conform to many of the tenets of the community development approach to health promotion, as outlined by Beattie (1991).

Given that a high degree of involvement in the gay subculture was found to be related to a high level of psychological well-being in the gay identity formation study, one way of promoting psychological well-being among gay men would be to facilitate social involvement with other gay men among those who, for whatever reason, lack such involvement. One reason why some men may not be involved in the gay subculture is that they have only recently reached a stage in the construction of their gay identities where they feel capable of adopting such an identity in a public domain. In the London area, groups exist which offer these men support and the opportunity to discuss shared concerns and to socialise with others who are negotiating similar identity tasks. However, such provision is limited in other parts of the country. In these areas, it might be useful to establish discussion groups for men who are actively constructing their gay identities, with the facilitation of entry into the gay subculture constituting an optional activity within this context. Some of the men may feel apprehensive about entering a gay social context because they are unsure about what they will encounter or about how they should behave and they may feel self-conscious about entering this environment by themselves. Such apprehensions may be mitigated by involving more experienced gay men in the discussion groups firstly to answer participants' questions about the gay subculture and then to accompany them to a local gay social venue. This strategy may help dispel any fears that the men have and may give them the confidence to attend gay social venues without group facilitators. Progress towards independent functioning in the subculture may be facilitated by suggesting that several of the men arrange to visit gay social venues together. Specific issues related to socialising in a gay context may subsequently be addressed through discussion and role play at future meetings of the discussion group.

Group exercises

Although gay men may accrue considerable psychological benefits from the straightforward sharing of experiences, some problematic issues may be dealt with in a more directive way within a group context through the use of group exercises and role play. This strategy is located within a broadly educational model of health promotion, although the exercises that will be outlined owe more to a self-empowerment educational approach than to a didactic one. To take an example of a situation in which group exercises could prove useful health promotion tools, if group members were discussing their experiences of disclosing their sexual identity and if some were considering engaging in initial disclosure or in disclosure to new audiences in the future, the facilitator could construct group exercises that might promote positive disclosure experiences.

Such an exercise might involve having group members choose a particular disclosure audience as their focus (for example, parents) and brainstorming a range of disclosure strategies or settings that might be appropriate for the disclosure of one's sexual identity to this audience. The group would then be subdivided. Each subgroup would be assigned certain strategies or settings and would be asked to identify the advantages and disadvantages of engaging in disclosure using those strategies or in those settings. Through processing feedback from this exercise, the group could reach general conclusions about the nature of optimal disclosure strategies and settings, allowing of course for variations in the circumstances faced by individuals. The facilitator would then elaborate an imaginary situation in which a gay man is about to disclose his sexual identity to the chosen disclosure audience. The group would divide into subgroups and, using the disclosure strategies that they have identified, participants would role play the disclosure situation and its consequences, with some playing the gay man, some playing the disclosure audience and some acting as process observers. Alternatively, the facilitator could seek volunteers to play the gay man and the disclosure audience: these volunteers could then begin the role play while the rest of the group observed. At various junctures in the role play, other group members could volunteer to assume the roles or else the role play could be repeated in order to enact different outcomes to the scenario.

The purpose of this exercise is to provide gay men with an opportunity to practise and refine disclosure strategies and to help them to cope with alternative outcomes to disclosure situations or at least to be aware of what these outcomes might be. This may then encourage some men to engage in self-disclosure, which may mitigate the strains of passing as heterosexual that respondents described in the gay identity formation study.

Participating in the exercise may help other men to realise that it is not feasible to disclose their sexual identity to certain people in their social world, perhaps because they are particularly unsure about how these people would react and/or because they could not cope with any rejection that might ensue. If, on the basis of the issues raised by the exercise, some men make an informed decision not to disclose their sexual identity to people whom they had previously been considering as potential disclosure audiences, the facilitator can initiate a discussion about strategies for passing as heterosexual and about strategies for coping with any negative feelings experienced when passing. The exercise can easily be adapted and applied to many potentially problematic situations that may be encountered in the establishment and maintenance of a gay identity.

Other group exercises can promote self-esteem by encouraging gay men to examine the negative social representations of gay men and homosexuality with which they were socialised. By portraying gay men as sick and abnormal, these social representations may encourage those gay men who have internalised them to attribute any identity-related difficulties they may have experienced or may be experiencing to personality or psychological defects. Exercises that permit the critical examination of the nature and effects of these social representations may help gay men attribute any identity-related difficulties not to internal factors but to the difficulty of constructing a positive gay identity against a backdrop of negative social representations of gay men and homosexuality. Any tendency towards self-reproachment may thereby be diminished. Some training materials that have been designed to raise awareness about HIV/AIDS contain exercises that permit the examination of issues related to sexuality and sexual stereotypes (for example, see Aggleton et al., 1989). Adaptations of these exercises may prove useful tools in helping gay men to explore the nature of negative social representations of gay men and homosexuality and to consider how these have impacted upon their gay identity formation experiences.

The value of HIV/AIDS awareness training in promoting the psychological well-being of gay men should not be overlooked. If gay men carry vestiges of internalised negative social representations of gay men and homosexuality, they may at least partly acquiesce in negative social representations of HIV/AIDS which have portrayed HIV as transmitted through the unnatural sexual practices of irresponsible, immoral, promiscuous gay men. Most HIV/AIDS training packs contain exercises that help those participating in training to examine these representations in a critical way and to identify the illogicalities and prejudices that underpin them (for example, see Aggleton et al., 1989, & Weisner & Grant, 1989). As gay sexuality features so prominently in social representations of HIV/ AIDS, the use of such exercises within an HIV/AIDS training context can help gay men to disentangle their sexuality from these social representations and may empower them to see their sexuality - and, by extension, themselves - in a more positive light.

It could be argued that rather than attempting to counteract the effects of the internalisation of negative social representations of gay men and homosexuality, a more proactive approach to promoting mental health among gay men would involve minimising the internalisation of these social representations in the first place and actively challenging them. Such a strategy represents what has been termed the 'radical' approach to health promotion (Tones, 1981). In this case, it would entail providing children with factual and positive education about homosexuality that presents being gay as a life choice of equal value to heterosexuality. However, the provision of such education has been forbidden by Section 28 of the 1988 Local Government Act which prohibits the teaching in any maintained school of the acceptability of homosexuality as a 'pretended family relationship'. The outrage caused by a gay rights group which distributed positive educational leaflets about being gay or lesbian to schoolchildren (O'Neill, 1991) suggests that mental health promotion among gay and lesbian students is not regarded as an important issue within the educational system. Without the co-operation of the educational system in providing positive education about being gay or lesbian, it is difficult to deliver a broadly-based challenge to negative social representations of homosexuality, which will continue to compromise the psychological well-being of gay men and lesbian women. Any mental health promotion interventions with gay men will therefore of necessity be reactive rather than proactive.

Improving clinical services for gay men

In considering the ways in which mental health issues among gay men can be addressed effectively, it is useful to examine the approaches adopted by other projects that have sought to address similar concerns. One such project is the Evelyn Hooker Center for Gay and Lesbian Mental Health, established within the Department of Psychiatry at the University of Chicago (Boxer, personal communication). The Center is primarily concerned with promoting mental health among gay men and lesbian women who have encountered mental health problems rather than proactively trying to prevent such problems arising. The clinical services that it offers include out-patient counselling and psychotherapy for gay and lesbian individuals as well as for gay and lesbian couples and for families in which one or more members are gay or lesbian. In-patient psychiatric services for gay and lesbian clients are also offered at a local hospital. Both out-patient and in-patient services are delivered by mental health professionals who are themselves gay or lesbian and/or who receive ongoing, in-depth, specialised training on gay and lesbian mental health issues. In the future, the Center plans to develop more specialised clinical services for gay men and lesbian women, including counselling and support programmes for perpetrators and survivors of domestic violence; family counselling for gay and lesbian youth and their families and for gay and lesbian parents and their children; treatment programmes for alcoholism; substance abuse and sexual dysfunction in gay men and lesbian women; support groups for gay men and lesbian women who have chronic mental illnesses; and specialised services for gay men and lesbian women with HIV/AIDS and for their caregivers. The Center also provides an array of training opportunities in gay and lesbian mental health issues for (mental) health professionals and students, social service providers, criminal justice authorities and other institutions that directly impact on the lives of gay men and lesbian women.

It is unlikely that any UK health authority would prioritise the establishment of a centre for gay and lesbian mental health which delivers specialised mental health services to this client group in a co-ordinated way. However, some of the strategies used at the Evelyn Hooker Center could be usefully promoted for adoption in the UK. Gay men and lesbian women who experience psychological problems may wish to consult a gay or lesbian counsellor or psychotherapist because these practitioners' empathic potential may be greater than that of heterosexual therapists by virtue of the experiences and understandings that clients and therapists may share. Health promotion workers could facilitate this process by devising a directory of gay and lesbian counsellors and psychotherapists in their area, and distributing it to local gay groups, public libraries and citizens' advice bureaux.

The fact that HIV/AIDS training has been provided to health care workers in many health authorities attests to the feasibility of promoting awareness of particular issues among staff in a systematic way. In the same manner, it would be possible to implement training programmes to promote awareness of gay and lesbian issues among mental health staff, possibly within a more general training programme on sexuality-related issues. Such training could increase staff's understanding of the psychosocial pressures faced by gay and lesbian clients and could heighten their empathic potential in their interactions with this client group. If health promotion workers and mental health professionals in a health authority perceived a need for such training on the basis of their experiences or on the basis of health needs assessments conducted with the local gay community, they might then be willing to lobby for funding to be made available for training.

Conclusion

In conclusion, the research on gay identity formation found a level of psychological well-being among the gay men who participated that was comparable to that shown by men from the general population who had undergone potentially traumatic life events. Much of the emotional trauma experienced by gay men can be attributed not to any inherent psychological defect but to the difficulties involved in constructing a positive sexual identity within a social context that devalues that identity and having to do so with often limited support from others in their social world. The health promotion interventions that have been outlined may help to increase psychological well-being among gay men by providing them with an opportunity to discuss their experiences and to learn from the experiences of others in a supportive, non-threatening environment; to increase access to social support from other gay men; to examine critically the negative social representations of gay men and homosexuality which may have sabotaged their attempts to develop a positive gay identity; to generate, practise and refine strategies for coping with some of the potentially traumatic tasks of gay identity formation; and to receive understanding and non-judgemental treatment from providers of mental health services, if they should require them.

However, in order for a programme of such interventions to be established, health authorities must recognise that the promotion of mental health among gay men is a legitimate and necessary area of work in which health promotion departments should become involved. It must be admitted that at present the likelihood of this occurring is small. Many health authorities appear reluctant to tailor health promotion projects specifically to the needs of gay men. For example, although gay men constitute the epidemiological group most affected by HIV/AIDS in the UK to date (PHLS AIDS Centre - Communicable Diseases Surveillance Centre and Communicable Diseases (Scotland) Unit, 1992), only ten per cent of health authorities have been adjudged to have conducted adequate HIV/AIDS health promotion work aimed specifically at this group (King, 1992). In such a climate, any health promotion worker may have difficulty firstly in establishing mental health promotion with gay men as health promotion priority in his/her health authority and secondly in securing adequate funding for his/her work.

Health promotion workers who wish to promote mental health among gay men are therefore advised to conduct assessments of the mental health needs of gay men in their local community. When lobbying their departments of public health in order to obtain permission and funding to undertake mental health promotion interventions with this client group, they could use their findings to support their case. Furthermore, the possible interventions that have been outlined are relatively small in scale and involve initiating projects through local gay contacts and social groups, enlisting gay men as co-workers and empowering gay men to promote their own psychological well-being. The adoption of this approach in mental health promotion projects with gay men represents an economical way of promoting mental health, which, at a time when concerns about cost-effectiveness are paramount, may increase the likelihood of such projects receiving official sanction.

References

Aggleton, P., Homans, H., Mojsa, J., Watson, S., & Watney, S. (1989). *Learning about AIDS: Exercises and materials for adult education about HIV infection and AIDS*. Edinburgh: Churchill Livingstone.

Armstrong, E., (1985). *Tabloids and taboo*. Unpublished literature review in part fulfilment towards the Diploma in Health Education: South Bank University, London.

Beattie, A., (1991). Knowledge and control in health promotion: A test case for social policy and social theory. In J., Gabe, M., Calnan, & M., Bury (Eds.), *The sociology of the Health Service*, (pp.162-202). London: Routledge.

Berridge, V. (1992). AIDS, the media and health policy. In P. Aggleton, P. Davies, & G., Hart (Eds.), *AIDS: Rights, risk and reason* (pp.13-27). London: The Falmer Press.

Boxer, A.M., Personal communication. Department of Psychiatry, University of Chicago.

Boxer, A.M., & Cohler, B.J., (1989). The life course of gay and lesbian youth: An immodest proposal for the study of lives. *Journal of Homosexuality*, **17**, 315-355.

Carlson, H.M., & Baxter, L.A., (1984). Androgyny, depression and self-esteem in Irish homosexual and heterosexual males and females. *Sex Roles*, **10**, 457-467.

Cass, V.C., (1979). Homosexual identity formation: A theoretical model.

Journal of Homosexuality, **4**, 219-235.

Coleman, E., (1982). Developmental stages of the coming-out process. In W. Paul, J.D., Weinrich, J.C., Gonsiorek, & M.E., Hotvedt (Eds.), *Homosexuality: Social, psychological and biological issues*, (pp. 149-158). Beverly Hills, California: Sage.

Cox, B., Blaxter, M., Buckle, A., Fenner, N.P., Golding, J., Gore, M., Huppert, F., Nickson, J., Roth, M., Stark, J., Wadsworth, M., & Wichelow, M. (1987). *The health and lifestyle survey*. Cambridge: Health Promotion Research Trust.

Coyle, A., (1991). *The construction of gay identity (Vols. 1 & 2)*. Unpublished PhD thesis: University of Surrey.

Coyle, A., (1992). 'My own special creation'? The construction of gay identity. In G.M., Breakwell, (Ed.). *Social psychology of identity and the self concept*, (pp.187-220). London: Surrey University Press/Academic Press.

Coyle, A., (in press). A study of psychological well-being among gay men using the GHQ-30. *British Journal of Clinical Psychology*.

Coyle, A., & Craig, M. (1992). *An additional burden? Service users' views of HIV/AIDS services in North East London*. London: Association of London Authorities/North East Thames Regional Health Authority.

Daniels, M., & Coyle, A., (1992, September). *'Health dividends': The use of co-operative inquiry as a health promotion intervention with a group of unemployed women*. Paper presented at the Second Annual Conference on the Promotion of Mental Health: University of Keele.

Feldman, D.A., (1988). Gay youths and AIDS. *Journal of Homosexuality*, **17**. 185-193.

Goffman, E., (1963). *Stigma: Notes on the management of spoiled identity*. Englewood Cliffs, New Jersey: Prentice-Hall.

Golan, N. (1981). *Passing through transitions: A guide for practitioners*. New York: Free Press.

Goldberg, D.P., (1978). *Manual of the General Health Questionnaire*. Windsor: NFER-Nelson.

Gonsiorek, J.C., (1991). The empirical basis for the demise of the illness model of homosexuality. In J.C., Gonsiorek & J.D. Weirich (Eds.), *Homosexuality: Research implications for public policy*, (pp.115-136). Newbury Park, California: Sage.

Harry, J. (1983). Defeminization and adult psychological well-being among male homosexuals. *Archives of Sexual Behavior*, **12**. 1-19.

Hart, M., Roback, H., Tittler, B., Weitz, L., Walston, B., & McKee, E., (1978). Psychological adjustment of nonpatient homosexuals: Critical review of the research literature. *Journal of Clinical Psychiatry*, **39**, 604-608.

Hencken, J.D., & O'Dowd, W.T., (1977). Coming out as an aspect of identity formation. *Gay Academic Union Journal: Gai Saber*, **1**, 18-22.

Herdt, G., (Ed.) (1992). *Gay culture in America: Essays from the field*. Boston: Beacon Press.

Herdt, G. & Boxer, A., (1992). Introduction: Culture, history and life course of gay men. In G. Herdt (Ed.), *Gay culture in America: Essays from the field* (pp.1-27). Boston: Beacon Press.

Hetrick, E.S., & Martin, A.D., (1987). Developmental issues and their resolution for gay and lesbian adolescents. In E. Coleman, (Ed.), *Psychotherapy with homosexual men and women: Integrated identity approaches for clinical practice*, (pp.25-44). New York: The Haworth Press.

Hirsch, D.A., & Enlow, R.W., (1984). The effects of the acquired immune deficiency syndrome on gay lifestyle and the gay individual. *Annals of the New York Academy of Sciences*, **437**, 273-282.

Hooberman, R.E., (1979). Psychological androgyny, feminine gender identity and self-esteem in homosexual and heterosexual males. *Journal of Sex Research*, **15**. 306-315.

Jacobs, J.A., & Tedford, W.H., (1980). Factors affecting self-esteem of the homosexual individual. *Journal of Homosexuality*, **5**, 373-382.

King, E., (1992, June 25). Letter to the editor. *The Guardian* (p.22).

Kitzinger, E., (1987). *The social construction of lesbianism*. London:Sage.

Lee, J.A., (1977). Going public: A study into the sociology of homosexual liberation. *Journal of Homosexuality*, **3**, 49-78.

Malyon, A.K., (1982). Biphasic aspects of homosexual identity formation. *Psychotherapy: Theory, Research and Practice*, **19**, 335-340.

Martin, J.L., (1988). Psychological consequences of AIDS-related bereavement among gay men. *Journal of Consulting and Clinical Psychology*. **56**, 856-862.

Minton, H.L., & McDonald, G.J., (1984). Homosexual identity formation as a developmental process. *Journal of Homosexuality*, **9**, 91-104.

Morin, S.F., & Batchelor, W.F., (1984). Responding to the psychological crisis of AIDS. *Public Health Reports*, **99**, 4-9.

Morin, S.F., Charles, K.A., & Malyon, A.K., (1984). The psychological impact of AIDS on gay men. *American Psychologist.* **39**, 1288-1293.

Noh, S., Chandarana, P., Field, V., & Posthuma, B., (1990). AIDS epidemic, emotional strain, coping and psychological distress in homosexual men. *AIDS Education and Prevention*, **2**, 272-283.

O'Neill, S., (1991, November 24). Gay group to leaflet schools. *The Independent on Sunday* (p.1).

PHLS AIDS Centre - Communicable Diseases Surveillance Centre and Communicable Diseases (Scotland) Unit (1992). *Unpublished quarterly surveillance tables, no.16, June 1992.* London: PHLS AIDS Centre - Communicable Diseases Surveillance Centre and Communicable Diseases (Scotland) Unit.

Pillard, R.C., (1988). Sexual orientation and mental disorder. *Psychiatric Annals*, **18**, 51-56.

Plummer, K., (1975). *Sexual stigma: An interactionist account.* London: Routledge & Kegan Paul.

Remafedi, G., (1987a). Male homosexuality: The adolescent's perspective. *Pediatrics*, **79**, 326-330.

Remafedi, G., (1987b). Adolescent homosexuality: Psychosocial and medical implications. *Pediatrics*, **79**, 331-337.

Richardson, D., (1981). Lesbian identities. In J. Hart., & D. Richardson, (Eds.), *The theory and practice of homosexuality*, (pp.111-124). London: Routledge & Kegan Paul.

Rizzo, A.A., Fehr, L.A., McMahon, P.M., & Stamps, L.E., (1981). Mosher guilt scores and sexual preference. *Journal of Clinical Psychology*, **37**, 827-830.

Sherr, L., (1989). AIDS. In L. Sherr (Ed.), *Death, dying and bereavement*, (pp.179-196). Oxford: Blackwell Scientific Publications.

Simmons, R.G., Blyth, D.A., Van Cleave, E.F., & Bush, D.M. (1979). Entry into early adolescence: The impact of school structure, puberty, and early dating on self-esteem. *American Sociological Review*, **44**, 948-967.

Skrapec, C., & MacKenzie, K.R., (1981). Psychological self-perception in male transsexuals, homosexuals and heterosexuals. *Archives of Sexual Behaviour*, **10**, 357-370.

Stulberg, I., & Smith, M., (1988). Psychosocial impact of the AIDS epidemic on the lives of gay men. *Social Work*, **33**, 277-281.

Tones, B.K., (1981). Health education: Prevention or subversion? *Royal Society of Health Journal*, **101**, 114-117.

Troiden, R.R., (1979). Becoming homosexual: A model of gay identity acquisition. *Psychiatry*, **42**, 362-373.

Troiden, R.R., (1988). Homosexual identity development. *Journal of Adolescent Health Care*, **9**, 105-113.

Van den Aardweg, G.J., (1985). Male homosexuality and the neuroticism factor: An analysis of research outcome. *Dynamic Psychotherpy*, **3**, 79-87.

Watney, S., (1987). *Policy desire: Pornography, AIDS and the media*. London: Comedia.

Weinberg, T.S., (1983). *Gay men, gay selves: The social construction of homosexual identities*. New York: Irvington.

Weis, C.B., & Dain, R.N., (1979). Ego development and sex attitudes in heterosexual and homosexual men and women. *Archives of Sexual Behavior*, **8**, 341-356.

Weisner, W., & Grant, L. (1989). *Working with HIV and AIDS*. Leicester: AVID Productions.

Williams, S.G., (1981). Male homosexual responses to MMPI combined subscales Mf_1 and Mf_2. *Psychological Reports*, **49**, 606.

16 'Health dividends': The use of co-operative inquiry as health promotion intervention with a group of unemployed women

M. Daniels and A. Coyle

Introduction

From the publication in 1938 of Eisenberg and Lazarfeld's classic work on the psychological consequences of unemployment, the adverse effects of unemployment upon psychological well-being have been well documented. With regard to the extent of these negative consequences, Jackson and Warr (1983) stated that twenty per cent of unemployed people experience a deterioration in their mental health as a result of unemployment. In more specific terms, the same authors reported increased anxiety, depression, insomnia, irritability, lack of confidence, listlessness, inability to concentrate, and general nervousness among the unemployed men whom they studied. This list succinctly summarises the biopsychosocial consequences of unemployment that other studies have also identified. Additional characteristics that others have noted include anomie, self-blame, anger, aggression, reduced life satisfaction, decreased motivation to work, and a feeling of helplessness and of not being in control of one's life (Kaufman, 1982); loss of self-esteem (Shamir, 1986); and disturbance in family relationships (Hill, 1977; Jackson & Walsh, 1987; Martin & Wallace, 1984). Some authors have sought to locate psychological reactions to unemployment within a stage framework and have identified stages of shock and disbelief; denial, optimism and the making of concerted efforts to secure re-employment; anxiety, distress, self-doubt, anger and pessimism; and resignation, fatalism, withdrawal and adjustment (Fagin & Little, 1984; Harrison, 1976; Hill, 1977; Kaufman, 1982).

Focusing on the benefits of paid employment that are lost when a person becomes unemployed, Warr (1983) outlined nine features of the unemployed role that may militate against psychological well-being, i.e., a decrease in income and, consequently, in the variety of one's life; a reduction in the number of one's goals; decreased scope for significant decision-making; reduced opportunities for the development and practice of skills; an increase in psychologically threatening activities and experiences such as rejection and social stigma; insecurity about the future; decreased variety in one's interpersonal contacts; and changes in social position. Others have itemised additional losses consequent upon unemployment, including the loss of the predictable temporal division of one's day; the potential for positive feedback on one's competence and worth; a sense of purpose; habitual activities; and one's role within the family context (Brenner & Bartell, 1983; Fagin, 1979; Fagin & Little, 1984; Fineman, Johoda, 1982).

In a more socially-oriented analysis, Breakwell (1986) pointed to the way in which the dominant social representation of 'the unemployed' threatens the identity of unemployed people. This social representation, which is expressed in various cultural forms and which exists in people's attitudinal and belief systems, is negative in tone. It equates unemployment with laziness and lack of motivation, representing unemployed people as 'social miscreants (Scroungers) who have failed in some way to comply with society's requirements and are being legitimately chastised through the loss of paid work' (Breakwell, 1986, p.57). There is evidence that people evaluate the unemployed negatively and that unemployed people believe that others despise and deprecate them, to an even greater extent than they actually do (Breakwell et al., 1984). If unemployed people believe that others perceive them in terms of this negative social representation, or if they view themselves in this way, their psychological well-being in general and their self-esteem and identity in particular may suffer.

Warr (1983) has listed various factors which may mediate the effects of unemployment, including gender. Research on the effects of unemployment has traditionally either ignored women or has studied them only as the spouses of unemployed men. There is evidence that women's psychological well-being is adversely affected when they themselves are unemployed (Hall and Johnson, 1988; Martin and Wallace, 1984). Some studies have reported similar psychological outcomes for both men and women following unemployment (Ensminger and Celentano, 1990; Gore and Magione, 1983), while others have suggested that unemployment has more serious consequences for men than for women (Fagin, 1979; Jahoda,

1982; Snyder and Nowak, 1984).

In 1991, a health promotion worker from Enfield Health Authority in north London decided to construct a project that would address the mental and physical health needs of unemployed women in her locality. However, she felt that the inconclusive findings reported by those studies which have attempted to describe the effects of unemployment on women's mental health were an unsatisfactory basis for a health promotion intervention. She therefore decided to undertake an assessment of the mental and physical health needs of unemployed women in Enfield so that appropriate health promotion interventions could be designed to address these needs. She wished to undertake this needs assessment in such a way that the research process itself would constitute a health promotion intervention with unemployed women. As the chosen method was somewhat innovative, a detailed account of the project's methodological content and process will be provided, partly to contextualise and explain the approach taken, and partly to guide those health promotion workers who wish to apply the method in their work.

Methodological issues

Co-operative inquiry

The health promotion intervention that was undertaken was based upon principles of co-operative inquiry, which has been characterised as a new paradigm methodology (Reason, 1988; Reason & Rowan, 1981). The prime characteristic of co-operative inquiry or - as it is also termed - participatory research is that the researcher interacts with those who, within an orthodox research approach, are construed as passive research 'subjects'. The principal aim of this interaction is to establish 'a dialogue between research workers and the grass-roots people with whom they work' (Reason, 1988, p.2) and to enable them to contribute actively to the research process at every stage as co-researchers (Heron, 1981). Such a method may also be located within the community development approach to health promotion, which operates when 'a group or groups of like-minded people, who recognise themselves as having common experiences in health matters, come together to discuss and review their concerns, to take stock of their situations, to identify mutual problems and to share in the process of clarifying options, working out appropriate joint action and setting about the process of trying to change their circumstances' (Beattie, 1991, p.176). In that the health promotion worker responsible for initiating the project operated within a community development framework, the adoption of a co-operative inquiry approach accorded with her theoretical assumptions about health promotion.

Recruiting participants

As the research issue that was to be addressed concerned the health needs of unemployed women, it was decided that women from this target group should be involved in the project as co-researchers with the project initiator, i.e. with the health promotion worker. One of the advantages of involving unemployed women as co-researchers is that they may more easily be able to contact other unemployed women through their social networks and motivate them to participate in the needs assessment research than would the project initiator if she were action as sole researcher. The difficulty of contacting unemployed women and of motivating them to participate in research or in health promotion projects - noted by Warr (1987) - was encountered in an earlier attempt to initiate a health needs assessment using a more traditional research framework. At the outset of this intended project, the health promotion worker assiduously visited local job centres and Department of Social Security offices and distributed handbills and displayed posters that outlined the nature of the research and sought participants. This strategy failed to elicit any response from the target group. From this experience, it was clear that a more innovative approach was required in order to contact unemployed women and to motivate them to participate in the needs assessment.

It was felt that the use of a co-operative inquiry methodology would motivate women to participate in the project as co-researchers by offering them many of the psychosocial benefits of paid employment, thereby helping to promote their sense of psychological well-being. For example, it was hoped that involvement in the project would provide the women with new goals; variation in their everyday routine; new social contacts; the opportunity to develop and practice new skills, to participate in significant decision-making and to receive positive feedback on their competence; and a renewed sense of purpose. These aims overlap considerably with what Warr (1983) considered to be the psychosocial characteristics of 'good unemployment', i.e., an unemployment situation which would help to maintain psychological well-being. Also, the women's psychological well-being could be boosted by their being involved in a meaningful project that would have demonstrable results, as their research findings would inform the design of subsequent health promotion interventions for unemployed women: Haworth and Evans (1987) concluded that involvement in meaningful activity can moderate the negative psychological consequences of unemployment. It was felt that involvement in the project might also allow the women to construct

210

an identity as a researcher or - if they became involved in resultant health promotion programmes - as a voluntary health promotion worker. The adoption of such an identity might prove less corrosive to psychological well-being than would an 'unemployed' identity, in that the women might cease to regard the negative social representation of 'the unemployed' as applicable to them. To the extent that this personally adopted social identity becomes recognised and accepted by others in the women's social networks, these others may cease to apply the negative social representation of 'the unemployed' to them. For the unemployed women who would participate in the project as co-researchers, the research therefore constituted a mental health promotion intervention.

In order to gauge the extent to which the intervention succeeded in promoting psychological well-being, the women completed the 30-item version of the General Health Questionnaire (GHQ-30) (Goldberg, 1978) at the beginning and at the end of the project. This instrument provides an indication of a person's psychological well-being on the basis of whether or not they have experienced certain symptoms or exhibited certain behaviours during the previous few weeks. The extent to which any psychological benefits persist after the completion of the research will depend upon such factors as the degree to which the women can become involved in further goal-directed projects, such as the establishment and maintenance of health promotion programmes that seek to address the health needs identified by their research.

The research can additionally be viewed as offering three potential psychological benefits to those who adopted the traditional role of research subjects. Firstly, their accounts of the ways in which unemployment has effected their mental and physical health will shape health promotion interventions that will address their health needs. Secondly, the process of verbalising their accounts of unemployment may prove cathartic. Thirdly, this process may help them to construct a coherent, interconnected, psychologically-pleasing account of the changes that have been demanded in their identity by their experiences of unemployment.

In selecting those women who would act as co-researchers and/or as participants in the research, it was impossible to employ techniques such as random or quota sampling, for various reasons. Firstly, the only way of gaining access to comprehensive information about women in the locality who were registered as unemployed would have been through the Department of Social Security, which properly regards this information as confidential. Secondly, even if access to such information were granted, it would be incomplete, as many women who are unemployed do not register as such because they are unable to obtain benefits if their partner is in paid employment or is in receipt of benefits.

In the light of the aforementioned recruitment difficulties, it was decided to adopt an opportunistic approach to the recruitment of co-researchers. Four women were therefore enlisted as co-researchers through various community health networks. All had attended discussion groups on a range of health-related topics that had been facilitated by the same health promotion worker who was responsible for initiating the co-operative inquiry project. All four women were unwaged and three were actively seeking work or further training. Three of the women were in their twenties and one was in her fifties. These particular women were recruited because they were involved in part-time voluntary work and were therefore deemed likely to have access to other unemployed women in the community.

The methodological process

The co-operative inquiry group met four times over a period of one month. The proceedings of each session were recorded and later transcribed. Edited versions of these transcriptions have been presented elsewhere (cf. Daniels, 1992). The group consisted of the four unemployed women, the health promotion worker who assumed the role of group initiator, and a female participant observer. The term 'initiator' is used rather than 'leader' or 'facilitator', as the person who assumes this role works actively with the group during the initial stages of the co-operative inquiry process in order to help establish the group's aims and methods of working. However, beyond this point, she transfers responsibility for the group onto the group members and moves towards adopting the role of a co-worker. the principal role of the participant observer within the group was to act as a debriefing partner for the initiator and to provide her with feedback on the nature of the group dynamics.

During the first group meeting, the initiator's role involved establishing rapport with the women, administering the GHQ-30, and conducting a minimally structured group interview to ascertain the various ways in which unemployment had affected the women. To reduce the likelihood of self-presentational effects occurring on the GHQ-30, the women were told that it was being used simply to supplement the data from the group interview. The discussion that arose in the interview was at first generic but then focused upon how unemployment had affected the women's health, attending particularly to its mental health implications. Through this discussion, the women identified their health needs in the light of unemployment. In consultation with the initiator, the group proceeded to design a research task that would identify the mental and physical health needs of other unemployed women. The women decided that they would contact other unemployed women in the locality and would talk to them in a loosely structured manner about the ways in which unemployment had affected them. They would then seek to identify the women's health needs, i.e., those health-related issues on which they would like information, training, or opportunities for discussion. With regard to data recording, the co-researchers decided to make notes about the content of their conversations after they had taken place. Over the next month, the four women contacted and interviewed six other unemployed women.

It may be legitimately argued that the implementation of health promotion interventions on the basis of the opinions and experiences of only ten subjects is unwarranted. However, the research was designed as a pilot study for a larger scale future assessment of the health needs of unemployed women. Lest the small sample should identify idiosyncratic needs, it was envisaged that the health promotion interventions established in the light of the research findings would be relatively small in scale and low in cost. This strategy was necessary to avoid channelling a disproportionate amount of funds into addressing the specific health needs of a small number of people.

The second and third meetings of the co-operative inquiry group focused on processing feedback from those women who had conducted interviews and on clarifying the research protocol in the light of their feedback. This procedure was continued in the fourth and final session during which key comments from the accounts of unemployment provided by the four co-researchers and by the six research participants were displayed on flipchart paper. The group then engaged in a collective thematic content analysis of the research findings. Having identified the main themes in the data, the group offered suggestions about how these could inform potential health promotion interventions and discussed the roles that they could play in these interventions.

At the close of this process, the initiator saw each woman individually and asked her to complete the GHQ-30 again, while the other women talked with the participant observer. In the one-to-one interview, each woman was given the opportunity to discuss any issues that had been raised by the research in general or by the GHQ-30 items in particular and which she did not feel comfortable in discussing with the group. Finally, before the group engaged in closure exercises, each woman completed an evaluation form which asked her to identify what, if anything, she had enjoyed about or had gained from her participation in the project. Six months later, a follow-up session was convened at which the health promotion worker shared her official written report of the research with the group and sought their feedback on this document. The preparation of this report was therefore also characterised by consultation, negotiation and co-operation with the group. At this session, the women were additionally given feedback on the progress that had been made in establishing health promotion interventions to address the health needs identified by their research.

Results

In considering the outcome of the co-operative inquiry project, we will first report the ways in which the ten women said that unemployment had affected them and examine the findings of the health needs assessment. Secondly, we will identify changes in psychological well-being among the four co-researchers during the project in order to determine how effective participation in a co-operative inquiry group might be as a mental health promotion intervention.

With regard to the interviews with the ten women, several thematic clusters were identified in the analysis of the replies given by the women when they were asked to describe the ways in which unemployment had affected them. Accounts of the practical effects of unemployment focused on the consequences of a reduction in income: the women spoke of constantly having to 'skimp' and of being unable to afford to take a holiday or to engage in meaningful time-occupying activities such as using leisure facilities or taking language classes. the somatic effects that were mentioned included reduced levels of sleep and activity and increased smoking. The psychosocial effects that were cited centred on feelings of depression; a lack of confidence; a lack of control over one's life; an awareness of the low value ascribed to unpaid and/or voluntary work (although some said that engaging in voluntary work made them feel better about themselves) and of other people's negative opinions of 'the unemployed'; having to 'keep up appearances'; isolation; loneliness; limited access to other people; segregation; and the stress of having to stay at home. The health needs that the women identified were diverse. Those directly relevant to mental health included the need for self-help groups, free and easily accessible psychotherapy, relaxation techniques and stress management skills. However, many of the other health needs that the women cited also incorporated a mental health component.

The mental health implications of involvement as a co-researcher in a personally relevant co-operative inquiry project were assessed through the pre- and post-project administration of the GHQ-30 - the results of

214

which are presented in Table 1 - and through the completion of evaluation forms at the close of the research project.

Table 1
The GHQ-30 scores of the four women co-researchers at the beginning and at the end of the co-operative inquiry project

	scores at the beginning of the project	scores at the end of the project
Woman 1	17	3
Woman 2	13	0
Woman 3	3	0
Woman 4	0	0

The establishment of a profile of psychological well-being for any group on the GHQ usually involves selecting a 'threshold score' above which a respondent is considered to have a low level of psychological well-being. From their review of studies that have used the GHQ-30, Goldberg and Williams (1988) reported that the most commonly chosen threshold score was five. Another method of interpreting the scores obtained by the four women is to compare them with scores obtained by women from the general population. In this respect, the mean score of 4.41 obtained on the GHQ-30 by the women studied by Cox et al. (1987) constitutes a useful yardstick. Two of the women in the co-operative inquiry group recorded scores above this mean and above a threshold score of five at the beginning of the co-operative inquiry project, whereas none recorded such scores at the close of the project.

Some of the comments that the women made in the evaluation of the project provide further insights into the ways in which their involvement in the group had affected their psychological well-being. One woman stated that 'it was good to have a regular activity to do and the sociable aspect'. Another said that 'it seems like a little job'. Another woman found that it was 'very encouraging to be asked views on health/community issues - from a self-esteem point of view'. One woman said that through her involvement in the group she had learned 'how much of the various problems/drawbacks I have had, being out of work, are similar to other people', while another said she had 'learnt about what employment can mean to other women'. Others emphasised the mental stimulation that they had gained through their involvement, saying that they had enjoyed 'talking about various topics with other women - especially in a friendly environment'; 'talking and listening to other women - working as a group, sharing experiences'; and 'sharing ideas/discussing common or differing views'. One woman said that after each session, she felt that she was 'left with something to think about, or an idea to challenge or reflections on the group processes and their discussion'.

Discussion

A significant degree of overlap was observed between the effects of unemployment outlined in the literature on the topic an the effects identified by the ten women who were interviewed. Their descriptions of feelings of depression, lack of confidence and reductions in their levels of sleep and activity mirrored Jackson and Warr's (1983) account of the mental health implications of unemployment. The women's inability to engage in meaningful time-occupying activities because of the financial cost of such activities may be seen as supporting Warr's (1983) claim that the reduction in income associated with unemployment leads to a decrease in the variety of a person's life, which may exert a detrimental effect on psychological well-being. The women also echoed Warr (1983) in their emphasis on the restriction in their social life caused by unemployment and on their resultant feelings of isolation, loneliness, segregation and stress. It appears that, for these women, the social ramifications of unemployment figured prominently in their hierarchy of those consequences of unemployment that militate against psychological well-being. The effects of unemployment that they identified did not differ significantly from the effects reported by those studies which investigated the experiences of unemployed men.

After the research project had been completed, attempts were made, where feasible, to construct health promotion interventions that would meet the women's explicitly expressed health needs and that would also try to counteract some of the negative psychosocial effects of unemployment that they described. These interventions often involved putting the women in touch with agencies and individuals that could meet their needs, with the health promotion worker facilitating this communication. For example, some women complained that it was impossible for them to go swimming with more than one child without another adult because of the difficulty of attending to their children simultaneously in the pool. The health promotion worker therefore contacted the local voluntary services council and arranged for volunteers to meet mothers at the pool in order to look after their children. This meant that the mothers felt comfortable in bringing all their children to the pool. They could also leave their children in the care of the volunteers and swim independently. Not only were they accorded access to the physical and psychological benefits of exercise but they were also able temporarily to transfer responsibility for their children onto others and to create time for themselves which they could use as they wished. Such an intervention may help to promote psychological well-being among women who have adopted a domestic maternal role since losing their job and whose scope for independent functioning had consequently become limited. By linking the women with the volunteers and by placing them in a context in which there is potential for social interaction, the intervention may also help to counter-act the social isolation of unemployment.

One of the aims of using a co-operative inquiry method was to provide the women with many of the psychosocial benefits that usually accrue from paid employment. Indeed, one of the women explicitly likened her involvement in the co-operative inquiry group to 'a little job'. However, Breakwell (1986) claimed that interventions which aim to replace the work-related psychosocial benefits that unemployed people have lost are inadequate in rectifying the psychological distress and social dislocation occasioned by unemployment. She regarded these consequences as resulting more form the effects of the application to the unemployed person of the negative social representation of 'the unemployed'. The themes that emerged from the analysis of the interview material provide examples of the effects of the application of this social representation: the women spoke of other people's negative opinions of 'the unemployed'; the low value ascribed to work that is unpaid and/or voluntary; and the pressure of having to 'keep up appearances' and to deny that unemploy-ment has had any adverse practical or psychological effects. Rather than trying to replace the psychosocial benefits of paid employment, Breakwell advocated that efforts should be channelled into modifying the negative social representation of unemployed people so that its judgemental character is mitigated.

However, this must be seen as a long-term goal, because, as she admitted, the attitudes which inform this social representation have evolved over a period of six hundred years. In the shorter term, any intervention should be welcomed if it offers unemployed people the psychosocial benefits that are usually derived from paid employment, and the opportunity to escape their identity as unemployed and to construct an identity which may be less detrimental to their self-esteem.

It could be claimed that the increased psychological well-being and the practical marketable skills and experience which the women gained through their involvement in the co-operative inquiry project may help them to secure paid employment and to escape the unemployed role on a long-term basis.

In that the co-operative inquiry project unearthed mental and physical health needs among unemployed women that could then be addressed through health promotion projects, it can be adjudged a useful tool for health needs assessment and for the design of subsequent interventions with this group. However, the use of co-operative inquiry proved to be more than an effective methodological tool. Of the four unemployed women who were involved in the project as co-researchers, three demonstrated increased psychological well-being on the GHQ-30 during the course of the project: the psychological well-being of the remaining woman, which was high at the outset, was unchanged at the close of the project. The comments that the women made in their evaluation of the project stressed that their involvement had increased their self-esteem and had given them the opportunity of exchanging their ideas about and experiences of being unemployed with others who were in similar situations, thus counteracting any sense of physical of psychological isolation that they may have felt. As the women were given the opportunity of becoming involved in the health promotion projects that resulted from their research, they could potentially continue to avail of the psychosocial benefits that they had gained from their involvement in the co-operative inquiry group and could construct a positively-evaluated identity as a voluntary health promotion worker.

Conclusion

On the basis of these considerations, it can be concluded that the use of the co-operative inquiry group itself constituted a valuable intervention in the promotion of the women's mental health. Furthermore, through the channelling of the results of the research on needs assessment into specific health promotion interventions, the project yielded considerable mental health dividends for all the unemployed women who participated in it.

References

Beattie, A. (1991). Knowledge and control in health promotion: A test case for social policy and social theory. In J. Gabe, M. Clanan & M. Bury (Ed.), *The sociology of the health service*, (pp.162-202). London: Routledge.

Breakwell, G. M. (1986). *Coping with threatened identities*. London: Methuen.

Breakwell, G. M., Collie, A., Harrison, B., & Propper, C. (1984). Attitudes towards the unemployed: Effects of threatened identity. *British Journal of Social Psychology*, 23, 87-88.

Brenner, S. O., & Bartell, R. (1983). The psychological impact of unemployment: A structural analysis of cross-sectional data. *Journal of Occupational Psychology*, 56, 129-136.

Cox, B., Blaxter, M., Buckle, A., Fenner, N. P., Golding, J., Gore, M., Huppert, F., Nickson, J., Roth, M., Stark, J., Wadsworth, M., & Wichelow, M. (1987). *The health and lifestyle survey*. Cambridge: Health Promotion Research Trust.

Daniels, M. (1992). *Health dividends? The use of co-operative inquiry as a health promotion intervention with unemployed women.* Unpublished MSc dissertation: South Bank University, London.

Eisenberg, P., & Lazarfeld, P. (1938). The psychological effects of unemployment. *Psychological Bulletin*, 35, 358-390.

Ensminger, M. E., & Celentano, D.D. (1990). Gender differences in the effect of unemployment on psychological distress. *Social Science and Medicine*, 30, 469-477.

Fagin, L. H. (1979). The experience of unemployment. I: The impact of unemployment. *New Universities Quarterly*, 34, 48-65.

Fagin, L., & Little, M. (1984). *The forsaken families: The effects of unemployment on family life*. Middlesex: Penguin.

Fineman, S. (1983). *White collar unemployment: Impact and stress*. Chichester: John Wiley & Sons.

Goldberg, D.P. (1978). *Manual of the general health questionnaire*. Windsor: NFER-Nelson.

Goldberg, D., & Williams, P. (1988). *A users' guide to the general health questionnaire*. Windsor: NFER-Nelson.

Gore, S., & Mangione, T. W. (1983). Social role, sex role, and psychological distress: Additive and interactive models of sex differences. *Journal of Health and Social Behaviour*, 24, 300-312.

Hall, E. M., & Johnson, J. (1988). Depression in unemployed Swedish women. *Social Science and Medicine*. 27, 1349-1355.

Harrison, R. (1976). The demoralizing experience of prolonged unemployment. *Department of Employment Gazette*, April, 339-348.

Haworth, J.T., & Evans, S. T. (1987). Meaningful activity and unemployment. In D. Fryer, & P. Ullah (Eds.), *Unemployed people: Social and psychological perspectives*, (pp.241-267). Milton Keynes: Open University Press.

Heron, J. (1981). Philosophical basis for a new paradigm. In P. Reason & J. Rowan (Eds.), *Human inquiry: A sourcebook of new paradigm research*, (pp.19-35). Chichester: John Wiley & Sons.

Hill, J. M. M. (1977). *The social and psychological impact of unemployment: A pilot study*. London: Tavistock Institute of Human Relations.

Jackson, P. R., & Walsh, S. (1987). Unemployment and the family. In D. Fryer, & P. Ullah (Eds.), *Unemployed people: Social and psychological perspectives*, (pp 194-216). Milton Keynes: Open University Press.

Jackson, P. R., & Warr, P. B. (1983). *Age, length of unemployment, and other variables associated with men's ill-health during unemployment*. MRC/SSRC Social and Applied Psychology Unit Memo 585: University of Sheffield.

Jahoda, M. (1982). *Employment and unemployment: A social-psychological analysis*. Cambridge: Cambridge University Press.

Kaufman, H. G. (1982). *Professionals in search of work: Coping with the stress of job loss and underemployment*. New York: John Wiley & Sons.

Martin, R., & Wallace, J. (1984). *Working women in recession: Employment, redundancy, and unemployment*. Oxford: Oxford University Press.

Reason, P. (Ed.) (1988). *Human inquiry in action: Developments in new paradigm research*. London: Sage.

Reason, P., & Rowan, J. (Eds.) (1981). *Human inquiry: A sourcebook of new paradigm research*. Chichester: John Wiley & Sons.

Shamir, B. (1986). Self-esteem and the psychological impact of unemployment. *Social Psychology Quarterly*, **49** 61-72.

Snyder, K. A., & Nowak, T.C. (1984). Job loss and demoralization: Do women fare better than men? *International Journal of Mental Health*, **13**, 92-106.

Warr, P. (1983). Work, jobs and unemployment. *Bulletin of the British Psychological Society*, **36**, 305-311.

Warr, P. (1987). *Work, unemployment and mental health*. Oxford: Oxford University Press.

17 Developing community resources for carers: A prevention model in practice (or the Rime of the Ancient Mariner)

L. Goodbody

Introduction

In this paper, I shall be describing and analyzing the development of the South Devon Carers' Helpline project as an example of a community approach to the prevention of mental health problems. Although the design of the project is well grounded in relation to theory and research, it is not my aim to make this a traditional academic presentation. Nor is it my intention to give a '1066 and All That' account of what happened on the basis that it was 'A Good Thing' which people ought to know about. Rather, it is my aim to find a way of telling the story of the Helpline that picks out themes to grapple with from the rich untidiness of the tale. A number of questions of practical and theoretical significance, to which I don't have many answers, arise from this exploratory analysis. These questions may stimulate discussion in this symposium on 'Promoting Community Resources for the Prevention of Psychological Distress' so that we can start to construct a discourse of ideas and experience around health-promoting community interventions.

The Ancient Mariner, you may remember, stops a guest on his way to a joyful wedding, and regales him with the story of his strange and eventful journey.

Theoretical context: community psychology and models of prevention

Community psychology is a fairly new discipline in this country, the subject of which is 'located at the interface between person and context'

221

(Orford 1992, p.14). It is a theoretical and practical endeavour to focus upon the interaction and reciprocal influence between individual and social forces (cf. Lewin's (1951) famous equation, $B=f(P,E)$) which has not been addressed adequately by either the individualistic models of conventional psychology or the collective analyses of the sociological tradition.

Orford (1992) sets out a number of principles of community psychology through which it can be defined. In addition to the fundamental concept of focusing on the interaction between people and their social settings as the origin of problems, he also points out that community psychology apples a range of research methods (e.g. qualitative and action research) operating at various levels of analysis but particularly at those of the organisation and community. Furthermore, community psychology is distinguished by its emphasis upon prevention rather than treatment, a proactive approach to service development and working in the relevant social settings. Through facilitation and collaboration, it seeks to encourage the development of voluntary and self-help movements, as the structure of social support and of power are seen as key determinants of transactions between the person and his or her environment.

A community psychology intervention would therefore be constructed around a recognition of the psychosocial nature of mental health and mental health problems, and would work through consultation and collaboration with different aspects of community systems to improve access to resources of social support and power.

The second context, that of the literature on the prevention of mental health problems, suggests similar directions. In her recent book, Newton (1992) tackles the old chestnut about the real effectiveness of preventive interventions. From her review, she proposes three main good practice criteria which can be summarised as follows:

1. Quality research findings should be used to identify 'at risk' groups for the efficient targeting of resources.
2. Interventions should be designed to increase individual control over life circumstances and reduce dependency on services.
3. Services should make maximum use of existing natural community resources and networks.
   (after Newton, 1992)

Although there are differences between these two fields of study, with prevention commonly assuming a fairly simple linear aetiology of disease which for the community psychologist is the product of complex multiple interactions between people and systems, they are affirming of one another in most other respects. The concept of the 'at risk' group is a

222

common one in prevention, and so I shall go on to make a case for carers being such a group to whom it is reasonable to direct resources with an expectation of significant health benefits.

Carers as an 'at risk' group

Demography

Recent census figures (Green, 1988) have given us a clear demographic profile of Britain's carers. There are about 6 million of them, and 6 out of 10 are women, who also tend to be looking after more dependent people for longer periods. So caring is an experience that affects many people and especially women. It cuts across social classes, ethnic groupings and rural-urban settings.

Haffenden (1991) has argued that it is important to extrapolate from these census figures in order to derive estimates which can then be used to raise awareness and lobby for resources. South Devon is a popular retirement area so the estimates given below are likely to be conservative

Table 1
Estimated Numbers of Carers in South Devon
(Adult population of South Devon = 253,000)
* 35,420 people provide for someone who is sick, disabled or frail
* 10,120 people care for some one in the same household
* 6,983 People do not receive visits from any services
* 5,364 people provide intimate personal care
* 4,554 people spend at least 50 hours a week caring

The cost of replacement care would clearly be very high, meaning that there is a strong financial argument for investing in carer support to maintain their ability to continue to care in the community if they wish to do so.

Social and psychological risk factors

Whilst the figures above indicate some of the demands of caring, there are particular social risk factors associated with the caring situation. Most carers experience some of the following:
- Financial hardship, loss of employment/earnings/pension (e.g. Rimmer, 1983; Nissel and Bonnerjea, 1982)
- Restricted opportunities for self-care and recreation (e.g. Ungerson, 1985)
- Social isolation and diminished social support through difficulty in

maintaining reciprocal relationships, stigma, mobility problems etc.

- Loss of intimate relationships and increased family tensions (e.g. Qureshi and Walker, 1986)
- Physical health problems, pre-existing and those arising from caring.
- Lack of recognition generally, and specifically lack of 'recognition through provision' of community services.
- The baffling complexity of benefits and uncoordinated services, and poor information about access and rights.

In an earlier qualitative exploration of the subjective experience of caring (Goodbody, 1988), I was able to identify a number of key psychological features which mirror the social factors. These include powerlessness, a negative sense of identity, conflict of needs and denial of needs and a restricted range of coping mechanisms. Whilst isolation, exhaustion, limited activities and relationships are objective consequences of the practical nature of caring, the corresponding subjective consequences are feelings of guilt, stress and impotence (e.g. Orford, 1987).

Carers and mental health

It has been shown that the caring role is heavily loaded with factors commonly associated with poor health. Caregiver burden (Zarit et al., 1986) has been one way of conceptualising the exposure to multiple and long term stressors, and it is not difficult to see the resemblance with the risk factors identified by Brown and Harris (1978) in their work on the social origins of depression, especially if the carer has lost a primary confiding relationship in the dependent person.

There have been numerous studies which generally show an enhanced prevalence of psychiatric and physical symptomatology among carers. For instance, George and Gwyther (1986) found that carers scored lower on mental health indicators than non-carers, and Gilhooly (1984) notes that some studies show that 50-60% of carers score on psychiatric screening devices in a way comparable to those who seek help.

Summary

There is a well established body of research which demonstrates that carers are at risk of developing mental health problems as a result of the interaction of the social and psychological processes characterising their situation. In terms of potential health benefit and the cost of replacement care, they are an appropriate group at which to target resources.

Rationale for designing an intervention

The emphasis on social support is a recurrent theme of the literature about carers. It is also one of the focal topics in community psychology, for these are numerous studies which indicate that people with good social support experience higher levels of well being (Heller et al., 1991; Gottlieb, 1987). The mechanisms whereby the health benefits are produced are still largely unknown but the most common model concerns the 'buffer' hypothesis which states that support (e.g. discussing problems with another) works by attenuating the impact of stress. However, there is a general need for further research to clarify which specific supportive functions are effective for which populations and psychological situations (Wills, 1991). Intervention research about social support is still at an early stage of development.

Whilst there is lack of consensus in the research on carers about the ways in which factors such as age, relationship to the dependent person, length of caring and degree of dependency interact to effect the level of strain experienced, a couple of studies have used multifactorial designs to explore the relationship between satisfaction with support and distress. Baillie et al., (1988) found a distinct and large main effect, so that satisfaction with support was associated with lower levels of depression independently of other factors. Likewise, in their two year study, Schultz and Williamson (1991) showed that perceived availability of support was a major independent predictor of carers' well being (i.e. as perceptions of available support declined, depression increased).

Therefore, in terms of a rationale for a preventive intervention with carers, both community psychology and the literature on carers indicate that social support of some kind should be a central feature of its design.

Newton's (1992) remaining two guidelines concerning increasing personal control over life and using existing community resources, point to the intervention processes through which improved social support for carers may be achieved.

Setting up the Carers' Helpline: a practitioner's notebook account

'Community psychology takes very seriously its obligation to apply theory in real-life settings.' (Schiaffino, 1991, p.99). Therefore, girded and supplied with a strong theoretical perspective, I was ready to tackle the real world. It is time to embark upon the story proper.

The beginning: Year 1

> The ship was cheered, the harbour cleared,
> Merrily did we drop below the kirk, below the hill,
> Below the lighthouse top.
>
> The Rime of the Ancient Mariner, Coleridge, 1970, p.174

Starting off was fun. It involved initiating, building alliances, assessing the setting conditions and mobilising interest around a common 'mission'.

I was in my first job as a clinical psychologist, and having done some academic research about carers, I wanted to 'give something back' by promoting service development. Remembering the principle of collaboration, my first step was to write a letter to all the people and agencies connected with carers to ask them if they were interested in meeting to discuss possible developments. The time seemed right. There were television programmes about carers and the Community Care Act was on the horizon. I also went along to meetings of the local branch of Carers National Association. However, I got a zero response all around, so rather puzzled, I decided that if I could not even mobilise initial interest, this was going to be a non-starter.

The initiative was resurrected six months later at a carers' day in a neighbouring district. Over coffee, a colleague said she had discovered my letter recently under a pile of papers and suggested that the South Devon people present should meet again. So we did and with some further networking, we were on our way. The group was made up of statutory and voluntary representatives, including the local Carers National Association (C.N.A.) branch, and both practitioners and managers. A good proportion had been or were carers although there was no one currently caring full time until a later stage. Carers' Action Group currently has 12 members and I am the chairperson. We have access to an enormous range of contacts at various levels in different organisations and a lot of complementary skills and experience.

In order to decide what our practical objectives should be, it was necessary to consult with carers about local needs. This gave us our first positive collective experience of what we could achieve through working together. A workshop for carers was organised, and through good use of local media, the workshop was oversubscribed, with almost a hundred carers attending. The purpose of the workshop was to derive an action plan from small group discussions. We ended up with a clear mandate to work on the provision of respite care and sitting services, improving representation, G.P. education and information about the availability of support services.

It became obvious that no one had the time to really take this work on as every one was struggling to protect even our monthly meeting times from competing demands. We networked again, holding 'Forum Meetings' with agencies and professionals throughout the district in order to continue the process of consultation and to see if any one would pick up a project with our support. The Forum Meetings dwindled and finally we decided that there were insufficient existing resources so we would have to apply for funding to pay a carer co-ordinator to work with carers' groups and local agencies to research information and build working links for the provision of support and services.

Every one was still very positive, so whilst we were writing up project proposals and funding applications, other small projects, not necessarily within our specific brief but which we could actually do, went ahead. These included:

- liaising with professional and voluntary workers in particular towns or small areas. One group did a 'benefits Jamboree' for carers as a result.
- getting representation for carers on the Health and Social Services joint planning committees. There are still a number of 'vacancies' but the co-ordinator of these committees now works on issues of carer representation.
- arranging for workshops and a performance of the play 'Carers' by a local company that works with social issues through engaging the actual protagonists in the production of theatre. Professionals and managers of services were also engaged in the process.
- working with the Carers National Association branch to strengthen its committee and solve problems of low membership of current carers.

The middle: Year 2

About, about, in reel and rout
The death-fires danced at night'
The water, like a witch's oils,
Burnt green, and blue and white.   Coleridge, 1970, p.176

This stage was not fun. It involved further networking, negotiating with funding bodies, sorting out messes and tensions, re-appraising our work and aims and apparently getting nowhere fast.

The Carers Action Group learnt that as a result of poor communication with organisations outside our area, some one else had put in for funding for a carers' project in South Devon. We worked hard to salvage the situation and our credibility, held yet more meetings with people outside

227

the group and took advice from the national office of Carers National Association. Social Services and the Health Authority were convinced that the funding ought to go to our locally based project.

Tensions between the different interests of members of the working group were becoming apparent, reflecting the dilemmas individuals experienced with the organisations they represented. Although united in the overall aim in relation to carers, it was underwritten by many different sub-texts. There were conflicting agendas from the organisations we represented. The group ceased to function well, with more energy in meetings being devoted to undercurrents than to the job in hand. As chairperson, I tried to work with this fairly unsuccessfully. Most people were having a horrible time and wishing they had never got involved, myself included.

With half of our funding secure and the other half promised, we were working on setting up the job of the carer coordinator. One of the voluntary organisations involved was asked to employ the person with the continuing support of the group. They felt unable to do so, but the Health Authority agreed to act as employing agent. We were about to advertise the post of carer coordinator when the membership of the voluntary organisation in question failed to support the final official motion to award the money promised to Carers Action Group. Our budget was reduced by half, the particular voluntary organisation representative's positions within the group and her own organisation were almost untenable, the group was in a state of angry shock. There was a lot of personal stress and distress for most people involved.

There followed a moratorium period along classic 'To be, or not to be' lines. No one wanted to give it all up even though by now we were aware there were tragic flaws in the structure and process of our working group. Now there were new agendas in the group, for instance, 'We've got to find a way of spending the money we have been granted or I'll lose all professional credibility', and 'We've got to do something for carers, the needs are still there'.

So when some one came up with a new suggestion to rescue the project and the group, we worked hard to tight deadlines to assess its feasibility. This was the Helpline project, a telephone service designed to provide accessible and coordinated information specifically relevant to carers. The project seemed feasible. I organised a 'day out' with an outside facilitator which helped us to focus on the project alone and to turn down new funding that was awarded to us to do developmental outreach work in the rural areas. It was much needed important work but we did not have the managerial resources to make it happen. The group had found a new modus operandi borne of resignation to the limitations of members and organisations rather than from resolution of conflict, and started to work on the Helpline project. Soon we were busy with negotiating roles and management structures, developing an information base and operational policy, training volunteers to staff the Helpline, implementing a publicity programme and making arrangements for financial accountability, support and quality assurance.

The end?: Year 3

> And now this spell was snapt: once more
> I viewed the ocean green
> And looked far forth, yet little saw
> Of what had else been seen -
> Like one, that on a lonesome road
> Doth walk in fear and dread,
> And having once turned round walks on,
> And turns no more his head;
> Because he knows, a frightful fiend
> Doth close behind him tread.   Coleridge, 1970, p.185.

The South Devon Carers' Helpline opened in November 1991. The service is provided on three days a week by two local voluntary agencies with whom we have service agreements. This means that we subcontract with these agencies that for an agreed sum they provide office premises, recruit, train and manage the volunteers who actually deal with the enquiries, develop the information resource etc. We retain overall responsibility as the management committee, including determining policy and standards, providing support and evaluation. Subject to satisfactory evaluation and future funding, the two agencies will take the project on jointly in their own right next year, at which point the Carers' Action Group I have been describing will disband and cease to exist. We have a transitional withdrawal programme which includes coordinating a meeting for carers and carers groups to look at what they want to do in the future.

The aims of the Helpline can be categorised in three ways as follows:

1. Overall long term aim - To reduce the risk associated with looking after someone at home by increasing potential access to support services, thereby limiting subjective and objective stress factors.
2. Immediate aim - To provide a coordinated, accessible information resource covering services, groups and issues relevant to carers.
3. Community development aims - a) To create new networks

between support services and carers. b) To monitor service gaps and advocate needs to relevant organisations. c) To increase public recognition of carers. d) To provide specialist information to other information agencies. e) To facilitate the development of voluntary agencies concerned with carers.

We are just starting to evaluate the project in relation to most of these aims so I can only make informal comments on the outcome of this work. We are not tackling the overall aim of risk reduction directly as this would involve research resources which are not available to us, but there will be a consumer evaluation which includes utilisation of information about services and how supportive the experience was perceived to be. We clearly have succeeded in the immediate goal of setting up the Helpline, but it remains to be seen how adequate the information resource is for carers. In relation to the community development aims, we have probably made some progress towards realising all of them.

I have left the most obvious area of evaluation until last in order to make the point that a preventive community project of this kind has a wide range of possible outcome effects as a result of the variety of sub-interventions involved in the overall process. However, this final area is probably the most serious one from the point of view of future funding. During the first 10 months of operation, the Helpline has only received 54 calls. We know it is a common experience of new helplines for uptake to be very slow, and we are always looking at ways in which the service is publicised and delivered is limiting its utilisation. Nonetheless, there is a real possibility that in spite of what carers were saying to us at the initial consultation workshop that either information is no longer a priority need or the Helpline is not a good way of meeting that need.

Discussion of issues in the community intervention process

And I had done a hellish thing,
And it would work 'em woe:
For all averred, I had killed the bird
That made the breeze to blow.   Coleridge, 1979, p.175.

The Ancient Mariner killed the Albatross, the bird that accompanied the ship, the good omen that he should have revered to ensure safe passage on his voyage. He then had to suffer torments of many kinds, including the agonised telling and re-telling of his tale. In spite of fair weather at the theoretical point of departure, the project which ultimately led to the Carers' Helpline cannot be regarded as a clear success. It has involved

230

over three years difficult and sometimes unrewarding work for quite a number of people, with fairly limited demonstrable benefits.

Was there an Albatross, something or some things that we failed to recognise for what they were and which would have made a difference? Even if I cannot answer this question, I can suggest some of the key themes that may be relevant to exploring it.

Assessment and consultation

As with work with individuals, assessment of potential and resistance to change, of strengths and weaknesses and contextual factors, is an important part of community interventions. In common with an action research model, there needs to be a continuous cycle of assessment and re-evaluation in a long-term project like this as new factors enter and exit. For instance, the points when no one answered my initial letter, when the members of the main voluntary organisation did not back their committee's support of the project, and when the difficulties in involving other workers to take on carers' issues were all times when different decisions about feasibility could have been made. Similarly, although carers were members of the working group, it may have made a difference to have had ongoing rather than one-off consultation with a wider range of carers and a more systematic assessment of both need and likely utilisation patterns.

The further you go into this kind of project, the more you have invested (both personally and professionally), and the harder it becomes to bail out or steer a radically different course. The working group is prone to all the vagaries of decision-making known to occur in groups and apparent solutions soon become the next generation of problems. Although I took supervision about my participation, supervision of the group by an external consultant was far more effective and would have been useful at an earlier stage.

Collaborative working in groups and networks

One of the great strengths of the project was the diversity of the multi-agency working group, with access to a wide range of competencies and networks. However, it was also an inevitable source of conflicting agendas and divided loyalties which underscored our collective goals. Power and responsibility was the theme here, with members from the voluntary sector indicating they though the better resourced statutory agencies should take more on, and statutory members having the aim of facilitating the development of voluntary organisations to provide support for carers. This was evident from one organisation's refusal to employ the carer coordinator. Furthermore, communication is a major issue in networks as was made forcefully apparent when some one else put in a competing bid for funding.

The group also went through clearly definable stages normal to the life cycle of any group. We had a great beginning united by our common if slightly idealised aims, a really rough middle phase where our differences threatened to undermine our capacity to pursue our goals, before coming to a more realistic appraisal of what could be achieved through our collaborative effort. The fact that nearly every one stuck it out to reach that point is admirable, but I wonder if there are quicker or easier ways to maximise multi-agency working.

Complexity and interactions between systems

Third party developments in the organisations we represented or in higher order systems also affected the group's functioning, for instance, the re-organisations and re-definitions of policy that took place in the statutory organisations due to political and legislative developments at a national level. As mentioned above, there was a kind of 'purchaser-provider split' between members of the group, with the macro-level socio-political systems issues being acted out at a more micro-level (cf. Bronfenbrenner, 1979).

The complexities of systems interdependence are a distinctive feature of the ecology of community work. Although the different transactions between systems can be very confusing and create feelings of lack of control amongst those expecting to implement an intervention according to linear procedure, they can also be exploited for the development of the project. It involves a reflexive style of working at which my voluntary sector colleagues generally seemed most skilled. An example would be our use of service agreements to run the Helpline, an idea belonging to a market culture which in other respects created major difficulties for us, but which could also be deployed to resource community organisation. However, I am sure some environmental opportunities were still missed.

Process and outcome

Although the evaluation of the project is only at an early stage, I pre-empted its conclusions by suggesting that the Helpline was not successful because of the limited number of calls that have been made to it. This is indisputable but misses other important benefits and developments that have accrued as a result of the process of the work. Taken from an eco-behavioural perspective, there have been a number of spin-offs and side effects in the community as a result, such as putting carers on the public agenda through a constant flow of publicity, improving representation, and general flag-waving and networking with other organisation.

This is a model borrowed from ecology, and an analysis of biological disasters brought about by human interventions in natural systems, for instance the Aswan Dam. It means that there will be unpredicted effects which will not, therefore, be caught by a narrow evaluatory trawl. Whilst we will not be able to say whether our interventions have led to improved services to carers from agencies we have not worked with directly for instance, it is clear that those we have tried to resource have developed their work considerably. Therefore, the process or means by which the ends were achieved was as important as the Helpline itself.

Conclusion

This paper has tried to illustrate the difficult relationship between theory and practice when using a community development model of mental health promotion, in this case, the process of setting up a carers helpline. Community psychology and the prevention literature can provide a convincing rationale for intervention, but there are only general guidelines for implementation (such as working collaboratively to strengthen community resources, governed by principles of empowerment). Community psychology in particular is in the realm of 'grand theory', which seeks to unify different levels of knowledge in a single explanatory framework about the world, and which is therefore difficult to operationalise directly. Whilst other mental health disciplines have theories about practice, for instance in the form of various therapies, community oriented workers have little to guide their practice other than an ideology.

Community intervention research is still in its infancy, and Vaux (1991) argues that it is appropriate at this stage to engage in broad programmes and to tease out the process and key ingredients which can be investigated more rigorously later. The alternative to this is to say that more detailed research into specific factors, in social support process for instance, is necessary first so that interventions can be more precisely targeted. In relation to the Helpline, the supportive functions it aimed to fulfil were certainly global and assumed. However, I suggest that as what is achieved through the process of intervention is as important as the specific outcome, then getting on with **doing** is probably the most relevant future direction. Working with a complex, messy world where many systems interact in seemly uncontrollable ways is most likely to make significant contributions to our understanding.

I conclude with two quotations: '- if anything has been learned, it is that the social support process is far more complex than initially thought, as is its relationship to well-being. It is essential that interventions reflect that complexity. The greatest threat is not that powerful and effective social support interventions will prove impossible to develop and implement, but that we may become disillusioned by misunderstanding our failures'. (Vaux, 1991, p.90)

A sadder and a wiser man,
He rose the morrow morn.   Coleridge, 1970, p.189.

References

Baillie, V., Norbeck, J.S. & Barnes, L.E.A. (1988). Stress, social support and psychological distress in the family caregivers of the elderly. *Nursing Research*, **37**, 217-22.

Bronfenbrenner, U. (1979) *The ecology of human development: Experiments by nature and design.* Cambridge: Harvard University Press.

Brown, G. & Harris, T., (1978). *The social origins of depression.* London: Tavistock.

Coleridge, S.T., (1970). *The Rime of the Ancient Mariner*, in Poems. London: Dent.

George, L.K. & Gwyther, L.P. (1986). Caregiver well-being: a multi-dimensional examination of the caregivers of dementing adults. *The Gerontologist*, **26**, 253-269.

Gilhooly, M.L.M. (1984). The Social Dimensions of Senile Dementia. In I. Hanley & J. Hodge (Eds.). *Psychological Approaches to the Care of the Elderly.* Bechenham: Croom Helm.

Goodbody, S.C.L. (1988). *Women's experiences for caring for a disabled relative at home.* Unpublished M.Sc. dissertation, University of Exeter.

Gottlieb, B.H. (1987). Using social support to protect and promote health. *J. of Primary Prevention*, **8**, 49-70.

Green, H. (1988). Informal Carers. London: HMSO

Haffenden, S. (1991). Getting It Right for Carers. London: HMSO.

Heller, K. et al. (1991). Peer support telephone dyads for elderly women: Was this the wrong intervention? *American Journal of Community Psychology*, **19**, 53-73.

Lewin, K. (1951). *Field theory in Social Science.* New York: Harper.

Newton, J. (1992). *Preventing mental illness in practice.* London: Tavistock/Routledge.

Nissel, M. & Bonnerjea, L. (1982). *Family care for the wlderly: Who pays?* London: Policy Studies Institute.

Orford, J. (1987). *Coping with disorder in the family*. London: Croon Helm.

Orford, J., (1992). *Community Psychology: Theory and practice*. Chichester: Wiley.

Quereshi, H. & Walker, A. (1988). *The caring relationship: The family care of elderly people*.

Rimmer, L. (1983). The economics of work and caring. In Finch, J. & Groves, D. (Eds.) *A labour of love: Women, work and caring*. London: RKP

Schiaffino, K.M. (1991). Fine tuning to the needs of the world: Responding to Heller et al. *Am. J. Community Psychology*, **19**, 99-102.

Schultz, R. & Williamson, G.M. (1991). A 2-Year longitudinal study of depression among Alzheimer caregivers. *Psychology and Aging*, **6**, 569-578.

Ungerson, C. (1985). Gender divisions and Community Care - A British perspective. Paper prepared for 'Comparitive Aspects of Gender Divisions and Community Care' conference, University of Kent, April 1985.

Vaux, A. (1991). Let's hang up and try again: Lessons learned from a social support intervention. *Am. J. Community Psychology*, **19**, 85-90.

Wills, T.A. (1991). Comments on Heller, Thompson, Tureba, Hogg and Vlachos-Weber: 'Peer support telephone dyads for elderly women'. *Am. J. Community Psychology*, **19**, 75-83.

Zarit, S.H., Reever, K.E., & Bach-Peterson, J. (1980). Relatives of the impaired elderly: Correlates of feelings of burden. *The Gerontologist*, **20**, 649-660.

18 Presenters' perceptions of mental illness

P. Hall, I.A. Brockington and C. Murphy

The worldwide discharge of formerly institutionalised chronically mentally ill individuals and the avoidance of hospitalisation of the newly mentally ill both, I think in part at least for financial reasons, have led to an ever-increasing contact between the mentally ill and the population at large. This de-institutionalisation seems to rest on a number of largely speculative assumptions. Perhaps the chief of these is whether, on the one hand, it is better for the patients and/or their kith and kin and, on the other, whether, in broad terms, the community does indeed care. That is to say whether de-institutionalisation promotes better mental health and obviously, therefore, this is an issue of mental health promotion importance. Despite a great deal of debate and acrimony, there has, in fact, been singularly little research into whether there is some sort of mandate from the community at large for these changes in mental health practice, let alone whether it is indeed capable of showing the skills and tolerance that were previously the province of large mental hospitals and their staff. Such rather limited previous research as has been carried out was carried out almost exclusively in North America, in institutional psychiatric services and is largely unpublished.

I have been asked to tell you, therefore, something about a fairly complex piece of research which was carried out recently in the Worcester Development Project. As you probably know, this was the Department of Health's Model Unit in Community Psychiatry.

The purpose of the research was to try to reach some sort of understanding of the views of members of the community in which our large mental hospital had been dismantled and replaced by a community-based psychiatric service. In planning such services, a good deal of homage is paid to the idea of multidisciplinary planning. Psychiatrists, general practitioners, a variety of other mental health professionals, managers politicians and all sort of other people are consulted, but there is no referendum, as it were, of the population at large, nor is all that much attention paid to the wishes of the patients themselves or their relatives, despite a great deal of talk about NHS consumerism. In many ways, it would have been best to carry out our research before the Worcester Development Project opened, but we felt that late was perhaps better than never. We wanted to compare the views of our community and of the patients with a similar community and similar group of patients in an area still served by a large mental hospital.

I should say that our own research is published in a paperback by the Health Promotion Trust and the technical details will also be published in the British Journal of Psychiatry in the next few months.

The World Health Organisation had called together a colloquium in Umea in Sweden in March 1985 to which I happened to be the United Kingdom delegate. It seemed to us that as well as the point I have mentioned, if a community's tolerance for mental illness was exceeded, there might be a backlash into even more repressive measures than was previously the case, thereby causing adverse effects not only on the mental health of patients (Julian Leff), but on their families and perhaps the mental hygiene or mental health or whatever you like to call it of the wider community.

When I got back to the United Kingdom, therefore, Ian Brockington of Birmingham University, Jenny Levings now of Nottingham University, Chris Murphy who is now a consultant psychiatrist in Shrewsbury, and I got together and planned an initial study. We decided to compare two demographically similar adjacent areas in Worcestershire - Bromsgrove which was served by an excellent but traditional mental hospital, and Malvern which was served by Chris Murphy and myself in the context of a fairly advanced and relatively well resourced community-based service. We had a great deal of co-operation from too many people to mention, but it would be impertinent of me not to mention the help of the Worcester and District Health Authority, the help we had from both the University of Birmingham and the West Midlands Regional Health Authority, and particularly the generous funding we had from the Health Promotion Trust.

Now, obviously, there are a good many 'methodological problems' in such studies, e.g. trying to equate what people say and what they might do, or such problems as that if there is an interviewer, it's very difficult to

238

express negative attitudes. As against that, a pilot mail shot we carried out into people's attitudes towards the mentally ill gave a very poor response and we decided to use three instruments. The first was derived from a modified version of the so-called Opinions About Mental Illness Scale which is a fairly standard scale; the second instrument was an Anglicised, greatly revised, modified and updated version of the so-called Star Vignettes which were some vignettes of mental illness first developed by Star almost 50 years ago in the States. The third instrument was based on the so-called Perceived Stigma Questionnaire (Bruce Link) which we administered to all the traceable in-patients discharged from the Malvern and Bromsgrove services during the preceding two years. The first two instruments were administered to about a thousand randomly chosen respondents in Malvern and another in Bromsgrove using a random sample of what are called Census Enumeration Districts each containing 150-200 households. We had one interviewer for each district who interviewed 10 respondents - 1 from each of 10 households.

Taking first the O.M.I.S., our version included some 31 statements and subjects were asked to consider each statement in turn and indicate how strongly they agreed or disagreed on a 5-point scale. The next couple of slides give you some idea of the sort of questions we asked and the data was condensed by a principal component analysis. This instrument and our second instrument was administered by MORI and its trained interviewers and we are, of course, most grateful to them also. The second instrument consisted of four vignettes of fairly typical psychiatric patients, and the slides give you some idea of these vignettes. Each respondent was asked to tell us the cause of the vignette-featured person's problems, to recommend which agencies might be helpful to the subject of the vignette and thirdly, to predict how they themselves might behave confronted by the subject of the vignette. So there are 2,000 respondents, each have 31 opinions about mental illness and whether they agree/ disagree, or how strongly, with the statements. Secondly, they are shown vignettes of typical patients and asked what the diagnosis is, what treatment the person needs and how they themselves would behave towards that person.

The perceived stigma questionnaire, which is exactly what it seems, was administered to just about 100 patients from each service and as well as this questionnaire they then had an unstructured interview with the interviewer to explore their answers on how much stigma they perceived, whether they agreed with it, how they dealt with it, or evaded it.

Now taking the opinions about mental illness first, complex statistical analysis seemed to show three factors: First of all there was a factor that we call benevolence and that was very widely prevalent in the community and had its highest loading on the question 'We have a responsibility to provide the best care for the mentally ill'. Only 2% of subjects had negative scores and the strongest predictor of benevolence was having a close family member with mental illness, which is hardly surprising, and others who were relatively benevolent were those with higher education. Any politicians in the audience may wish to note that nearly 80% of respondents agreed the statement that more tax money should be spent on the care and treatment of the mentally ill.

The second factor was concerned with fear of the mentally ill. Its highest loading was on the statement 'Residents have nothing to fear from people coming into their neighbourhood to obtain mental health services', that is to say, the theme is the exclusion of the mentally ill from residential neighbourhoods. It is very interesting - and we think very important - that most people in the community at large show an absence of fear of the mentally ill. Almost 85% of the scores were positive and, again, the highest predictor of a lack of fear was having a close family member with mental illness, higher education, or professional experience of mental illness. However, allowing the mentally ill to reside or be treated in residential neighbourhoods, obviously requires a more positive acceptance of deviance.

The third factor was what we called an 'authoritarian' factor. This had its highest loading on such statements as 'A person would be foolish to marry someone who suffered from mental illness' or 'The exclusion of mentally ill people from responsibility and public office'. Globally, there was an overall rejection of authoritarian attitudes, but about one-third of people had socially restrictive scores. Again, the major determinant of less authoritarian and restrictive attitudes was having a close family member with mental illness followed by higher education and the strongest association of restrictive attitudes were advanced age, which was the strongest predictor, lack of education and relatively low occupational status. We had expected that either tolerant attitudes would develop in areas served by community psychiatry because the public there would become more accustomed to mentally ill people or, alternatively, that such a population would develop adverse attitudes to the mentally ill. In the event, neither hypothesis was true, there was actually very little difference between Malvern, the community psychiatry district, as opposed to Bromsgrove. What differences there were actually showed greater theoretical tolerance and benevolence in Bromsgrove where mentally ill people were still relatively tucked away in the mental hospital.

As you may remember, the second instrument had to do with the vignettes, what the diagnosis was, who should help and what the person themselves might do or not do. It was interesting that only about a quarter of respondents identified any vignettes as due to mental illness, although they were to any mental health professional of clearly described psychotic individuals. Females and the better educated members of the population fared slightly better, but most respondents postulated the problems as due to stress, unemployment, insecurity or childhood experience. One could of course, suggest that while for the mental health professional identification of a person as mentally ill might seem positive and tolerant, for the lay person, identification as neurotic indicates being weak, manipulative or ineffectual and identification as psychotic may equate with worthlessness, dirtiness, dangerousness or unpredictability. Our results suggest, however, that those perceived as mentally ill by the population at large and the media seem to only represent a small proportion of the mentally ill, that is to say, those who are perceived as such by the community, do not equate to those so regarded by professionals and this can obviously lead to mutual misunderstanding. We felt that it probably led to relative intolerance of a small, highly visible proportion of patients and by tolerance or indifference, or over-tolerance to the majority of the ex-residents of mental hospitals. Obviously, intolerance has to be distinguished from a legitimate concern over a lack of adequate facilities and tolerance from indifference. There are possible mental health promotion responses to this situation of narrow and selective stereotypes by health education campaigns, etc. As to the recommended agencies, we were chastened to find that only about 60% thought that a psychiatrist could be helpful and psychiatrists were even less often mentioned by those who had been mentally ill. About half thought a GP or social worker could help and we were surprised by the low public profile of community psychiatric nurses, whom we would have rated much more highly. It was interesting that while Bromsgrove residents were theoretically more tolerant in their opinions about mental illness scales, Malvern residents seemed much more enterprising in recommending more helpers and perhaps they were more competent at handling mentally ill people because of their greater exposure to them. Finally, as to the actions predicted by the respondents, it is possible to arrange these predictions into a simple gradient from, say, a close personal relationship or marriage at one end to 'willingness to speak in the street if I know them' at the other. From that, it is possible to derive simple, arbitrary action scores for each vignette and these could be of value to clinicians, social workers and others, and the next slide just gives you one or two examples of these action scores. It was interesting that, although respondents were predictably more tolerant of obsessionality

241

than a paranoid illness, the differences actually were not great. The practical overall tolerance of a community is, of course, raised because individuals holding very negative views would probably completely avoid the mentally ill if they could. Almost all of our sample would speak to the vignette subjects in the street, about half would join the same club, work alongside them, live next door or allow their children to speak to them, about a third would go to a party in their home, 11% would be prepared to have a close relationship and 6% would have been prepared to marry them.

Now, finally, as to the patients. We felt that in a community-based service patients are nearer their home and they are therefore at increased risk of being identified as mentally ill. We also felt that perhaps not only the patients would be found to be stigmatised, but also their illness and those who were associated in some way with them. There was some anxiety amongst our own staff about the survey because they felt that if our group homes and other facilities were, as it were, identified as such, they might have problems. In fact, it was our experience that hostels, day centres, etc are much less obtrusive than mental health professionals believe. Eighty-five percent of our community knew where the mental hospital was, about half knew where the local day centre was, but the identification of hostels, group homes, etc, was only about 10%, even in those who lived very near them, so that was good news. In our patients we used Bruce Link's questionnaire and also his views about labelling, that is to say, that mentally ill individuals behave in various ways to avoid unpleasant contacts with others. They may be secretive about their own history, they may try to educate those around them, or they may socially withdraw completely. These behaviours may themselves adversely influence the course of their illness and their expectations influence the level of stigma that they perceive. Again, the two areas were very similar, except that in the community treatment area, patients reported no jokes about the local 'bin' - perhaps that was important. About three-quarters of our patients felt there was prejudice towards those who had been mentally ill, two-thirds felt that their social life had changed - one or two for the better since being mentally ill - and about half found that people had difficulty knowing what to say, found people to be embarrassed and about a quarter thought they were being avoided. Respondents were as likely to mention their relatives as others, as being those who treated them differently, and that was interesting because our survey of the community suggested that they were more tolerant, or thought they were more tolerant. Respondents felt that people were fearful of mental illness and, again, that conflicts with the community's views that they were not afraid of mental illness and our average respondent answered positively to about half the devaluation and discrimination statements in the scale. About that number - that is, half - endorsed strategies of secrecy, attempts at education and withdrawal. Obviously, the higher their perception of stigma, it must be said that many of the ex-mental hospital patients agreed with the stigma themselves and stigmatized each other. There is a cosy view that mental patients support each other, 'let's group them together, let's put them in hostels, they understand each other', I don't think that is true. I think, if anything, they are more rejecting of each other than other people. It is also important that we found that perceived stigma was highly associated with what one might call 'real life experiences' such as unemployment and poverty, so that one of the stigmatizing things about the ex-mentally ill which, of course, we all know, is that they are poor and often unemployed.

Now I have tried to be careful not to produce too much in the way of indigestible bits and pieces of facts and figures because our actual full report is several hundred pages, but I hope that I have been able to communicate the essentials of a study which, although its results were somewhat trite, they were, I think, modestly re-assuring. It seems to us that health promotion/health education campaigns which in the past have proved rather unsuccessful, should perhaps be focused on relatives and workmates of the mentally ill rather than globally and although community psychiatry is not going to solve the intractable problems of prejudice against the mentally ill, we emerged from our study fairly confident that the closure of asylums will probably not result in a backlash of increased community rejection. Nevertheless, even in the most ad-vanced services we have at present, there obviously is a lot of perceived stigma and I believe that this, rather than the alleged indifference of mental health professionals could partly explain why so many mentally ill people prefer even living in 'Cardboard City' to being stigmatised by their nearest and dearest.

19 HOME-START: Support, friendship and practical help for young families under stress

M. Harrison

Many young families under stress are unable to provide an emotionally stable home background from which their young children can develop their full potential. Some parents find these early years exhausting, frustrating and overwhelming. They can lack a sense of mental or even physical well-being.

HOME-START is a voluntary organisation which provides support, friendship and practical help to any parent with at least one child under the age of 5 years, who is experiencing such difficulties and for whom the regular visit in their own home of a HOME-START volunteer can offer a lifeline. HOME-START, which is home-based, was used by more than 20,000 children and their families in 1991.

HOME-START volunteers, normally parents themselves, can simply respond to whatever a parent needs during regular visits - 'Let's sit and talk'; 'Why don't I look after the children while you catch up with some sleep?'; 'Let's go out and kick leaves/have a picnic'; 'Why don't we all go down to the Health Centre together?'

Although the majority of families are referred to HOME-START by Social Workers and Health Visitors, volunteers and professionals perform quite different tasks. HOME-START can respond to individual family members as people rather than to their problems. HOME-START volunteers can support the parents in whatever the circumstances, for as long as is needed, without taking away their responsibilities.

By offering their time, flexibility, optimism and a sense of fun, HOME-START volunteers can enable families with young children to cope better, preventing family or parental breakdown. Many parents who have had

HOME-START volunteer themselves, and find inevitably that being a volunteer is in itself rewarding.

The late Mia Kellmer Pringle said that children need love and security, praise and recognition, responsibility and new experiences if they are to develop healthy minds and bodies. In HOME-START, very often, we first have to help parents experience these things themselves. They need praise and recognition. They need love and security. Maybe, just the knowledge that the HOME-START volunteer will turn up when she says she will. They need to know they matter. They need new experiences and, of course, responsibility.

Ann Dally, in her book 'Mothers - Their Power and Their Influence' says that children go through three stages of development:

(i) **Enclosure**, when children, up to about the age of two years, need to be nurtured and are very dependent on the care-giver (usually a parent).

(ii) **Extension**, when the children are increasingly, influenced by other people and by the world at large. As children are extended by their parents, they in turn, extend their parents.

(iii) **Separation** begins with adolescence and proceeds quite naturally to the point where, as young adults, children need their independence.

This model, I believe explains much of the HOME-START approach. When families are referred, they are at the 'enclosure' stage. They need to be cherished and nurtured in their own homes where their problems exist. They need a time of dependency where they know another 'mum' will come and respond to what they need. The trick, then, is to move them on to 'extension'. There they can begin to seek and use other resources in the community -such as a drop-in centre, a family centre or a health clinic. Other myriad services exist, but so often at first, these families are not aware of their presence, or have insufficient confidence to contact or use them. Finally, they 'separate'. They no longer need HOME-START. However, families very often return, perhaps a couple of years later, saying 'I'm going through another bad patch. Can I have my volunteer back?' HOME-START is available to respond to such a request.

HOME-START schemes are organised in a unique way. There are currently more than 120 throughout the UK. Each is rooted firmly in its own community with local funding, volunteers and management committee members. All HOME-START schemes share a common ethos and constitution. The structure of HOME-START requires a multi-disciplinary management committee, at least one paid organiser and a group of up to 30 committed HOME-START volunteers. In 1991, the average cost of HOME-START per annum was £430 per family and £177 per child visited. There are at least another 80 areas in the UK seeking to launch HOME-START schemes once local funding becomes available.

HOME-START also exists in Israel, Australia, Canada, Germany, Cyprus and Gibraltar. Schemes are currently being set up in Hungary and in the Netherlands.

Clearly the HOME-START approach which is simple, is acceptable to young families under stress, irrespective of political, religious, geographical, cultural, financial or educational differences. HOME-START can contribute to the mental well-being of everyone involved.

For more information,contact:-
HOME-START Consultancy
2 Salisbury Road
Leicester LE1 7QR
Tel: (0533) 554988
Fax: (0533) 549323

20 Communicating in print

J. Hartley

Much material in the field of mental health promotion comes in print - leaflets, posters, letters, reports, questionnaires, etc. In this talk I want to focus on three aspects of presenting printed text: layout, language, and effectiveness. These considerations are reflected in Figures 1, 2 and 3. Here we can see a piece of text first in its original format, then with a revised layout, and then further revised in terms of its language.

The layout of text

One of the first decisions that a designer makes when considering how to present a document concerns which page-size to use. Today this decision is helped by a choice from an array of standard paper sizes (A4, A5 etc.). This first decision about the size - and the orientation - of the page on which the material is to be printed affects a host of other decisions about, for example, margins, column widths, interline spacing, the choice of typesizes, and the positioning of illustrations, diagrams, tables and graphs.

Once the column widths are decided another major decision concerns the choice of typefaces, typesizes and whether to use 'justified' or unjustified' composition.

The original text in Figure 1 is set in what is technically called 'justified type'. Here the left-hand and the right-hand edges of the text form straight lines. To achieve this the spacing between the words (and sometimes between the letters in the words) is varied, and sometimes words are broken in two by hyphenation. An alternative approach is to range the text from the left hand margin and to have a ragged right-hand edge for each column of print. This approach is technically called 'unjustified' composition (and is typical of typescript). Here the spacing between the words is regular and consistent, and hyphenation is (usually) avoided.

In some texts (e.g. long passages of continuous prose as in this book) the effects are small, but in other text (such as that shown in Figures 1 and 2)

The Patient's Charter

The rights and standards set out in this leaflet form *The Patient's Charter.*

The Charter is a central part of the programme to improve and modernise the delivery of the National Health Service to the public, while continuing to reaffirm its fundamental principles.

The Patient's Charter puts the Government's *Citizen's Charter* initiative into practice in the health service.

Seven existing rights

Every citizen already has the following National Health Service rights:

to receive health care on the basis of clinical need, regardless of ability to pay;

to be registered with a GP;

to receive emergency medical care at any time, through your GP or the emergency ambulance service and hospital accident and emergency departments;

to be referred to a consultant, acceptable to you, when your GP thinks it necessary and to be referred for a second opinion if you and your GP agree this is desirable;

to be given a clear explanation of any treatment proposed, including any risks and any alternatives, before you decide whether you will agree to the treatment;

to have access to your health records, and to know that those working for the NHS will, by law, keep their contents confidential;

to choose whether or not you wish to take part in medical research or medical student training.

Figure 1 Shows the original layout of the first page of The Patient's Charter, published by H.M.S.O. Note that in this original text the title, and the heading 'every citizen already has ...' were printed in green, and there was a marginal side heading, also in green.

250

The Patient's Charter

The rights and standards set out in this leaflet form *The Patient's Charter*.

The Charter is a central part of the programme to improve and modernise the delivery of the National Health Service to the public, while continuing to reaffirm its fundamental principles.

The Patient's Charter puts the Government's *Citizen's Charter* initiative into practice in the health service.

Every citizen already has the following National Health Service rights:

- to receive health care on the basis of clinical need, regardless of ability to pay;

- to be registered with a GP;

- to receive emergency medical care at any time, through your GP or the emergency ambulance service and hospital accident and emergency departments;

- to be referred to a consultant, acceptable to you, when your GP thinks it necessary and to be referred for a second opinion if you and your GP agree this is desirable;

- to be given a clear explanation of any treatment proposed, including any risks and any alternatives, before you decide whether you will agree to the treatment;

- to have access to your health records, and to know that those working for the NHS will, by law, keep their contents confidential;

- to choose whether or not you wish to take part in medical research or medical student training.

Figure 2   Shows a revised layout of the same text as that shown in Figure 1

one might argue that the unjustified setting is more appropriate. Furthermore, there are subtle advantages for unjustified composition. With unjustified text there is no need to fill the line with print just because the space is there. One can consider other rules for determining the ending (and even beginnings) of lines. In Figure 2, for example, the percipient reader may see that I have chosen to stop each line in accordance with its underlying grammatical structure, and to group and separate related parts within lines.

A more subtle difference between Figures 1 and 2 may not be so readily apparent. In most books (as here) the text on each page starts and finishes at the same point on each page. The text is vertically justified. To achieve this there is variation and inconsistency in the spacing between the elements going down the page. If, however, the internal spacing is consistent, the stopping point on each page may vary. In Figure 2, to achieve consistent internal spacing, there is one unit of space below each item, one below the secondary heading and two above it, and four units of space below the main heading. And these rules of spacing would be used consistently throughout the document. Elsewhere I have argued that both the vertical and the horizontal spacing needs to be consistent in this way if together they are to indicate to the reader at a glance the underlying structure of the text (Hartley, 1985).

The case is perhaps clearer with more complex text than that shown here. It can be developed, too, to encompass the presentation of other elements in text, such as tables and figures. Here there also needs to be a consistent amount of space above and below a caption, and such spacing needs to be specified in advance and adhered to consistently throughout the text, and not varied from page to page.

Finally in this section we may note that in the original of Figure 1 colour was used to enhance the headings (where I have used bold and italic). Such colour has a decorative effect and it is worth considering from this point of view. I would maintain, however, that the spatial arrangement of the text is more important, and should be considered first. Colour, or other typographic cues (italic, bold, capital letters) can be added to strengthen the message, but they should not be allowed to confuse it. The use of multi-coloured or multi-cued text is to be avoided if one is trying to convey information clearly.

The language of text

I am assuming that in the field of mental health promotion there is a need for the language of written communication to be appropriate for the situation at hand. However, much written text - and figure 1 is no exception - is more difficult than it needs to be.

There are several guidelines on how to write clear prose, and there are also guidelines on how to revise existing text in order to make it easier to understand. However, there are no firm rules, accepted by all, that are routinely applicable (despite what some computer-aided writing programs state). Nonetheless, it is possible to make useful suggestions that writers can consider with reference to their own work. The guidelines that

I currently advocate for both writing and re-writing can be considered under two headings - textual and procedural - as follows:

Textual

- . Think of your reader.
- . Use the active voice where possible.
- . Use simpler wording if possible.
- . Shorten long sentences (say, over 40 words long), or expand them into two or three simpler sentences.
- . Divide long paragraphs into shorter ones.
- . List actions and procedures (and put them in their temporal sequence).
- . When in difficulty, think of how you would explain to a friend what you are trying to say - or actually explain it to one. Write down what you say. Polish it.

Procedural

- . Read the text through and ask what changes do I need to make to make the text clearer?
- . Consider making big or **global** changes, as well as small or **minor** changes.
- . **Global** changes you might like to consider in turn are:
  re-sequencing parts of the text
- . adding in examples
- . changing the original examples for better ones more appropriate to your reader
- . deleting parts that seem confusing
- . **Minor** text changes involve things like:
- . checking punctuation
- . looking for split infinitives
- . checking for consistency in verb tenses
- . checking for consistency in spellings (particularly of people's names)
- . removing vague modifiers
- . You can ask colleagues to help you to simplify drafts, either by simplifying them further themselves, or by pointing out where they think other readers will find difficulties.
- . You can also try out the text with a sample of the intended readers. Ask them to circle any parts they think readers less able than themselves will find difficult.
- . Finally, leave each draft for at least 12 hours, and then repeat as many of the above procedures as you can as often as time allows.

As already noted above, these guidelines are suggestions, not firm rules. There are, however, some data to support their application (Hartley, 1985).

Figure 3 shows what happened to Figure 1 when I applied some of the above guidelines. I am not saying that Figure 3 is the 'correct answer'. Different readers will have different ideas for improvement. However,

The Patient's Charter

This leaflet describes your rights as a patient in the National Health Service.

Our aim is to let you know what you can expect from the National Health Service in our efforts to improve it.

The *Patient's Charter* says:

- You have the right to medical attention, whether or not you are able to pay for it.

- You have the right to any emergency treatment.
  This may be given by your doctor, the emergency ambulance service, or a hospital.

- You have the right to have your own doctor.

- Your doctor can, if necessary, send you to a consultant, but this consultant must be acceptable to you.

- You have the right to receive a clear account of what will happen to you before you decide whether or not to have any treatment.
  This account must describe the risks involved and outline any other possible treatments.

- You have the right to see another doctor or consultant for a second opinion, if you and your doctor agree.

- You have the right to choose whether or not you wish to take part in medical research, or in the teaching of medical students.

- You have the right to see your own medical records, and to know that they are confidential.

Figure 3 Shows the contents of Figure 1 revised in terms of both its wording and its layout

I would maintain that the text in Figure 3 is more effective than that in Figure 1. How can I tell whether this is the case or not is the subject of the next section of this paper.

Measuring the effectiveness of text

Several tools can be used to evaluate the suitability of a text for its intended audience. They can be used by **authors** when they are producing text, and by **judges** when they are assessing the suitability of published texts for others. Let me consider just some of them here.

Readability formulae

Readability formulae aim to predict the suitability of text for children of different reading ages. Typically a readability formula contains two main measures combined with a constant to predict a reading age. The two main measures are the average length of the sentences in samples of the text, and the average length of the words (usually measured in terms of the number of syllables) within these sentences. Clearly the underlying notion is that the longer the sentences and the more complex the vocabulary then the more difficult the text will be to read. Such a notion is obviously sensible but, of course, it has limitations. So readability formulae provide a rough guide to difficulty.

Today, with the advent of word processing systems, it is easy to apply some fairly complex readability formulae. For example the style program of the IBM Xenith text formatting system can be applied to text to provide four sets of readability data (derived from four different formulae). When this program was run on the text shown in Figures 1 and 3 the following results emerged:

Formula	Figure 1 Reading Age	Figure 3 Reading Age
1	16.7 yrs	14.0 yrs
2	16.3 yrs	14.0 yrs
3	16.6 yrs	14.0 yrs
4	18.8 yrs	15.3 yrs

As can be seen the two texts do differ slightly. My textual revisions have made the text easier to read. But the changes are not enormous. Indeed, we still might think that the reading age level required to understand the text in Figure 3 is too high. (And, as an aside, I might observe that the reading age for sections of the North Staffordshire **Patients' Charter** is even higher, with a suggested reading age of 17 years.) So, when we remember that the reading age level of **The Sun** is 12 years (and that of **The**

Times is 18 years) we have to reflect on that fact that in producing written materials for mental health promotion we are likely to be trying to reach populations with greater reading difficulties than we think.

Readers' preferences

Another way to evaluate the effectiveness of two or more tests is to ask readers which ones they prefer. However, here it is always useful to consider using a baseline text which readers can refer to when judging another text. We could rate Figure 1 out of 10 for clarity, but this would only be meaningful if we compared it to other documents. Figure 1 is not (in my view) as successful as Figure 3, but compared to much government prose it is quite well done. Preferences then are relative measures, but they can provide useful information.

Experimental tests

Few readers of this paper will probably want to bother making experimental comparisons between different versions of the same piece of text, or between different texts. But should they wish to do so there are a number of measures that could be made. For example, one might compare the texts in terms of

- readability
- preferences
- reading speed
- amount of information conveyed
    - as measured by recall tests, comprehension tests, or using the text to carry out procedures or instructions, etc.
- costs

In my view it is important to use as many measures as is appropriate, and to consider the combined results, rather than to rely on one measure on its own.

Cyclical testing and revision

Finally, in this section, we should note that the idea of writing a piece of text, trying it out, revising it in the light of the information obtained, trying it out again, and then revising it again, and so on, until the text achieves its stated objectives, is perhaps the most effective way of producing a piece of information text. Examples to illustrate this are provided in Hartley (1985).

So in this section of this paper I have discussed briefly a number of different approaches to assessing the effectiveness of text. The issues are too complex to describe in detail here, but fuller descriptions of these and other methods can be found in the references.

Acknowledgements

I am indebted to Margaret Woodward for assistance in the preparation of this paper and to John Morin for help with the production of the figures.

Useful references

Cutts, M. & Maher, C. (1986). *The Plain English story*. Plain English Campaign. Outram House, Whaley Bridge, Stockport, SK12 7LS.

Hartley, J. (1985). *Designing instructional text* (2nd Ed.). London: Kogan Page.

Hartley, J. (1989). Tools for evaluating text. In J. Hartley & A. Branthwaite (Eds), *The applied psychologist*. Milton Keynes: Open University Press.

Miles, J. (1987). *Design for desktop publishing*. London: Gordon Fraser.

Misanchuk, E.R. (1992). *Preparing instructional text: Document design using desktop publishing*. Englewood Cliffs, N.J.: Educational Technology Publications.

21 Laughter: The best medicine

R. Holden

'The best doctors in the world are Doctor Diet, Doctor Quiet, and Doctor Merryman.' Jonathan Swift

Some people will admit to owning false teeth; others will casually confess they do not wash thoroughly behind their ears. Some people are happy to broadcast their latest implant, lift or tuck; others are quite prepared to divulge they are penniless, poor and bankrupt. Some people tell of ghastly addictions to garlic, chocolate or pasta; others will openly say - in either pounds, ounces or kilograms - exactly how much they weigh. We will all of us admit to many things, but, *nowhere, ever at any time, have I ever heard anyone admit to not having a sense of humour.*

Humour is a core condition of *humanness*. Laughter, smiles and a happy sense of humour are our passports of entry into the human race. We each of us grow, develop and unfold through laughter, happiness and humour. The greatest wisdom schools in the world have advocated a balanced ploy of both seriousness and joy. Laughter can also be a medicine - a medicine with tangible, physical benefits as well as therapeutic emotional, mental and spiritual benefits.

At the *Laughter Clinic*, I advocate happiness as a foundation for health: *'Be happy be healthy'* is one of our mottos. *Laughter Medicine* is used as an umbrella term for exploring some of the most fundamental issues of health, happiness and wholeness, such as, the language of laughter, the art of joyful living, the therapeutic power of play, the human need to celebrate life, the pursuit of personal happiness, re-creation, and, the quest for our inner fun child.

259

There is now a wealth of orthodox medical research from around the world which supports the idea that, humour heals! In particular, the exciting research of *psychoneuroimmunology* proves conclusively that a happy, joyful approach to life can inspire energy, vitality and health - on every level. This view is also supported by some of the more creative and imaginative schools of counselling and psychotherapy, such as, *Rational-Emotive Therapy, Transactional Analysis and Existentialism.*

Laughter and relaxation

Have you ever asked yourself why you laugh the way you do or why you smile the way you do? Generally speaking, laughter has a two-step action on the physical body: step one, it *stimulates*; step two, it *relaxes*. During laughter, the body is stimulated and exercised; after laughter, the body relaxes and calms itself. Laughter is often, therefore, a most effective method for inducing physical and mental relaxation - *laughter is a medicinal relaxant.*

The relaxing effects of laughter, as discovered by medical research, include, lowering muscle tension, relaxed sympathetic nervous system, better circulation and a full, deep and healthy respiration pattern. In particular, humour, merriment and mirth are acknowledged as devices for discharging surplus nervous energy. According to modern research, laughter serves as a form of 'safety-valve' for the body's energies.

Laughter is often a social signal for calm, for relaxation and for confidence. There is an old English proverb that says, *'Laugh to let go'* - laughter really can help us to let go of the physical, emotional and mental tensions. Indeed, the therapeutic benefits of one minute of genuine laughter is thought to be equivalent to approximately forty-five minutes of deep relaxation, according to one piece of recent research. For this reason, laughter is sometimes described as a form of internal massage.

Pain: 'laugh it off'!

Although laughter has been advocated as the best medicine since time immemorial, it was not until the late 1970's that the medical profession began to take laughter seriously. In particular, it was the experience of one man, Norman Cousins, that really underlined the potential medicinal powers of mirth. In 1978, the *New England Journal of Medicine* published an article by Norman Cousins which outlined his recovery from a painful, crippling disorder known as ankylosing spondylitis - his chief medicine was regular prescriptions of *Candid Camera* episodes and *Marx Brother* movies.

In his book, *Anatomy of an Illness*, Norman Cousins *'made the joyous discovery that ten minutes of genuine belly laughter had an anaesthetic effect that would give me at least two-hour of pain-free sleep.'* Norman Cousins found that laughter could help to relieve pain - probably because of its ability to relax muscles and nerves. Norman Cousins is now a professor of medicine. He has actively helped to pioneer much of the research of *Psychneuroimmunology* - one of the major findings of which is that laughter and happy, positive attitudes can effect a release of *endorphin* hormones into the body - endorphins are our body's natural pain-killers.

Smile away your stress

It was Herman Melville, author of *Moby Dick*, who wrote, 'A laugh's the wisest, easiest answer to all that's queer.' One of the inspirations for starting the *Laughter Clinic* was the number of people attending my NHS Stress Buster Clinics who would testify, 'the turning point came when I started to laugh'. It is so often true that during times of stress, laughter, smiles and humour can offer light relief and personal release.

Psychologists have posited over eighty different theories as to why we laugh. One major theory states that laughter has a profound effect on personal perception - we change the way we look at the world, when we laugh. Therefore, one reason why we laugh is to change perceptions, alter perspective and create a new view. This is so important for successful stress control because, as the old saying goes, 'People are disturbed not by things, but by the view they take of them, ' Epictetus, 1st century, A.D.

Laughter is such a capable healer when it comes to stress - laughter can fizzle fear; laughter can help us to see the folly of our anxieties; laughter is often a wonderful release during times of mental tension; we laugh to increase our tolerance and understanding. Another major theory of laughter suggests that laughter is an act of liberation and self-superiority: as a medieval poet once penned, *'Laughter takes us up, way up high; from a dark bottomless pit, to the fresh, clear blue sky'*.

Fun for fatigue

Mind, body and soul light up like a bright neon light whenever we laugh. Laughter, humour, happiness and play can all create chemical changes in the body so as to effect energy, vitality and strength - *when we are laughing we are truly alive*. We each of us have an abundant store of energy which we are occasionally denied, not because of a poor diet of food or drink or breath, but because of a poor diet of attitude, thought and belief.

Energy is first and foremost a product of mind; not of body. Laughter tends to inspire enthusiasm, fresh resolve, positive outlook and the ability to start over again. Laughter is a form of zest, and as the philosopher, Bertrand Russell, once wrote, *'What hunger is in relation to food, zest is in relation to life'*. Laughter, happiness and joy fire the 'energiser hormones', noradrenaline and cortisol, through the body, and in so doing, laughter helps us to embrace life with all of the intensity, application and enthusiasm we require.

Conclusions

For so long, the medical profession has tended to dismiss laughter as being something that merely makes people feel good.. The whole point is, however, that 'merely' making people feel good is an essential requirement of health, happiness and wholeness - when we **feel** well, we tend to **be** well. This is increasingly apparent with the advent of modern mind/body research, psychosomatic medicine and psychoneuroimmunology research.

Laughter is a medicine - it has tangible, physical effects as well as subtle, therapeutic emotional, mental and spiritual effects. The recent upsurge of medical research into mirth, merriment and laughter supports an holistic model for health that proves health can be supported and enhanced by a person's sense of happiness and wholeness. Learning to allow yourself to laugh, to smile, to play, to be joyful and to be happy are essential talents and skills that can create a more permanent foundation for well-being. **Humour heals!**

Robert Holden is a stress consultant to NHS, BBC, Local Government and to trade and industry. In 1989, he opened the first **NHS Stress Buster Clinic** in Britain, and in 1991, he launched the first **NHS Laughter Clinic**. He has recently accepted a contract to teach laughter medicine to doctors and health professionals. His books, **Stress Busters** and **Laughter, the best medicine** (March 1993) are both published by Thorsons (Harper/Collins). For details of **Laughter Clinic** Workshops across the country, contact Robert Holden at, Personal Empowerment Programmes, 34 Denewood Avenue, Handsworth Wood, Birmingham B20 2AB, Tel & Fax: 021 551 2932

References

1. 'Laughing Possible!' - How Tibetans reach wisdom through laughter, Ngakpa Chogyam, Caduceus, Winter 1990, pp 14-16.

2. Intangibles in Medicine, Norman Cousins, Caduceus, Spring 1989, pp 15-17.

3. Fun as Psychotherapy, Albert Ellis, audio-cassette, Institute for Rational-Emotive Therapy, 45 East 65th Street, New York, NY. 10021.

4. Games People Paly, Eric Berne, Penguin Books, 1964.

5. Individual Therapy, edited by Windy Dryden, Open University Press, 1990.

6. The Physiology of Laughter, H. Spencer, Macmillan's Magazine, 1. pp 395, 1960.

7. Neuroendocrine and Stress Hormone Changes During Mirthful Laughter, Lee S. Berk, et al, Am. Journal of the Medical Sciences, Dec 1989, volume 298, Number 6, pp 390-396.

8. Eustress of mirthful laughter modifies natural killer cell activity, Lee S. Ber, et al, Clin Research 37: 115A, 1989.

9. The Respiratory Components of mirthful laughter, Fry WF, J Biol Psychol, 19: 39-50, 1977.

10. Laughter and Relaxation, John Wicker, Journal of Research in Personality, 11, pp 359-363, 1968.

11. *Moby Dick*, Herman Melville, pp 39, 1851.

12. The Conquest of Happiness, Bertrand Russell, Penguin, pp 10, 1930.

22 Staff care in the work community

J. Hopkins

Introduction

This paper draws together the practical experience of staff working within Social Service Departments who have been engaged with the Staff Care Unit at the University in the provision of staff care. It explores the theme of the workforce as a community and shows how staff care has been delivered at different levels within the community. The paper then introduces the concept of a staff care practice serving the community, collaborating with other services within the organisation, and drawing on members and groups within the community as service providers as well as service users. It concludes with a model describing the roles that are necessary to provide an integrated service within the work community.

The work organisation as a community

The perspective of the workforce as a community is not a new one but it is one that is relatively neglected in the literature. The history of work communities and communes is a long one, and more recent attempts have been made to examine residential care organisations as communities. However, most work organisations are viewed as a social entity only when the whole community is threatened by closure or divided by industrial conflict. The literature on employee assistance services largely ignores the work community and focuses on meeting the needs of individuals and groups; the notable exception being the 'promotion of health' campaigns targeted at all members of the workforce. The literature on community work, as a method of social intervention, is focused on communities of place, usually neighbourhoods or on communities of identity, usually seeking to empower under-represented groups to redress their grievances.

To view work organisations as a social entity is to recognise that members of the workforce are linked to each other by the common conditions of life at work, are organised under the same authority and live alongside other members of the same community, sometimes for a large number of their waking hours. Within this communal life individuals and groups co-operate and conflict, but do not transgress the boundaries of accepted behaviour, and sustain their own culture.

Levels and types of intervention within the work community

We give below some examples of staff care in Social Service Departments with which we have worked.

(i) Community based projects

Staff Care workers have initiated and supported a number of community wide services. They have encouraged the Personnel Department to develop flexible working arrangements including career breaks, job sharing, paternity leave and term time working. They have taken a key role in monitoring equal opportunities policies and worked closely with the Personnel Department in developing and monitoring the policies in relation to sexual harassment and violence towards staff. They are also involved with occupational health in developing non-smoking policy, stress management training, the Department's sickness policy, alcohol policy, extending the provision of well person checks and counselling staff who become terminally ill. They have set up a staff 'hardship fund' and assisted at events organised by members of the community to raise monies for it.

Some staff care workers in Social Service Departments have also played a key role in the agency's response to traumatic events in the community. Their role is to support counsellors working with victims and their families, and to debrief those involved after a critical incident. They have responded to a local fire and were an integral part of the arrangements to deal with casualties in the Gulf War. What is more confusing is their role when their own organisation is thrown into crisis by threatened reorganisation and redundancies. Their own service becomes vulnerable and their role has so far been limited to picking up individual anxieties through the counselling provision. Interest however, is developing on their role in helping to mitigate the effects of organisational crisis, but the collapse of morale and the perceived threat to livelihood overshadowed the community and preoccupied most of its members. The response of the staff care service was essentially reactive and the decision made that staff who wanted help would be able to use the existing provision when they needed it.

(ii) The patchwork of groups

An initial survey of staff care needs conducted in a Social Service Department highlighted reported different levels and types of stress at different worksites, among different occupational groups and at different workplaces. This information allowed the differential targeting of staff care services e.g. the workers ensured that they introduced themselves to the staff of residential children centres at an early stage. A survey in the Social Services Department of a neighbouring authority addressed the stress levels among staff providing services to clients with physical disabilities and sensory impairment. This confirmed that although the work was perceived as rewarding and challenging by all staff, there were significant differences between reports of stress experienced by staff directly involved in service provision and the staff who supported their work. This has implications for staff care planning.

What emerges is a picture of the organisations as a patchwork of work groups, some built around the workplace, others involve reaching across to their peers in different parts of the organisational structure and others reflect particular work interests or seek to provide support to particular populations within the work community.

(a) Services provided for particular populations within the community include setting up services for staff with dependants, including workplace nurseries and establishing support groups for staff caring for elderly parents. Workers have also set up a help line for staff with a physical disability or sensory impairment, support groups for black staff in the predominantly white organisation, a programme of preretirement courses and facilitated a network of former employees who have taken voluntary redundancy.

Services for women include courses for women returning to work after a career break, assertiveness training for women who wish to enter management and self support groups for women managers.

(b) Development work with workbased teams has been a crucial part of staff care. In particular, work with the Senior Management Group is seen as enabling them to find time to take the measure of their own wellbeing and the way that stress impinges on their performance and to find ways of addressing this. Staff care workers have been able to respond to crisis situations immediately or to minimise the effects of traumatic events. They have helped staff in residential home work cope with the death of a colleague on duty, and brought together staff involved in a closure some weeks after they were dispersed across the Department, in order to acknowledge the value of the life that they had shared and which had been ended in frustration.

(c) Occupational groups have proved to be particularly useful targets for developing staff care in Social Service Departments. The programme of training courses provided by the training staff of Social Service Departments, brings together staff from across the organisation, who share the same occupational group. Co-working with the trainers the staff care workers have developed the support as well as the training needed to deliver effective service. They have also provided their own training programme to raise awareness of staff care issues among line managers. Training programmes that draw their membership from different workplaces create a new set of personal links across the work organisation.

The evidence of the surveys suggests that there is also merit in working with staff providing the variety of services to a particular client group. It would appear the work with each client group presents particular challenges to staff, and their shared experience makes staff sensitive to the needs of colleagues who may be providing a different service, based at a different worksite to the same client grouping. The challenges vary from coping with the death of elderly clients to being cross examined in the witness box in cases of child protection.

(d) Other groups are targeted according to the worksites. These include the managerial, professional, administrative, clerical and manual workers. Staff care is on the agenda of meetings of the various staff groups and minuted for action. Matters that concern other staff beyond their own worksite are fed into District based staff care groups. The staff care workers attend the District meetings on a regular basis and the worksite meetings on request.

The interlocking relationship between these various staff groups means that intervention in one part of the network may influence others. The informal communication network that emerges has proved particularly important in establishing the credibility of the staff care service within the community. Personal reports of positive experiences of the work of the staff care workers overcome the initial suspicions of the new service, and support the proactive approach taken by the staff care workers.

(iii) Personal services

These are primarily personal counselling and consultancy services, and take the form of a telephone service, short term counselling or longer term counselling. However, there is an informal tradition of mentor support, usually provided by someone who was a line manager, early in the service career. In one department a senior manager is offered as mentor to staff who are subject to disciplinary procedures, this is in addition to the counselling service. Developments in other organisations have led to consideration being given as to how to manage a monitoring provision within the service. Initial targets are the support of black staff and women in management.

A staff care practice

The flexibility of the service provided within the framework of staff care and the engagement of staff members in the service at different times at different levels and in different roles led to the concept of a staff care practice within the work community. This has proved central to the development of a community based approach.

Service provision

The services provided broadly fall into three categories.
  (a) Preventive Services:
    Anticipating events and circumstances that cause stress and distress among staff, taking measures to address the cause of stress and ensuring arrangements are in place enable staff to deal with the situation effectively when it occurs.
  (b) Problem solving services
    This focuses on existing problems. Helping staff to define their immediate problem and to find alternative solutions to it.
  (c) Post incident services
    Helping staff to rebuild the social fabric of their life after a traumatic or disruptive event.

Service resources

  (a) It is not the purpose of this paper to discuss the infrastructure that supports a staff care service, although it is possible to elaborate on each function in the light of experience. Essentially the set of requirements will be similar whether the service provided is a personal counselling or a more extensive staff care provision. The requirements are shown in the diagram below as differentiated functions to demonstrate that the roles may be distributed among the various personnel and are not necessarily vested in the staff care workers.

(b) The fact that the staff care practice is rooted in the work community means that the members of the community are involved at different levels of the service and in different ways. They become actively engaged with the staff care provision both as service provider, in supporting the service and as service users. In this way staff care is more likely to permeate the organisation.

(c) A model of a community based staff care service is outlined below. (Fig 1) It is a first step in refining our experience of the past year, and illustrates the way in which the concept of staff care has moved beyond a personal counselling service to one that permeates the social fabric of the work community.

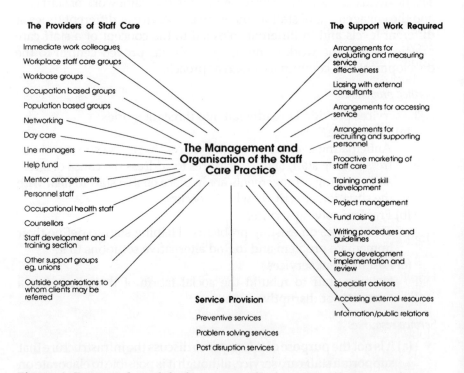

Figure 1 Proposed model of a community based staff care service

Conclusion

This paper set out to draw a theoretical model of a staff care service based on the practical experience of staff who have engaged with the Unit in providing staff care in Social Service Departments. What has emerged is a model based on the concept of the workforce as a community containing a patchwork of interlocking groups and personal experiences. The concept of a staff care practice within the work community is a particularly useful one. The service provision includes personal counselling but goes beyond this to address shared experiences among the various groups of staff and among members of the community as a whole. Much of this work is done in partnership with staff in other parts of the organisation and the model opens up the way for members of the community to become service providers, support staff and service users.

Further research is needed to develop the model and to test it out in other organisations.

Reference

Recent publications by members of the Unit arising from work with Social Service staff include:-

Code of Practice for Staff Care in the Health and Personal Social Services. Published jointly by Keele University and the Local Government Training Board 1990.

Hopkins, J. (1991). Managing risks in child protection. *Child abuse review*. 5 (2) 3-6.

Hopkins, J. (1992). Trial and error: Social workers as witnesses in cases of alleged ritual abuse. *Social Work Today*, 23 (8) 21.

Hopkins, J. (1992). Ch. Secondary abuse. A. Bannister (Ed.), From Hearing to Healing (pp.148-164) Longmans

Hopkins, J., & Grimwood, R. (1992). Staff care in a residential children's centre. *The Journal of Training and Development*, 2 (3) 7-18.

Hopkins, J., & Waterman, M. A pilot study of Staff care in services for people with physical disabilities and sensory impairment. (to be published)

Sloboda, J. & Hopkins, J. (1992). Promoting Mental Health in the Workplace: The staff care Concept. In D. Trent, (Ed.), *Promotion of Mental Health*, 1 (pp.297-304). Avebury.

23 The development of Flexicare

P. Horridge

In the mid 1980's, a new and flexible method of providing community care for people with learning difficulties was developed in South Glamorgan. The original idea for a vocational training scheme was put together by an interagency working group and taken forward by Barry Frost, then a Social Services development officer. The basic concept drew on a number of ideas which were being debated at that time in Social Service circles. Pioneering community care developments in other counties suggested some elements. The scheme which emerged became known as Flexicare. Although the elements of the scheme are all found elsewhere the particular blend is believed to be unique to Flexicare.

The original scheme was funded by the Welsh Office under its strategy for mentally handicapped people. It has been described in detail by Newman and Cox (1987) and has been identified by the Audit Commission in its report; Making a Reality of Community Care (1985) as a useful model for innovative services.

The success of the Mental Handicap Flexicare Scheme led to proposals for a similar scheme for clients of the mental health service. In 1988, the South Glamorgan Social Services Department and South Glamorgan Health Authority agreed to jointly fund a small initiative, to be administered by Social Services. It is the progress of this latter scheme that is reported in this paper.

The primary objective of the Mental Health Flexicare Scheme is to enhance the quality of life of individuals whose opportunities have been damaged by mental illness or other persistent mental health problems. Priority is given to Flexicare programmes which assist discharge of patients from hospital or maintain them in the community and those which relieve stress on carers, and minimise damage to normal social relationships which may be a consequence of mental illness. All these objectives are of course shared with other services.

The Flexicare scheme is designed around four main elements:

a) An individual client programme which emphasises client's interests and strengths.
b) A flexible budget.
c) An approach which emphasises opportunities and resources available within the local community.
d) Flexicare workers employed on a contractual basis to assist individual clients.

How the Flexicare scheme typically operates

As the scheme was initially established, requests for Flexicare support are made by social workers, community nurses and other members of the local multidisciplinary teams on behalf of their clients. These key workers draw up proposals with their clients. Typically, these are requests to help the client take part in some activity in the community, for example, to join a sporting activity. The proposals are sometimes similar to familiar rehabilitation programmes. However, whilst the client's problems and disabilities are not ignored, the main focus is on the client's abilities, interest and aspirations. All those involved are encouraged to put forward imaginative proposals where possible using the normal facilities in the community open to all, rather than using specialised mental health services.

The proposed programme is presented to the Principal Social Services Officer for that area, who holds the local budget. An agreement is negotiated to provide financial support. This most usually is in the form of an agreement to pay a contractual worker for a fixed number of hours usually on a weekly basis for up to a maximum of three months. Short term and one off help may also be given. Clients can be given financial assistance in certain circumstances, but generally it is considered more appropriate that they meet reasonable travelling and other costs themselves.

The next stage is to find a suitable Flexicare worker. This person may be known to and have already worked with a few clients. However, not infrequently, Flexicare workers are recruited to work with a particular client. The matching of the client to the worker is important. Some workers may be recruited because of previous knowledge of mental health problems or because of abilities, such as music teaching, or because of ethnic background or familiarity with the client's own language. The client and the Flexicare worker are then introduced. If both are in agreement the Flexicare worker and the Principal Social Services Officer sign a contract for up to three months. The contract sets out the basic terms of the agreement, the rate of pay and the weekly hours. The keyworker maintains contact over the period of the contract and at the end of the period the client, Flexicare worker and keyworker review progress. Where appropriate programmes can be approved for further periods. Assistance can also be given in other ways that meet the general objectives of the scheme, for example, providing expenses to volunteers who do not wish to act as paid workers. Assistance has also been given to self help groups. As the scheme has progressed, variations on the standard procedures have occurred. These will be discussed below.

The progress of the Flexicare scheme

The scheme, which began in December, 1988, has now been in operation in all parts of the County, since April, 1989. The first Flexicare workers were recruited during 1988 and after interview, acceptance and a short induction programme were available to assist clients. During the initial period, progress has been assisted by using the payrolling system set up for clients with learning difficulties. During the first year, a total of £10,000 was available. Half of this was provided by the Health Authority. This increased to £11,000 in year two and £12,000 in year three. In the present financial year £14,000 is available, with additional finance to assist elderly mentally infirm clients and clients with problems of alcohol and drug dependence.

The uptake of the scheme was patchy over the early months and this led to some frustration amongst Flexicare workers already recruited. However, as the scheme has progressed it has won increasing numbers of converts amongst keyworkers. Over the last two years budget holders have had to exercise some prioritisation of schemes and limitations on hours to stay within budget.

Flexicare programmes and other assistance

Over the first three full years of its operation, there have been 110 individual programmes in the County. Many of the schemes progressed along the lines of the typical form described above, with clients attending sports clubs, visiting the library etc. However, there were other imaginative schemes, and variations on the standard approach as described above. Some examples which illustrate the range of interventions are given in appendix I. Further details are given in Appendix II: tables 1-3.

It will be seen immediately from Appendix I that some programmes e.g. those for Mr. A and Mr. B. are close to the original concepts and the model form described above. However, new elements were involved in other programmes: For Mrs. C. a behaviour modification element under the guidance of a psychologist was involved at the first stage, introducing an explicit therapeutic objective into the programme. Mrs. C and her family had of course been fully involved in deciding on this programme which took place in her own home.

For Mrs. D. the most important element was recruiting a Flexicare worker able to communicate in Cantonese. Mrs. D's participation at the planning stage of the programme was not as full as for the other clients because of communication problems related both to depression and language. Gaining her participation became a goal of the programme.

In the case of Mr. E. the activity agreed with him, which involved taking car trips out from the residential home, provided the opportunity for counselling.

For Mr. F. there is perhaps a paradox in that taking responsibility for some part of his life, his budgeting, has created the basis for keeping Mr. F in the community, and increasing his opportunities to be involved in normal community life.

These examples show something of the range of ages of clients and types of problems involved. Tables 1-3, in Appendix II give further details of the programmes over the first 3 years. It will be seen from Table 1 that a substantial number of schemes were carried over between years. This reflects a strong tendency for programmes to be continued for at least a second 3 month contract. There was overall, a tendency for more women than men to receive Flexicare, with a wide spread of ages. However, there was some variation in this in the different local areas. This is perhaps because keyworkers having seen Flexicare succeed with one client, have tended to apply for similar programmes for clients with similar backgrounds.

Mental health history of clients

As Flexicare is not established primarily as a form of treatment, detailed mental health history taking and recording of diagnosis were not given as much significance, as would be the case in standard forms of rehabilitation. However, this issue may be of interest to those who wish to learn about the scheme. Fund holders in particular are concerned that in financing schemes such as Flexicare, public money is being directed to priority groups.

276

It was not possible to analyse the backgrounds of all 110 clients who had programmes throughout the County. However, sufficient information was available to draw some tentative conclusions about the backgrounds of 47 Clients living in the Vale of Glamorgan area. Information on record, or from the keyworkers was available for 43 of these clients. Of these, twelve had histories of chronic mental illness, (generally schizophrenia), and four more had recent psychotic episodes. The largest group were 19 suffering from depression. In about half these cases, this followed a bereavement. Two individuals were known to be suffering from some form of dementia and two more had suffered traumatic brain damage. Four individuals were dependent upon alcohol.

At least 18 of these individuals had been treated in psychiatric hospitals during the previous year, and eleven were known to have spent at least one year as inpatients at some stage in their lives.

This information is perhaps sufficient to give a broad picture of the client group. In the view of the author it is a very typical cross section of clients seeking help from community mental health services.

Activities undertaken during programmes

The examples given in Appendix I give some idea of the range of activities undertaken. The scheme was set up to encourage imaginative responses, and its very success in this makes it difficult to present a systematic analysis without losing the quality of individuality in the process. However, it is possible to make some broad general observations.

Firstly, the frame of reference of Flexicare as hinted above, is one which is influenced strongly by a philosophy of normalisation. In the Flexicare scheme, the notions of promoting client choice, enhancing quality of life, bringing about changes in the client's support network, and using the normal facilities of the community are linked together. In practice tension can arise between these elements and one or other may come to the fore in particular programmes: In some cases, clients chose to use specialist services, but wanted help with transport and confidence building to attend. In other cases, the role of the Flexicare worker as change agent was important. Direct provision of care was an element for some clients, particularly the more elderly.

A review was carried out on the 47 programmes for the clients of the Vale of Glamorgan area. The scheme records (applications and reviews) were examined for common elements. The most important general feature reported to be a factor in 27 programmes, was confidence building. In 20 cases, the aim of overcoming isolation and building new friendships was a feature. In 15 cases their programmes specifically included taking part in sports or other leisure activities in the community. Shopping was a specific feature of nine programmes. In 5 programmes, counselling was identified at the outset and in 9 the importance of learning new skills was recorded. In five of the cases, (mainly elderly clients), there was an element of direct care provision, with the Flexicare workers role close to that of a specialist home help. Relationships with other family members were relevant to 10 cases, where Flexicare assisted in relieving carers or improving family relationships.

A feature of many of the programmes was befriending of the client by Flexicare workers. This was not in itself an objective of the scheme, rather a means to an end. However, in a number of programmes it may have been the most important element and have become an end in itself.

The recruitment and support of Flexicare workers

As indicated in the section above, the importance of matching of clients and Flexicare workers was recognised from the outset. Practice showed the importance of building confidence, and of befriending. These point to the significance of a relationship of trust, built up with the Flexicare workers. This in turn indicates the importance of considering how Flexicare workers are recruited.

In total, 46 Flexicare workers have been used over three years. The initial group was selected from individuals who had answered advertisements in the local press and been interviewed by Health and Social Service Staff. They were given a one day induction to the scheme. It rook about six months for applications to come in regularly, in all the local areas, and a number of the recruits were not offered work at the time. Despite emphasis given during the recruitment on the likelihood of delays and the probability of only a few hours work each, for each week, there was disappointment to some of these individuals. Many did however go on to take part in the scheme. Over three years many Flexicare workers have left the scheme for a variety of reasons, though six of the original group remain working with the scheme.

It became necessary to recruit further Flexicare workers at an early stage. This was a result partly of the registered workers leaving the scheme, but also because of the importance of matching the clients and workers and of finding Flexicare workers in the right locality. Since that time recruitment has been the responsibility of the local teams and has mainly been through personal contacts of the key workers and other area staff.

The Flexicare workers come from a wide range of backgrounds and have varying experiences of mental health issues. A number, including some who answered the original advertisement had no previous knowledge of mental health problems. Those in this group have tended to work with a number of clients simultaneously. For these workers, Flexicare has been important as a source of income although it is not ideally suited to those wishing guaranteed earnings. Flexicare workers have also included four people who have themselves been mental health clients, including one who had had Flexicare help. Quite a large proportion of the new recruits have been individuals who have had some professional experience in the mental health field. This has included retired social workers, individuals on professional training courses wanting part time work, and women with young children who want to retain some links with their profession. A number of Flexicare workers have been recruited from volunteers already helping mental health clients. Finally, some have been recruited because of special abilities.

All Flexicare workers are paid at the same rate, which is tied to the home care aide rate of pay. The support to Flexicare workers is primarily from the key workers for each client. The programmes cannot proceed unless the key worker agrees to undertake this function. In addition, the Flexicare workers in each local area are encouraged to meet as a group. Multidisciplinary staff in each local area are responsible for helping Flexicare workers in their area to share experiences and develop their understanding and skills.

Evaluating Flexicare

There are a number of key questions which need to be considered relating to how far Flexicare has achieved its objectives, whether it holds together as a coherent scheme and what its relationship should be to other services provided by the statutory and voluntary sectors.

Has Flexicare achieved its objectives for clients?

The sources of information available on this are firstly from clients themselves, secondly from others involved with them; keyworkers etc. In the original design of the scheme it was intended that reviews would take place at the end of the contracted period, with clients being asked to give their opinion. This has not happened as comprehensively as might be wished. (Inconsistency in record keeping has perhaps been the unavoidable price of emphasising local initiative). Where clients have completed these reviews they have been generally highly complimentary of the Flexicare workers. However, not all clients have been satisfied. About 25% of programmes did not run for the whole 3 month period. Although there were also other reasons for programmes ending early, client dissatisfaction was a factor in some cases.

Conversely clients have frequently expressed strong wishes for the scheme to continue at the end of the contract period. A high proportion of programmes were renewed for at least one further period. There is clear evidence that the programmes were valued by these clients, though this is not quite the same as saying the original objectives of the individual programmes were achieved. A further, more comprehensive, evaluation of clients views needs to be conducted. As indicated in preceding sections, Flexicare has won many advocates amongst professional staff. Whilst this does not necessarily indicate that it has met its objectives it does suggest that it must be doing something right!

The significance of the components of the scheme

As described in the introduction, the scheme is designed around four main elements; individual programmes, flexible budgeting, using community resources and employing contractual workers. In evaluating Flexicare, questions arise about the significance of each of these components, and whether they hold together to form a coherent service.

At the time of the development of the original Flexicare Scheme, flexible budgeting, whilst not new, was a somewhat more radical departure from traditional community care funding than it now appears. The White Paper, Caring for People - Community Care in the Next Decade and Beyond (1989), proposed flexible budgets covering the community care and residential care needs. The implementation of the National Health Service and Community Carer Act (1991) will make such budgeting essential at least for those disabled enough to be candidates for residential care.

The White Paper's proposal for flexible budgeting crucially depend upon this being tied to individual plans based upon needs assessment. Individual care or treatment planning is not new. It can be seen to be inherent in the medical model, and is at least implicit within the welfare responsibilities of local authorities since the National Assistance Act (1948). However individual programmes for care or for rehabilitation, provided by both the Health Service and Local Authorities have been dominated by approaches which have emphasised problems only and have tended to provide stereotyped solutions. Flexicare tries to make positive use of the client's interests, strengths and hopes. In doing this it follows thinking which has been taken further in the learning difficulties field. Mainline Mental Health services have been curiously indifferent to this issue at least for the more disabled, even though the idea of stimulating self curative action is an old one in medicine and psychotherapeutic thinking. However, under the guidance for assessment recently issued to local authorities an important place is given to this issue. Indeed, it is hard to see how client self determination can have any real meaning unless both the client's needs and strengths are taken into account.

If the client's internal resources have often been neglected in social care provision and rehabilitation, so too have the resources of the community. There are however, at least three strands of thinking which point to the wider community, rather than specialist facilities, as sources and locations of help. Firstly, the 'theory' of normalisation helps us to see this issue in terms of values. (In a recent article Ramon (1991) reviews the relevance of these ideas within the mental health field). Secondly, in the social welfare field, community work has traditionally tried to draw on potential sources of help in the community. (The position for social work was extensively reviewed in the Barclay Report). Thirdly, groups studying social networks, at least for the most disabled groups, and to the importance of confiding relationships, which, may be with professionals or through ordinary relationships with other members of the community. (The Taps Project; Dunn et al (1990) and Leff et al (1990) gives a recent view from this perspective).

Flexicare has shown that it is possible to make use of community resources in two senses. Firstly, there has been little difficulty in recruiting Flexicare workers with appropriate skills, amongst those who do not want full time employment in the mental health field, and secondly, it has emphasised the value of ordinary activities, such as shopping, sporting activities etc. These can be seen to have enhanced the quality of clients' lives and are therefore an end in themselves, but also to have often provided opportunities for learning, including social skills learning. However, at this stage, it can only be claimed that Flexicare has taken a few small steps. It has shown that it is possible to promote community support with appropriately designed and funded projects. These developments could be taken much further.

For example, the importance attached to shopping, discussed above, should perhaps be no surprise. Soap opera may be ahead of the social welfare agencies in recognising the corner shop as a source of support and contact. It should not be beyond the wit of service planners to find a way to form links with local shopkeepers, who benefit from the custom of this client group.

The Flexicare workers are the keystone of Flexicare as it currently operates. The only real impediment to establishing a similar system elsewhere is the need for a payrolling system. In South Glamorgan this was set up as a separate development. There is however, no reason why local authorities could not make use of existing Home Care payrolling systems.

No all individuals who have offered their services to Flexicare have wanted to be paid. At the present time a local MIND association is looking at the possibility of establishing a link between Flexicare and volunteers.

Given that each of the four components described above can be found separately in other services, does Flexicare hold together? It does seem to work as a coherent system. It is easily grasped and understood by clients and professionals, and although at times it may depart from is original emphasis, this can be seen as a strength as much as a weakness. It remains an open question whether Flexicare should continue as a distinct method of service provision or be absorbed into a wider flexible budgeting system for providing for the community care needs of the more disabled clients.

What relationship should Flexicare have to other types of support to clients?

In the preceding sections, comments have been made about variations from the standard form of Flexicare. At times, programmes have been closely similar to befriending schemes, social skills training, behavioural programmes or specialist home care. This in some measure reflects local service deficits.

Befriending schemes, good neighbour schemes and other voluntary support to clients all have a part to play alongside Flexicare. The needs for a long term supportive role like Flexicare for more disabled individuals is also shown by the demand for the renewal of programmes. However, where long term support is required the community workers may perhaps be more appropriately employed on permanent contracts, either as outreach workers from specialist facilities, or as specialist home care staff.

As Flexicare is jointly funded by Health and Social Services, a final question remains as to its value to each agency.

Flexicare can be seen as falling within the area of overlapping statutory functions of Health and Social Services in the field of prevention and aftercare. In this context further research on its effectiveness will clearly be required. For Social Services Flexicare can also be seen as an alternative to traditional methods of meeting welfare responsibilities. In this perspective the user view of the service should clearly be a significant factor in determining the future of Flexicare.

References

Audit Commission (1986). *Making a Reality of Community Care*. London: HMSO.

Barclay, P.M. (Working Party Chairman) (1982). *Social Workers, Their Role and Tasks*. London: National Council for Voluntary Organisations.

Department of Health (1989). *Caring for People: Community Care in the Next Decade and Beyond*. London: HMSO.

Dunn, M., O'Driscoll, D., Dayson, D., Wills, W., & Leff, J., (1990). The observational study of the social life of long-stay patients. *British Journal of Psychiatry*. **157**, 842-848.

Leff, J., O'Driscoll, D., Dayson, D., Wills, W., & Anderson, J., (1990). The structure of social-network data obtained from long stay patients. *The British Journal of Psychiatry*, **157**, 848-852.

Newman, A., & Cox, S., (1987). Your flexible friend... South Glamorgan's Flexicare Service: *Social Work Today* 18/26.

Ramon, S., (1991). The background dimensions of normalisation worker 1-Principles and conceptual knowledge. In S. Ramon (Ed.), *Beyond Community Care* (pp 6-33). London: MIND/Macmillan.

Welsh Office (1991). *Managing care: Guidance on assessment and the provision of Social and Community Care*. Cardiff: Welsh Office.

Appendix I

Examples of Uses of Flexicare:

a) Single payments:

   1. A client with long term mental illness wished to travel to a family funeral in the North of England, but lacked the confidence to travel. A volunteer travelled part of the way and helped the client make a rail connection. The volunteer's expenses were paid.

   2. A community psychiatric nurse took a group of his patients on holiday to the West Country. Additional finance was given to assist this.

b) Flexicare Programmes:

[Note: The costs of the schemes given, are the direct costs; administrative costs are not included].

1. Mr. A.

This young man came to South Glamorgan from the London Area to be near his mother who subsequently left the area. During his adolescence he had been in care and had spent two years in a psychiatric hospital for treatment of a recurrent psychosis. He presented as very immature, withdrawn and lacking social skills. He was, not surprisingly, socially isolated. A Flexicare worker was recruited specifically to work with Mr. A. The programme helped him to become involved in community activities, playing pool etc. The scheme has been renewed on three occasions. Mr. A. has shown a marked improvement in social skills and has taken initiatives in making new relationships in the community.

     Dates of Programmes: Cost of Programmes:

     18.09.91-20.01.92   £196.83

2. Mr. B.

This sixty year old man had been an inpatient at Whitchurch Hospital for some years. He had an interest in music and had played the piano in his earlier life. A Flexicare worker who had had experience as a volunteer with mental health services, and was also a music teacher was recruited and helped Mr. B. regain his confidence and music skills. He has on occasions played the piano in local pubs since that time.

     Dates of Programmes: Cost of Programmes:

     20.04.89-04.08.89   £149.00

3. Mrs. C.

Mrs C. is a young married woman with two small children. She has suffered periods of depression and is of below average intelligence. She had marked obsessional traits which interfered with normal life, including child care. Two Flexicare programmes were agreed. During the first, the Flexicare worker under the supervision of a clinical psychologist, assisted Mrs. C. to reduce obsessional behaviour in her home. In the second programme Mrs. C. was helped to get involved in activities outside the home including attending Mother & Toddler Groups.

Dates of Programmes: Cost of Programmes:
20.06.89- 27.06.90   £515.76

4. Mrs. D.

This 40 year old married Chinese woman came to this country as an adult, and has no English. She has three children, and suffered a prolonged depressive illness after the birth of the third child. There were concerns over the safety of her children. A Cantonese speaking Flexicare worker was recruited to support Mrs. D. and received guidance from the Consultant Psychiatrist and the keyworker. The Flexicare worker also liaised closely with Social Workers in the Children and Family Services.

Although this programme had to be brought to an end early because the Flexicare worker took up full time employment, she made a valuable contribution to the help the family were receiving.

(Fifty per cent of the costs of this programme was funded by Children and Family Services).

Dates of Programmes: Cost of Programmes:
01.06.90-14.0990   £147.47

5. Mr. E.

This fifty eight year old man was suffering from presenile dementia. Following the breakdown of his marriage, he was living in a residential home, but was very unsettled. A Flexicare worker was recruited who had skills in loss counselling. Mr E was taken out on car trips. These presented an opportunity to counsel Mr E who responded well and became more settled.

Dated of Programmes: Cost of Programmes:
11.01.90-09.08.90   £429.71

6. Mr. F.

Mr. F. is a man in his early fifties who has a history of mental health problems. He is of below average intelligence and has spent a number of years in a mental handicap hospital, and other institutions. He had a long history of offending, mainly theft. He had great difficulty managing his finances. A Flexicare worker was appointed to become a D.S.S. appointee and to help Mr F budget. He is not known to have re-offended during this period.

Dates of Programmes: Cost of Programmes:
23.07.91-28.11.91   £260.76

Scheme currently continuing.

Appendix II
Table 1
Numbers of Clients Receiving Flexicare Programmes

	1989-90	1990-91	1991-92	3 years
New Clients	43	24	43	110
Continuing Clients	-	13	6	-
Total Number of Clients	43	37	19	-

[*This excludes clients receiving help on a single occasion]

Table 2
Sex of clients

MALE	FEMALE	TOTAL
45	65	110

Table 3
Age of clients* at begining of programme

AGE	Under 20	20-29	30-39	40-49	50-59	60-69	70-79	Over 80	Total
NUMBER OF CLIENTS	2	19	19	17	17	11	13	5	103

(* Information not available on 7 clients)

24 Attitudes towards mental health promotion by health and social care workers

G. Humphris

Abstract

Attempts to promote mental health will be strengthened by active support of the major disciplines already providing initial help or more specialist interventions with those experiencing mental health problems. A study was conducted to develop a questionnaire to assess mental health workers' views towards mental health and its promotion. Additional scales on the preventability of a series of mental health problems (20 items) and the suggested coping skills required to abate difficulties arising from a crisis were also included (26 items). The questionnaire was completed by four distinctive groups, nurses undergoing mental health training (n=54), trained mental health nurses (n=43), delegates at a regional mental health promotion conference (i.e. representatives from health and social services, n=43) and a group of general medical practitioners (n=21).A number of internally consistent scales were constructed from preliminary analyses. The groups varied in their opinion of what constituted mental health. GPs adopted a more biological approach, while conference attenders viewed mental health as a more positive emotional-state. GPs were less favourable to mental health promotion programmes than the rest of the sample. There was remarkable consistency across the groups in the view of the coping skills the public should engage in during a crisis. Preventability of mental health problems was affirmed strongly by nurse respondents for anxiety-related and dependency problems. Conference attenders were more optimistic abut preventing severe mental health problems. These results suggest that various occupational groups have wide ranging opinions abut what constitutes mental health and this partially extends to their views on associated preventive approaches. However high agreement appeared to be evident across the disciplines on the success of self-help approaches to cope with crises and this finding may point a way forward to promote consistent, multi-disciplinary messages to the public.

Introduction

It has been argued that there should be an emphasis on action rather than a detailed focus on definition of mental health, prevention or promotion (Fernando, 1988). This approach is unlikely to serve satisfactorily the field of mental health promotion. When a loose agreement and poor definition is applied there is a distinct possibility of programmes being devised and implemented without a clear formulation of the predicted processes that require change. To achieve common aims and arrive at consensus when developing a local strategy the study of opinions towards mental health health promotion has merit. Health workers' views towards mental health and mental illness constitute an important area of concern, as our improved understanding of their views will make us more effective in arguing for the finite resources which need to be transferred to prevention but are currently used mainly for treatment services.

Therefore in order to have an influence within the current UK health service organisations, i.e. purchasers and providers in the planning of innovative health promotion initiatives it would be prudent to explore the views of major staff groupings within the health and caring agencies.

Previous work by Roskin, Carsen, Rabiner and Morell (1988) has reported their attempts to assess attitudes of mental health professional groups towards their target of service provision, namely patients. They quote studies which have been weak in devising measures and lacking in scope in the assessment of mental health workers' views towards individuals with mental health problems. Roskin et al. (1988) have developed an 'attitudes Towards Patients' questionnaire which consists of a series of items split into several sub-scales with known reliability. They then present in their study a comparison of the attitudes of four different professional groups (psychiatrists, psychologists, social workers and nurses) towards the aetiology and treatment of psychiatric illness and aspects of the doctor-patient relationship.

In this paper a description of the Mental Health Promotion Attitudes Questionnaire will be given, detailing the rationale of its construction, development into specific named scales and a summary of some of its properties, i.e. reliability and variability across a number of health worker groups.

To devise a broad assessment instrument, a model of attributes which helps to describe mental health is referred to (see Figure 1). This crude construction refers to two major sets of variables believed to be important in determining mental health, namely constitutional or biological factors and environmental factors. The interaction of these two sets of factors is considered an additional precursor to predicting both mental health and

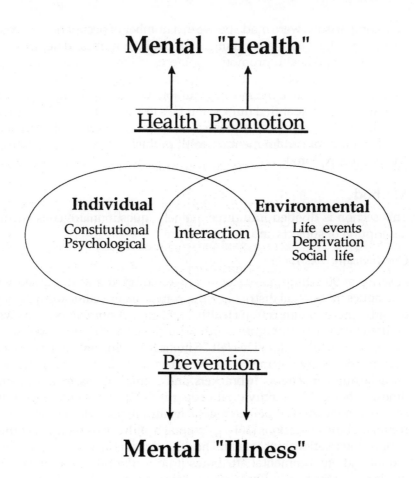

Figure 1 Schematic framework for the construction of questionnaire

mental ill health. Note that the terms mental health and mental ill health are located in different areas in the schematic diagram and reflect recent proposals to consider health and ill health as separate components (Trent, 1991). The advantage of separating these constructs deliberately in this way avoids confusing the related actions of promotion and prevention. Although there may be overlap between the two endeavours of promotion and prevention, on occasion they may require very different approaches.

The aim of this study was to devise a questionnaire that was broad enough in scope to assess health workers' views towards mental health promotion following the conceptual framework just outlined. In addition, comparisons were made between a number of occupational groups including fully qualified nursing staff, trainee nurses, delegates to a regional mental health promotion conference (held in September 1990) and general medical practitioners. It was predicted that the conference attenders would have the most favourable views toward mental health promotion, with qualified nurses and GPs less enthusiastic. In addition the relationship of these attitudes towards these workers' opinions of the preventability of certain mental health problems and coping strategies will also be explored.

Method

This section is divided into three, namely: questionnaire construction, description of subjects and the procedure.

Questionnaire construction

A series of 90 attitudinal statements were drafted and discussed with colleagues in the local district health promotion and clinical psychology departments of South Sefton Health Authority. A number of items were omitted because of ambiguity, or they produced a uniform response (i.e. no variation in attitude). This left 76 items for inclusion[1]. Each item had been purposefully grouped into five areas. The areas were as follows, with the number of items, in brackets, and example items: mental health/illness is based upon individual properties (23) e.g. 'mental health is a state of emotional well-being', mental health/illness is based upon environmental considerations (16) e.g. 'mental health can be retained without supporting relationships', mental health/illness is an interaction of individual and environmental attributes (6) e.g. 'the provision of material needs can be the best buffer to those at risk to mental illness', prevention procedures in the mental illness field are worthwhile (12) e.g. 'there is little evidence to show that prevention of mental health problems works', promotion procedures in the mental health field are worthwhile (10) e.g. 'mental health promotion has many fine ideals but little substance in practice'. All items were responded to by a standard 5 point scale with verbal anchors ranging from 'strongly agree' to 'strongly disagree' with a central 'undecided' category. An additional set of scales was included. A preventability scale was designed which listed 20 mental health problems e.g. 'depression', 'anxiety state', 'anorexia nervosa', 'schizophrenia' and invited respondents to indicate on a five point scale the degree to which each of these problems was preventable. The scale points included 'cannot prevent' - scored 1 to 'prevent completely' - scored 5. The purpose of this scale was to determine whether attitudes to promotion and, in particular, prevention were reflected in all areas of mental health problems, or were limited to a discrete set of difficulties.

A 26 item scale completed the questionnaire and asked respondents to show what an average member of the public would do to cope when faced with a major crisis (e.g. bereavement, loss of job, relationship breakdown etc.) and then to indicate what this member of the public should do. The items comprised of a list of coping strategies including 'talk with relative', 'take regular exercise', 'minimise problem', 'drink alcohol' etc. The answering scheme for both sets of 26 items ranged from 'never' - scored 1 to 'always' - scored 5. The purpose of this section was to find whether those who advocated general coping skills were also positive about promotion and prevention.

All questionnaires were returned anonymously. No reminders were sent. Details of age group, sex and duration of employment in current job and time since qualification were also collected. The GPs were not invited to supply employment information.

Subjects

Four groups of subjects were selected. Three groups were homogeneous in occupation, nurses in training, trained nurses and general medical practitioners. The fourth group comprised a variety of workers who were delegates to a regional day conference on mental health promotion and included nursing staff, psychologists, occupational therapists, social workers, health promotion officers, counselling staff, community nurses and users of mental health services, voluntary service members and organisers. Approximately 70% of the conference delegates returned their questionnaires.

The nurses in training group included all nurse candidates on RMN courses at two sites in Merseyside. Both courses were presenting a prevention and healthy life-style content as required of the new curriculum recently adopted by these two centres.

The trained nurses were employed by South Sefton Health Authority and worked in one of the wards of an acute 80 bedded-plus psychiatric unit which had been recently purpose-built. This group also included the community psychiatric nurses, of which the majority were RMN trained. The staff who were selected were regarded by local unit management to possess a general interest in the field of prevention. This was demonstrated on visits made by the author to these staff members, who were starting to implement preventive practices in their service. The interventions were mainly information giving.

The general medical practitioners were sampled from two Family

Health Services Authorities, namely: Sefton and Chester. The question-naires were mailed including a covering letter and s.a.e. Official endorse-ment in the covering letter by the relevant FHSA was hoped to improve the return rate. Of the 40 questionnaires posted to individual GPs replies were received from 22, of which 21 were complete. A similar response rate of approximately 50% was found from both areas.

Procedure

Somewhat different methods of inviting the members of the different groups to reply to the questionnaire were adopted. The tutors of the nurses under training were contacted and a research assistant was employed to administer the questionnaire. The trained nurses were invited to participate and given instructions, also by the aid of the research assistant. Some of the ward staff on alternative shifts completed the questionnaire under the supervision of the charge nurse. The conference delegates were invited to complete the questionnaire via an announce-ment at the conference. A letter of instruction was included. A similar letter was utilised for the GPs group, although only postal contact was made.

Results

The questionnaire items were submitted to factor analysis to establish unidimensional scales. Standard conventions were applied, including principal component solutions, orthogonal factors with varimax rotation. Items that loaded 0.4 or greater on interpretable and significant factors and were low on the remaining factors were retained in the analyses. The items were grouped into broad sets as indicated by the model which has been described at the item construction stage, so that a number of separate analyses were conducted. This approach was adopted as the procedure functioned more as a confirmatory analysis. It was predicted that certain items would correlate with constructs that were assumed to be inherent in the content of the questionnaire.

However it was apparent after a preliminary run of analyses that the simple structure expected was not fully supported. For example the 6 items which were expected to load on a separate factor to assess the extent that mental health was a product of an interaction between qualities of the individual and the environment was not found. These specific items were mixed with other factors or loaded very poorly on all factors. A summary of the scales that were constructed is contained in Table 1. From the number of items, the internal consistency (Cronbach's alpha) was calcu-lated. The F statistic and p level from the analysis of variance conducted

Table 1
Summary of scale description, internal consistency and results of significance testing across four occupational groups

	Scale	No. of Items	Alpha	F	P
	Mental Health associated with individual factors				
1	Positive State	5	.81	1.54	.20
2	Personal Vulnerability	4	.64	2.41	.07
3	Brain Function	2	.71	5.72	.001
4	Emotional Happiness	3	.55	2.70	.05
5	Ability to cope	2	.68	0.82	.48
6	Genetic Composition	4	.53	11.85	.0001
	Mental Health associated with environmental factors				
1	Deprivation	7	.56	0.59	.62
2	Early Experiences	2	.65	0.95	.42
3	Supportive Relationships	7	.64	2.17	.09
	Action to Promotion				
1	General mhp programmes	7	0.73	0.98	.006
	Attitude to Prevention				
1	Prevent more than treat	3	0.58	1.04	.37
2	Resources to Prevention	3	.50	1.95	.12
3	Evidence of Prevention	2	.48	2.52	.06
4	Self-Help Methods	3	.48	1.66	.18
	Coping skills public should adopt				
1	Avoidance Behaviour	4	.74	1.27	.28
2	Seek Professional Help	5	.71	0.28	.84
3	Minimise Problem	3	.64	0.87	.45
4	Friends or Logic	3	.58	0.80	.49
5	Get More Involved	3	.53	1.48	.22
6	Physical Outlet	4	.54	1.36	.26
	Mental Health Problem Preventability				
1	Anxiety Related	8	.89	4.41	.006
2	Dependency - Addictive	6	.85	7.70	.0001
3	Severe	6	.78	3.67	.01

on the scale values generated for the four occupational groups studied was completed for each scale.

Four main areas were identified which correspond broadly with the conceptual model presented in Figure 1. Two of these areas relate to explanations employed by mental health workers to understand mental health/illness, namely individual factors and environmental factors. A number of discrete scales were included under each area. The other two major areas described general attitudes towards promotion of mental health and the prevention of mental health problems. Only one scale in the promotion area was sufficiently well defined to function as a reliable measure.

The coping skills items and the preventability of mental health problems were introduced into the questionnaire as independent variables from the formulated model. The factor analyses with these items produced simple solutions with easily interpretable scales.

Analysis of variance showed there was significant variation of opinion

Table 2
Means and sd's of attitude scales which vary significantly across the four occupational groups

	Trained Nurses (n=54)	Nurses in Training (n=43)	Conference Attenders (n=43)	GPs (n=21)	P
Scale	M (sd)	M (sd)	M (sd)	M (sd)	
Mental health is associated with individaul factors					
Personal Vulnerability	13.04 (2.38)	12.76 (2.58)	12.47 (2.34)	14.51 (1.89)	*
Brain Function	5.65 (1.62)	5.31 (1.55)	4.84 (1.70)	6.60 (1.67)	****
Emotional Happiness	9.58 (1.37)	9.17 (1.79)	10.18 (2.04)	9.90 (2.10)	**
Genetic Composition	10.33 (2.14)	10.26 (2.34)	10.07 (2.34)	13.30 (1.62)	****
Attitude to Promotion/Prevention					
General mhp programmes	26.48 (3.13)	25.92 (2.89)	24.17 (5.33)	21.28 (5.93)	***
Evidence for Prevention					
Preventability					
Anxiety Related Disorders	27.00 (6.09)	25.33 (6.18)	24.17 (5.33)	21.28 (5.93)	***
Dependency-Addictive	19.35 (4.32)	18.31 (5.05)	18.12 (3.81)	13.62 (4.76)	****
Severe Disorders	12.37 (3.80	11.75 (4.22)	13.59 (3.89)	10.38 (2.59)	**

*	p<.07
**	p<.05
***	p<.01
****	p<.001

Notes:
1. High scores show strong agreement
2. High score shows greater likelihood that problem is preventable
3. Identical suffix letters against means denotes significant difference p<.05

across the occupational groups. However, before focusing on the differences, of note was the similarity of opinion held by the disparate staff groups in the influence of the environment on mental health and also the coping skills that mental health workers would advise people to use during a crisis.

Attitudes to four of the six individual qualities that help determine mental health were found to vary across the occupational groups studied (see Table 2). Post hoc comparison tests (Tukey HSD, alpha level=.05) were conducted. GPs were more disposed to the attitude that mental health was a product of an individual's personal vulnerability, their brain function and genetic make-up. Conference attenders and GPs were more inclined to rate emotional happiness as a feature of mental health than the nurse groups.

GP attitudes towards mental health promotion programmes were far less positive than the other three groups. In addition GPs expressed somewhat greater indifference to the available evidence for the efficacy of prevention and were the least optimistic about the likelihood of preventing mental health problems overall. The trained nurses were found to

	Attitudes					
	Mental Health					Promotion
	Individual Factors			Environmental Factors		
	Positive State	Brain Function	Ability to Cope	Lack of Relationships	Deprevation	MHP Promotion
Coping skills public should adopt						
Minimise Problem	.148	.223*	.231**	.017	-.050	-.003
Get More Involved	.198*	.116	.203*	.162	-.031	.101
Physical Outlet	.222*	.062	.070	.188*	.253**	.326***
Preventability of mental health problems						
Anxiety Related	.154	-.316***	-.009	.174*	.182*	.393***
Dependency/ Addictive	.181*	-.197*	.065	.130	.049	.240**
Severe	.178*	-.379***	.051	.135	.267**	.299***

*   p<.05

**   p<.01

*** p<.001

exhibit the most positive attitudes towards mental health promotion programmes and were especially strong in their beliefs that anxiety related and dependency-addictive problems were preventable. The conference attenders were the most positive in their beliefs that the severe disorders such as schizophrenia and manic depression were preventable.

Pearson product-moment correlations were calculated between some of the attitudinal variables and the scales to assess advocated coping skills and the preventability of certain types of mental health problems (see Table 3). Some notable associations were found. Respondents with strong views to the presence of mental health based upon an individual's positive nature were more likely to exhort the public to benefit themselves by getting more involved in their current difficulties ($r=0.198$, $p<.05$) or to seek a physical outlet ($r=0.222$, $p<.05$). Likewise this view of the positive nature of mental health was associated with beliefs that dependency ($r=0.181$, $p<.05$) and severe mental health problems ($r=0.178$, $p<.05$) were preventable. An anatomical view (i.e. brain function explanations) of mental health was related to the attitude that problems should be minimised in order to cope ($r=0.223$, $p<.05$), and that pessimism was expressed about prevention especially of severe disorders ($r=-0.379$, $p<.001$). Other relationships of note include the views of those who rate deprivation as explaining mental health levels were associated with the recommendation of a physical outlet to improve coping ($r=0.253$, $p<.01$) and an optimistic view to the preventability of anxiety related ($r=0.182$, $p<.05$) and severe mental health problems ($r=0.267$, $p<.01$) Positive views held concerning mental health promotion were associated with benefits of a physical outlet as a coping skill ($r=0.326$, $p<.001$) and the preventability of the three clusters of mental health problems.

Discussion

This study was designed to construct a questionnaire of broad scope to assess mental health workers attitudes towards mental health promotion and the prevention of mental health problems. The items that were devised were wide ranging and designed to fit into a conceptual structure. The resulting structure obtained from the data collected from a disparate sample of respondents only partially resembled the pre-conceived model. However a number of reliable and homogenous scales were found. Considerable differences of opinion between the various occupational groups involved in the study were found although some caution should be raised as the sampling methods for the groups were not identical.

The GP group were found to differ consistently from the other staff groups in their view concerning the constituents of mental health and the influence of individual factors. The GPs believed that mental health could be explained more successfully by the vulnerability a person possessed, a dysfunctional brain and a genetic predisposition to mental health difficulties. In summary this pattern of findings reflects a more biological position compared to other mental health workers' views and is consistent with Roskin et al. (1988) who found psychiatrists (i.e. specialist medics) expressing a clear preference to a biological aetiology of psychiatric disorder over psychodynamic explanations. However among the GPs (i.e. primary care medical specialists) the strong biological views expressed may be considered disappointing especially when the Royal College of General Practitioners (1981) over 10 years ago presented a Special Report on the prevention of 'Psychiatric Disorders' which concentrated on environmental issues to help predict the increased incidence of psychological problems such as anxiety and depression. Among the views concentrating environmental factors influencing mental health including poor social relationships and deprivation it was found that GPs did not differ from other staff. Therefore the GPs stronger biological bias in comparison with other disciplines had not influenced them to the extent that GPs reduced the significance of environmental pressures.

It was disappointing to find the comparatively low opinion that GPs held towards general mental health promotion campaigns and programmes, and also their limited endorsements of the effectiveness of prevention activities as presented in the literature. Only when evidence of preventive programmes are reported more widely in the GP journals will traditional views begin to be challenged.

A similar argument may be proposed from the findings of the preventability of mental health problems scales. In each of the three problem areas identified, GPs recorded the lowest optimism in preventing mental disorder. The conference attenders were predicted to score most favourably on this set of three scales, in fact they were most positive on only one of the three areas. The prevention of severe disorders (senile dementia, schizophrenia, etc.) was regarded as more preventable amongst conference attenders than the other three groups. However the trained nurses including ward staff and CPN's were the most optimistic in the prevention of anxiety-related and dependency problems. This was unexpected and may have been due to a selection bias although it was known at the time that the details of the new Project 2000 curriculum (ENB, 1989) were being discussed throughout the local nursing services. The curriculum includes significant coverage of prevention and the promotion of mental health problems.

Some of the relationships found between the coping skills which mental health workers suggest members of the public should adopt and attitudes towards mental health and promotion were revealing, and provide convergent support to the above findings. For example those who believe brain function was a key explanatory variable of mental health also believed that attempts to minimise crises is to be advocated and in addition views towards prevention were negative.

A consistent pattern of relationships was found when relating the two attitude scales: views about deprivation and mental health promotion campaigns with coping skills and preventability. Recommendations to use physical exercise as an outlet and optimism to the prevention of mental health problems is a very consistent profile for those who consider deprivation as a cause for poor mental health and likewise for those who agree that mental health promotion programmes are effective. It is interesting that perhaps more mechanistic coping skills are believed to be effective such as physical exercise rather than psychological methods e.g. relaxation, counselling. It would be very illuminating to invite members of the public in a representative survey to rate what they actually do in a crisis compared to the recommendations of 'experts'.

A new climate exists within the NHS, by virtue of the division of the service into purchasers and providers. This new situation presents health promoters, and specifically mental health promoters with new challenges. Hopefully opportunities will present themselves for health promotion activities to be included in a wide variety, if not all, of service contracts. The expansion of GP fundholding practices presents probably the greatest challenge to those wishing to encourage resources from these GP practices for mental health promotion.

The findings from this study of GP attitudes towards mental health promotion being somewhat unenthusiastic should act as a trigger to focus GPs as an appropriate target to persuade and encourage their interest. The targeting of GPs should be regarded a priority as it is within the clinics of the general medical practices where there is, arguably, the greatest expansion in the NHS of health promotion activities. Mental health promoters may need initially to concentrate their efforts with GPs by advocating programmes with practical interventions focusing on coping strategy methods. This approach of course reflects Fernando's pragmatic position quoted in the introduction. However once this important primary care level has been engaged in operating mental health promotion activities, it is hoped that the complex issues of mental health causation will be explored and potential differences of opinion relaxed to develop a more comprehensive model of mental functioning and hence improve promotional efforts.

Acknowledgements

The efforts of those who advised on various items of the questionnaire, especially Toni Lewis, are gratefully acknowledged, as well as the help received from the FHSA's in South Sefton and Chester. Finally, my thanks to the respondents.

References

ENB (1989). *Project 2000 - A new preparation for practice - Guidelines and criteria for course development.* English National Board for nursing, midwifery and health visiting, London.

Fernando, S. (1990). *Mental health promotion - the way forward.* In Proceedings of National Mental Health Promotion Conference. Salford. Health Education Authority.

NHMA (1987). Commission on the prevention of mental-emotional disabilities. National Mental Health Association. *Journal of Primary Prevention,* 7, 175-243.

RCGP (1981). *Prevention of psychiatric disorders in general practice.* Royal College of General Practitioners, London.

Roskin, G., Carsen, M.L., Rabiner, C.J., & Marell, S.K. (1988). Attitudes toward patients among different mental health professional groups. *Comprehensive Psychiatry,* 29, 188-194.

Trent, D. (1991). Breaking the single continuum. *The promotion of mental health volume 1,* Avebury: Aldershot.

A copy of the questionnaire and further details are obtainable from the author on request.

Acknowledgements

The authors wish to record their gratitude to ... the Queen charging agency ... support ... the help ... provided ... for ... of the recording.

References

FORD (1996), Arena 2000. ... recreation for private ... obtained and strategic conservation ... habitat, national flora ... fauna, inland waters and coastal waters. La Plata ...

Hunnable (1996), Atkins flora ... aquatic ... British Isles. Peterborough, English Nature, ...

NMA (1991) Recommendations ... mental disorders. Australian Mental Health Association. Darval, Germany ...

MCCLUSKY, Anderson ... aquatic invertebrates, water ... general ... Building, ...

BATE, C., Griffin, M.E., BR...on, C.T. & Wood, A.S. (1981) ... more dispersed aquatic health professional services. Psychiatric Psychiatry, 39, 156-176.

Smart, S. (1991) ... The association of mental health ... Prevention ... in Medicine ...

25 The implication of using Women Centred Therapy in the provision of positive mental health care

C. Jebali

Introduction

Throughout history up to the present day, women's emotional needs have been undervalued and consequently inadequately attended to. Statistical evidence to date points to the fact that women far outnumber men in the usage of mental health facilities and more women than men are receiving psychological treatments, whether this be drugs or counselling (Davis 1985). Two questions arise from this evidence, firstly, why is it that women appear to be so susceptible to emotional distress at this level? and secondly, if women are so prevalent within the mental health system, are there adequate and relevant resources to effectively deal with them?

Within this paper an exploration of women's mental health will be made with emphasis being placed on the inadequacies of existing mental health practice in relation to women. This argument will be made in the context of advocating the need for Woman Centred Therapy, in which aspects of women's day to day experiences are viewed from very different perspectives. The essence of Women Centred Therapy is that an understanding of a woman's psychology must be sought from their experience in society, and not as it is traditionally viewed, that a woman's social role flows as a natural consequence from her psychology, which in turn is determined by biology. The analysis of women's psychology has developed as a result of the Women's Movement and has transcended the earlier presuppositions that sex differences would be explained through the differing conditioning processes, whereby behaviourist social learning theories were drawn on to illustrate how women were conditioned into emotional and cognitive subordination.

As Lynn Segal states:

'Women's liberation involved throwing off much of this false conditioning, relearning assertiveness, self confidence and the whole array of skills which had served men so long and so well, so well indeed that men could destroy women's active involvement in the shaping of their own destinies' (Segal 1983).

The consciousness raising group has been identified as the practical means through which attempts at feminist psychotherapy began. This paper will continue in an attempt to overview the beliefs and theoretical underpinning of feminist psychotherapy, looking mainly at the construction of the feminine personality as it has been perceived by Freudian psychotherapy, and the theory of object relations, which has served feminist psychotherapists as the fundamental basis for Women Centred Therapy.

It may be useful first of all to examine the extent to which women are exposed to mental health problems, and the nature of those problems. As stated earlier, women figure more highly than men in estimated statistics of mental health involvement e.g. almost 60% of the population of British psychiatric hospitals are women, and women have a 1 in 6 life chance of entering a psychiatric hospital; for men it is 1 in 9 (D.H.S.S. 1977). The majority of women patients are diagnosed as suffering neurotic or depressive type disorders. It is also estimated that these figures are not representative of the vast numbers of women that do not even reach specialist services, but are treated by their GP. Twice as many female as male patients are believed to be diagnosed with having mental health problems (Davis 1985).

It is at this point that it is quite feasible to question the diagnostic process, which presents the dual argument as to whether it is that GPs and psychiatrists are more likely to apply psychiatric labels to women, or is it that women are more likely to seek help with emotional problems than are men. The answer to this may lie in looking more closely at the psychological role of women. One of the first psychological demands that emerges from a woman's social role is that she must defer to others. This form of deferential behaviour is in keeping with the way in which woman's social role is developed.

The primary role for women continues to be that of wife and mother. Being a wife, creating a home and caring for babies involves extensive social preparation, as they are not inevitable consequences of women's biology (Eichenbaum & Orbach 1985). Women are expected to be the emotional gate-keepers within the family; emotions are felt to be a woman's concern. Throughout all this women are not expected to receive anything in return and as a consequence come to believe that they are not important in themselves for themselves, this being a typical feature of any victim of oppression.

'The... subtle denigration women encounter daily through personal contacts, the impressions gathered from the images and media about them, the discrimination in matters of behaviour, employment and education which they endure, should make it no very special cause for surprise that women develop group characteristics common to those who suffer minority status and a marginal existence' (Millett 1977).

Many women retreat to their GP, not expecting to be given understanding or constructive help as this would be perceived as being over demanding. Instead they are seeking a method to enable them to continue in their existing role, a form of crutch, which is usually offered in the form of medication and a psychiatric label (Johnstone 1987).

This may explain the above mentioned dilemma; In keeping with their psychosocial note it is possible that women are more likely to seek out their GP, which enables the medical profession to make gross assumptions about the fragility of women's psychology in comparison to men's, which in turn perpetuates the myth that women are in some way naturally more predisposed to mental illness than are men. It is, however, becoming increasingly well documented that many GPs have a tendency to devalue women's specific medical problems such as pre-menstrual syndrome, miscarriage and the menopause as facets of women's imagination, thus depriving them of appropriate scientific investigation, and instead conveniently applying psychiatric labels.

The unsatisfactory process by which women tend to fall within the parameter of experiencing mental health problems is only matched in its complexity and inadequacies by the equally unsatisfactory process of how women are treated by traditional mental health practices.

One of the major reasons for the development of the Women's Therapy Centre in London by Louise Eichenbaum and Susie Orbach was the realisation that most current theory and practice of psychotherapy is imprisoned within conventional patriarchal ideology and in order to properly serve women there was a need to articulate a radically new psychological theory of women, based within feminist principles (Eichenbaum and Orbach 1985). When examining traditional psychiatric treatment of women as inpatients and within the community - it is evident that Doctors' and Nurses' understanding of women's psychology is based firmly within biological determinism and the patriarchal social structure. It can be argued that these assumptions, supported by both Medical and

Nurse education have a great impact in perpetuating and colluding with women's low self esteem and devalued self-image.

Historically the management of women's minds through the regulation of their bodies has been a major preoccupation of the medical profession. Victorian Psychology of women was directed mainly by the theories of sexual difference, as reinforced through Darwinian Science, which upheld that not only were there fundamental physical differences between the sexes, but the mentalities of the sexes differed as well. It was therefore the combination of the physical and mental differences that made up the essence Doctors confidently called woman's 'nature'. Mental breakdown was believed to occur in women when they attempted to defy their nature e.g. by trying to be equal to men as opposed to subservient or by seeking alternatives or additions to their maternal functions. With consideration of the ethos which belied the diagnosis of women at this time, it comes as no surprise to find that the treatments available to women ranged from ineffective to barbaric and were always in keeping with the Victorian ideology of how women should behave.

'Victorian psychiatry silenced women as effectively through its ideology as the 'scolds bridle' had muzzled noisy women in Bedlam before reform' (Showalter 1982).

It is believed that the 'moral management' of women with mental illness as described during the 19th century is indeed part of women's history, and that the theories which it was based upon were convenient ramifications of existing social relations between the sexes. However from contemplation of the treatments of women in psychiatric institutions during the 19th century, it becomes increasingly disturbing to see that there are many parallels to be drawn between that time and the present day. An integral part of the programme of moral management of women in Victorian asylums was to impose ladylike values of silence, decorum, taste, piety and gratitude. Activities would involve, cleaning, baking, laundry work, serving and reading. Perhaps the most emphasis was placed on appearance.

Women were expected to take more care of the way they looked than men and their sanity would often be judged in conjunction with their compliance to middle class standards of fashion.

It would be a simple process to equate all these expectations of 19th Century women with those expressed in psychiatric wards today.

Therapies which are presently offered to women are very much in keeping with their expected social roles, in that Occupational Therapy generally consists of shopping, cooking, sewing and staff use their observations of how make up is applied and how clothes and hair are worn, in their nursing assessment of a woman's mental health. Rarely, if ever, are these criteria applied to men. Johnstone (1989) attributes this negative treatment of women to lack of knowledge and understanding of women specific issues within both nursing and medical professions.

There is currently no specialised training for nurses available in dealing with women's specific problems, such as rape, miscarriage, postnatal depression and certainly no emphasis placed on gender psychology or women centred counselling.

As Johnstone States:

'It is only to be expected, therefore, that psychiatric staff will unwittingly reinforce the values of the society they come from, even where this actually makes the problem worse, since they have not attained any higher degree of critical awareness than their patients' (Johnstone 1989).

Jebali (1991) argues for the necessity of incorporating relevant aspects of feminist theory and practice into Nurse Education in order that women should receive a more appropriate service than is available at present, by raising awareness of sexuality and gender issues.

It can be argued therefore, that in order for a clearer and more beneficial understanding of women's emotional problems to be achieved, there is a need to be aware of the psychology of women, which is not directed by pseudo biological imperatives to justify domesticity and the inferiority of women. This became an important issue within the Women's Movement during the 1970's, when it was felt that there was a need to understand how social expectations were affecting women on a psychological level. Consciousness raising groups were a major and vital component of the Women's Movement but after several years many women realised that changes in society were not keeping pace with their changing perceptions of their role at home, at work and in their relationships. Due to this inconsistency, women would find that many aspects of their behaviour, instead of being continually challenged and reshaped, seemed to stand still (Orbach and Eichenbaum 1985). A further implication of the consciousness raising process was that it initiated powerful feelings such as envy, competition, and anger, that many women could not cope with on a conscious level. These issues highlighted the limitations of the consciousness raising groups and led women to ask far deeper questions about their inner feelings, their capacity to change how they felt, and their ability to understand unconscious processes.

It would seem logical that women would look to psychoanalysis and psychotherapy as a detailed way of thinking about the construction of femininity and the psychology of women.

Psychoanalysis is a complex theory of human behaviour pioneered by

Sigmund Freud at the turn of the century which has evolved into the western world's most influential theory of the development of personality and behaviour (Williams 1979). The basis of the theory rests on the concept of unconscious motivation, forces and drives of which we are unaware, which originate in early childhood and are fraught with conflicts. Should these conflicts not be successfully resolved and integrated into the personality, neuroses and other maladaptive behaviours will be the result. The psychology of women, however was not a central concern of Freud's psychoanalytic theory, indeed he had stated that the mental life of women was less accessible than that of men and it was therefore impossible to know what women were really like.

The Women's Movement originally fiercely denounced the whole psychoanalytic tradition, viewing it as a bastion of male supremacy in our society (Segal 1983). Feminist objections to psychoanalysis are focused mainly on its phallocentric bias, the implicit assumption that the male is the model human being. Despite Freud's dismissal of women's psychology, he did in fact write three papers about this very issue, which became influential in developing and directing future work in this area.

'Femininity' was the third of these papers, and looked at how a woman develops out of a child. It was concerned with how normal female development in relation to sexuality occurs in women and reveals a great deal of negativity inherent in Freud's attitudes to women. Freud's theory of penis envy was well established when he wrote 'Femininity', and he continues this theme by focusing on the necessity for women following their bisexual stage in their early years to abandon masculine clitoral sexuality in favour of feminine sexuality of the passive receptive vagina. A further need of normal female development would be the abandonment of the mother as love object in favour of the father. This change of feelings grows from the girl's castration complex, for which she blames her mother. These developmental tasks, Freud believed, occurred at great psychic cost to a woman, resulting in early termination of psychic development and thus leaving her rigid and less open to the possibility of further growth and development. This was believed to be also due to the girl's entry into the Oedipus Complex, driven out of her attachment to her mother through the influence of her envy for the penis.

'Girls remain in (the Oedipus Complex) for an indeterminate length of time, they demolish it late, and even so incompletely. In these circumstances, the formation of the super-ego must suffer, it cannot attain the strength and independence which give it its cultural significance and feminists are not pleased when we point out to them the effects of this factor upon the average feminine character' (Freud 1905).

Freud also openly acknowledged his position of determining women's psychology from a biological reproductive position.

'I have only been describing women in so far as their nature is determined by their sexual function. It is true that influence extends very far, but we do not overlook the fact that an individual woman may be a human being in other respects as well' (Freud 1905).

It is clear from this type of statement why feminists felt that psychoanalytic theory was detrimental to women, but it gradually became evident, particularly through the work of feminist writers such as Juliet Mitchell, that feminists were wrong to dismiss Freud, however misogynist his work may appear, Mitchell believed that in order for women to ever understand the deeper discontents of their identity as something intrinsically problematic as opposed to something they acquired, there was a need to better understand the importance of Freud's discoveries about the central importance of the unconscious in adult life and the persistence of infertile desires and conflicts (Mitchell 1974). For feminists, a new project of feminist psychoanalytic theorising unfolded.

It has been the Object-relations school of psychoanalysis which has had direct influence on informing the practice of feminist therapy, and in particular the work of the Women's Therapy Centre formed by Louise Eichenbaum and Susie Orbach in 1976. The major objectives within this approach were to recognise the importance of Freud's discovery of the unconscious, in order to understand the importance of the integration of psychic life and the politics of everyday experience and to understand girls' psychological development. (Eichenbaum and Orbach 1985).

Guntrip and Winnicott, two major influences within the object relations school, have had particular impact on the development of Feminist Therapy. Their observations about the construction of personality were based within a relational context. Object relations theory is a materialist psychoanalysis, in that it recognises the need to become a human being and that this will occur through relationships, this being in direct contrast to classic Freudian theory. The object relations theory argues that babies are object directed from birth and that the later distortions and repressions of sexuality arise from distorted object relations which can occur in the earliest years. (Segal 1983) The object relations approach was seen to be compatible with feminism. It posited a materialist view of psychological development based on an individual's need for relationships and contact with another human being, and it stated that the first two years of life are the most important time for the development of the inner core of the person, the psyche and the personality together, referred to as the ego. It also places the importance on the mother-child relationship. Eichenbaum and Orbach's work extends this further, by focusing on the mother-daughter relationship as central to womens' lives. They see women as emotionally bereft, men are incapable of nurturing women as adults; and as the daughters of their own mothers they were taught to put their needs second, as indeed their mothers did as little girls. Consciously and unconsciously mothers teach their daughters to put away their needs for emotional care and attention, leaving them with feelings of deprivation and unworthiness.

'We would say that women are very emotionally deprived. Women are always appearing both to themselves and to others as having tremendous needs. This is because they are actually starving.' (Llewelyn 1981).

From this overview of women's mental health and its treatment, past and present, it is clear that many damaging assumptions have been made about the nature of women's minds which have had negative repercussions not only for how women are treated but also for the way that professionals and 'experts' are educated. Most traditional psychiatric practice, even if not consciously aware, recreates Victorian type ideology of women and echoes Freud at his misogynist worst, in that women's psychology continues to be assessed in relation to their biology. Consequently many women's lives are mapped out for them, and to stray from the acceptable route is viewed as deviance which is rationalised as mental illness. The feminist movement has made great advances in raising awareness and giving women hope in the knowledge that there are new and positive pathways to tread in rediscovering women's psychology, and the object relations approach has been a significant factor in this development.

As Segal (1983) states 'feminist therapy is about combining feminism and therapy to heal the damage done to women growing up female in a male dominated world'.

If, as health professionals, we are committed to the notion of promoting positive mental health I believe it is crucial to develop a far deeper understanding of women's psychology in relation to their social experience as a separate issue in order to prevent the concept of mental health being defined within patriarchal parameters.

References

Davis, A., Llewelyn, S. & Parry, G., (1985). Women and Mental Health, towards an Understanding. In E. Brook, A. Davis (Eds.) *Women, the family and Social Work*. Tavistock, London.

Eichenbaum, L., Orbach, S., (1985). *Understanding Women*. Penguin, London.

Freud, S., (1905). Femininity. In J. Williams (Ed.) *Psychology of women. Selected readings*. Norton & Co., New York./

Jebali, C., (1991). Working together to support women with postnatal depression. *Health Visitor Journal*. 62 (12).

Johnstone, L. (1987). *Users and abusers of psychiatry*. Routledge, London

Llewelyn, S., (1981). *No turning back*. Penguin, London.

Millett, K., (1977). *Sexual politics*. Virago Press, London.

Mitchell, J. (1974). *Psychoanalysis and feminism*. Penguin, London.

Segal, L., (1983). *Is the future female?* Virago Press. London.

Showalter, E., (1982). *The female malady*. Virago Press, London.

Williams, J. (1979). Psychoanalysis and the woman question. In J. Williams (Ed.) *Psychology of women. Selected readings*. Norton & Co., New York.

26 Mental health promotion in the workplace

R. Jenkins

Introduction

Chairman, Ladies and Gentlemen I'm delighted to be here to talk about promoting mental health at work. It's a subject close to my heart, partly from the perspective of the major Department of Health concern with prevention of mental illness, and partly from my own standpoint as a psychiatrist and epidemiologist with a long standing interest in mental health in occupational settings.

In order to clarify the opportunities for prevention and health promotion in the workplace, it is helpful to cover the different kinds of psychological illness, what they look like, how common they are, how long they last, their prevalence in work settings, their causes and consequences and implications for the workplace, and then to deduce potential strategies for primary, secondary and tertiary prevention.

It always helps to say what one isn't going to cover, and this talk is not about alcohol or drugs. That's not to say they're not important - they obviously are. But they have already received quite a lot of attention in industry. In this talk I want to focus on the **psychological illnesses**, the commonest of which are depression and anxiety, and which are mostly caused by environmental stresses.

In a conference such as this on mental health promotion, several disciplines, both practical and academic, converge, and each brings with them their own terminology and jargon, and this can cause considerable confusion.

The meaning of stress

So first of all, I would like to discuss what we mean by stress and by mental or psychological illness. The issue is an important one for two reasons. Firstly, while stress is a much abused term, with several different meanings, nonetheless in the sense of external pressure it is something most of us are happy to admit to having a little of. However, by contrast, psychological illness, while having more precise meanings such as depression or anxiety, is generally associated with a great deal of stigma, and most of us would not remotely wish to be thought mentally ill.

So, what do these terms mean, is there an overlap, and, dare one suggest it, should we dispense both with the pride of being stressed or pressured and with the stigma of being mentally ill?

The Oxford English Dictionary describes about 15 meanings of the word stress, several dating from the fourteenth century but for our purposes it helps to concentrate on three. The first is an external challenge (which can be a good thing). See figure 1. The second is external hardship and

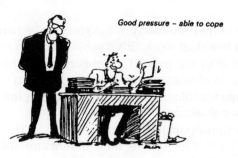

Good pressure – able to cope

Figure 1

advertising which when intolerable is (a bad thing). See Figure 2. and the third is the internal state induced within the individual by the external

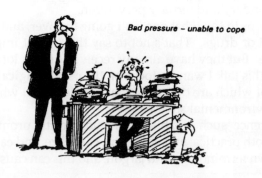

Bad pressure – unable to cope

Figure 2

adversity i.e. the **distress** or reaction of the person under stress. Thus the term 'stress' being used to refer to either cause or effect, and this is the cause of much confusion in the literature, and in our own understanding

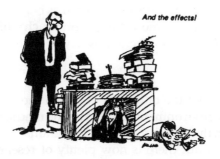

And the effects!

Figure 3

of the concept. See Figure 3.

We therefore need to emphasise the distinction between stress which refers to environmental demands and pressures on us (what the OED calls external hardship and adversity) and to stress which refers to the psychological and physical symptoms to which are the consequences of those environmental demands and pressures on us. The former sense is used in academic literature on the causation of mental illness, the latter sense is greatly used in the occupational literature.

What kinds of external stresses are there? There are many ways to classify stress, (see table 1) but a useful way to categorise it is into the different **broad social domains**, of marriage or intimate relationship: the other members of the immediate family, including children; social life,

Table 1
A classification of external social stresses and support

DOMAINS	STRESS	SUPPORTS
Marriage		
Family		
Social Life/Friends		
Housing		
Finance		
Work		

that is friends and acquaintances, and leisure activities; housing and living conditions; finance and occupation. All these different domains can be stressful.

A second useful categorisation of stress is by **duration of the event**. Thus we sometimes refer to **acute** life events such as bereavement, or job loss, or failing an exam, while more **long term or chronic** stresses would include loneliness, unemployment, poverty or illiteracy.

Social support

However, stress is not the only way in which the environment has an impact on us. **The environment can also be the medium of considerable support**. It is often thought that only close relationships have the capacity to provide support but there is now plenty of research evidence, and indeed it is commonsense that all the different social domains have the capacity to be supportive, as well as to be stressful. The concept of social support refers to information leading the individual to believe that he or she is cared for, liked and loved, to believe that he or she belongs to a network of communication and mutual obligation (Cobb 1976). This support is accessible to the individual through their social ties to other individuals, groups and the larger community. House (1981) has extended Cobb's definition of social support to include

(1) emotional support (esteem, affection, trust, concern, listening)
(2) appraisal support (affirmation, feedback, social comparison) which is associated with information relevant to self evaluation
(3) informational support (advice, suggestion, directives, information)
(4) instrumental support (aid in kind, money, labour, time, help in modifying the environment).

Why am I bothering to mention support? Surely it is really only stress that counts? Well, the reason is that we have evidence that support, not only protects us against the effects of stress but also that it has a beneficial effect in its own right. Social support can have a beneficial effect on normal growth, physical diseases such as infections and heart attacks, and mental illness.

Reactions to stress

Let us take a look now at the **different ways in which we react to stress**. We respond by gearing our body and mind up for appropriate action. However, if the stress goes on for too long then physical and psychological symptoms can occur. Physical symptoms can include backache, headache, high blood pressure, indigestion or even ulcers. Psychological symptoms can include fatigue, poor concentration, irritability, low or depressed mood, anxiety, obsessional thoughts or actions, poor sleep, poor appetite, depersonalisation and derealisation.

When does a symptom become an illness? In general when it occurs with a cluster of other symptoms, when it lasts more than a couple of weeks and when it is interfering with normal daily activities.

So what happens if we use epidemiological screening techniques, firstly in the general population at large, and secondly in the working population? We find that there are some psychological symptoms which are extremely common, and some which are relatively rare (see table 2). The symptoms which are extremely common are fatigue, irritability and poor concentration. A little less common are depression, anxiety, impaired sleep and appetite. Somewhat more unusual are obsessional thoughts, and activities and depersonalisation. Much rarer still are abnormal beliefs, abnormal perceptions, extremes of mood, and thought disorder. Table 3 shows the prevalence of these symptoms in a population

Table 2
Classification of psychological symptoms

Minor	(non psychotic)	Major	(psychotic)
1.	Excessive concern about health e.g. heart disease, cancer	1.	Abnormal beliefs
2.	Fatigue	2.	Abnormal perception
3.	Irritability	3.	Abnormal perception
4.	Poor concentration	4.	Thought disorder
5.	Low mood/depression		
6.	Anxiety		
7.	Obsessional thoughts and actions		
8.	Poor sleep		
9.	Poor appetite		
10.	Depersonalisation Derealisation		

of executive officers.

How do we categorise psychological illness? We make several broad distinctions (see Table 4). Firstly, there are the common illnesses of depression and anxiety, (rather akin to the common chest and gut diseases such as colds, flu, bronchitis, and tummy upsets). These occur in 15-30% of the population.

315

Table 3

Comparison of the frequencies of symptoms and manifest abnormalities reported at the first clinical assessment by interviewed male and female executive officers (weighted to represent all respondents)

% with	Men	Women
Somatic symptoms	13.3 (24)	33.1 (46)
Excessive concern	10.2 (19)	16.4 (23)
Fatigue	29.3 (54)	36.7 (51)
Sleep disturbance	14.7 (27)	15.1 (21)
Irritability	21.6 (39)	26.4 (36)
Lack of concentration	37.0 (68)	26.9 (37)
Depression	28.0 (51)	38.9 (54)
Depressive thoughts	24.1 (44)	26.9 (37)
Anxieties	34.5 (63)	32.2 (44)
Phobias	12.8 (23)	15.6 (21)
Obsessions	18.5 (34)	16.2 (22)
Depersonalization	8.9 (16)	6.1 (8)
Slow, retardation	12.1 (22)	6.9 (10)
Suspicious	2.6 (5)	3.3 (5)
Histrionic	1.9 (4)	0 (0)
Depressed	22.9 (42)	25.1 (35)
Anxious	10.8 (20)	5.9 (8)
Elated	1.9 (4)	0 (0)
Flat	0 (0)	0 (0)
Delusions	0 (0)	1.8 (2)
Hallucinations	0 (0)	0 (0)
Intellectual impairment	0 (0)	0 (0)

The numbers of subjects are shown in parentheses

Secondly, there are the much rarer and generally more severe illnesses such as manic-depressive psychosis, depressive psychosis and schizophrenia, (akin to the rare severe diseases of chest and gut such as pneumonia, cancer, ulcerative colitis etc) and these occur in 2-3% of the adult population.

Thirdly, there are the organic diseases which result from permanent damage to the brain, and these include senile dementia, (of unknown

316

cause) arteriosclerotic dementia (from arteriosclerosis of the blood vessels), and the dementia associated with AIDS and alcohol. Senile and arteriosclerotic dementia combined occur in 10% of the population aged over 65.

Fourthly, there are the personality disorders which are life long attributes of the person, life long traits, which are termed disorders if and when they are severe enough to handicap the person in some way. We do not know how prevalent these conditions are.

Table 4

Categories of psychological illness

		Prevalence in Adult Population
Psychoses	Affective Psychosis Schizophrenia	1%
Dementia	Senile) Arteriosclerotic) AIDS Alcohol	10% over age 65
Neuroses	Depression) Anxiety) Phobias) Obsessional)	15-30%
Personality Disorders	Cyclothymic) Anxious) Shy) Schizoid) Obsessional) Hysterical) Psychopathic)	?

This talk is mostly about the first group of illnesses, depression and anxiety.

The epidemiological studies

Most epidemiological work has been done on the general population in the community, and there are now a plethora of good epidemiological studies over the last 20 years showing that about 100-250 per 1000 adults have a psychological disorder in any one year (see Tables 5 and 6). By far the majority of these are depression and anxiety. Only 1-3% of this is psychosis of some kind, mostly schizophrenia and affective psychosis.

317

Table 5
Community studies

Author	N	Place	Instrument	Prevalence per 1,000
Myers et al 1984	3,481	USA	DIS	267
Goldberg, Kay and Thompson (1974)	213	South Manchester	GHQ	184
Finlay, Jones and Burvill (1977)	2,342	Perth, Australia	GHQ	120
Ingham, Rawnsley and Hughes (1972)	300	Industrial Wales (Rhondda)	CMI	175
	581	Rural Wales (Vale of Glamorgan)		103
Dilling 1979	1,231	Bavaria, W Germany	CIS	193
Weissman, Myers and Harding 1978	511	Newhaven USA	SADS-RDC	178
Orley and Wing 1979	191	Uganda Village	PSE	241
Duncan Jones and Henderson 1980	756	Canberra, Australia	PSE	90
Brown and Harris 1978	458	Camberwell, London	PSE	170
Brown et al 1977	154	North Uist, Outer Hebrides	PSE	120

Reproduced with kind permission from D. Goldberg and P. Huxley (1980): Mental illness in the community: the pathway to psychiatric care, Tavistock Press.

Table 6
Prevalence rates per 1,000 population at risk for random samples of the general population for all psychiatric illness in the past month; recent surveys based on direct assessment by standardised research interview

Author	N	Place	Instrument	Total Rates
Hodiamont et al 1987	486	Nijmegen, Holland	GHQ/PSE	73
Duncan-Jones and Henderson 1978	157	Canberra, Australia	GHQ/PSE	90
Bebbington et al 1981	800	London, England	PSE	109
Reiger et al 1988	18,571	5 sites USA	DIS	112
Vazquez-Barquero et al 1987	425	Cantabria, Spain	PSE	147
Mavreas et al 1986	489	Athens, Greece	GHQ/PSE	160
Weissman, et al 1978	511	Newhaven, USA	SADS/RDC	178
Dilling 1980	1,231	Bavaria, W Germany	CIS	193
Vazquez-Barquero et al 1981	415	Batzan Valley, Spain	CIS	239
Orley and Wing 1979	191	2 villages: Uganda	PSE	241
Cheng 1988	489	3 areas: Taiwan	CHQ/CIS	262
Overall rates				164

Abbreviations:

GHQ = General Health Questionnaire   SADS = Schedule for Affective Disorders and Schizophrenia

CHQ = Chinese Health Questionnaire   RDC = Research Diagnostic Criteria

PSE = Present State Examination   CIS = Clinical Interview Schedule

DIS = Diagnostic Interview Schedule

Reproduced with kind permission from D. Goldberg and P. Huxley (1991): Common Mental Disorders - a Biopsychosocial model, Routledge.

The numbers of epidemiological studies carried out in industry is much lower, and is far lower in this country than in the US (see table 7). However, they tend to show roughly what you would expect, namely that those disorders which are common in the general population, i.e., depression and anxiety, are also common in people at work while those disorders which are rare in the general population are even rarer in working populations. So occupational doctors, like GPs, will tell you that the bread and butter of their work is depression and anxiety.

Table 7
Occupational studies

Author	N	Population	Instrument	Prevalence per 1000		
				M	F	Total
Fraser R 1947	3,000	Light and medium engineering workers	Medical assesment	283	360	300
Heron and Braithwaithe	184	Colliery workers,	MMQ			
		Sedentary		334		
		Surface manual		452		
		Surface and underground		522		
Jenkins, MacDonald, Murray & Strathdee	162	Times Journalists 1 month after receipt of redundancy notice and	CIS (GHQ)	.		378 (360)
		2 months prior to closure date. At sale of newspaper when redundancy notices, revoked, and new proprietor arrived.				378 (369)
		12 weeks after threat of redundancy had been removed.				324 (243)
MacBride, Lancee and Freeman 1981	274	Air traffic controllers during an industrial dispute	CHQ			480
		4 months later				270
		10 months later				310
Jenkins 1985	184	Executive officers in Civil Service	CIS	362	343	
McGrath, Reid and Boore 1989	171	Nurses	GHQ			270
		Teachers				310
		Social Workers				370
Stansfeld, Marmot et al 1991 (unpublished)	10,314	Whitehall civil servants (administrative unified grades 1-7)	GHQ	248	353	
		SEO, HEO, EO,		247	331	
		Clerical		216	252	

How long do depression and anxiety last? Research studies show that while a half are better in 6-12 months, a third to a half last longer than a year. The longer lasting illnesses tend to be those which are associated with particular social stresses and sometimes with physical illness. (Mann et. al. 1981, Jenkins 1985). These were people who kept a daily health diary for 3 months, 84 days of physical and psychological symptoms:

a. well
b. depressed
c. backache
d. multiple symptoms

And what causes psychological illness?

The very severe psychotic illness have a strong genetic contribution (up to about 50%), and we know that from studies of identical and non identical twins who were adopted at birth. However, the non-psychotic illnesses, depression and anxiety don't have a genetic component. They are caused by environmental stress of one kind and another, and by physical illness.

It's sometimes said, well why should industry worry about these illnesses? Surely work doesn't cause them. Well, we have seen that work is one of the six social domains in which stresses and support occur, and in some people, it is a very dominant domain where we may spend more than eight hours a day, and to that extent is a potent medium, for better or for worse. But I must emphasise that the cause of depression and anxiety is nearly always multifactorial. There will always be a number of causes operating.

The causes of psychological illness can be classified into psychological, social and biological and it is helpful to think of them in terms of **predisposing factors** i.e., factors which may have been operating literally years ago to make one more vulnerable to illness, **precipitating factors** i.e., which precipitate the onset of illness and **maintaining factors** i.e., which prolong the illness (see Tables 8,9 and 10).

Again, it can be helpful to adopt a parallel with physical illness. Predisposing factors to chest infection may be a low immunity, smoking or allergy or exposure to chemicals. Precipitating factors may be a chill combined with exposure to a virus. Maintaining factors may be not resting, or a poor diet etc.

So you can see that the working environment is one of the environmental influences, operating for better or worse, on the predisposition, precipitation and maintenance of psychological illness. The important stressors and supports in the occupational setting, can be broadly categorised into

Table 8
Causes of mental illness

<u>PREDISPOSING FACTORS</u>

PHYSICAL	-	GENES, INTRAUTERINE DAMAGE, BIRTH TRAUMA, PERSONALITY DISORDER
SOCIAL	-	PHYSICAL AND EMOTIONAL DEPRIVATION IN CHILDHOOD, DUE TO BEREAVEMENT, SEPARATION, FAMILY DISCORD, CHRONIC SOCIAL DIFFICULTIES AT WORK AND AT HOME, LACK OF SUPPORTIVE RELATIONSHIPS
PSYCHOLOGICAL	-	POOR PARENTAL MODELS, LOW SELF ESTEEM

Table 9
Causes of mental illness

<u>PRECIPITATING FACTORS</u>

PHYSICAL	-	RECENT INFECTIONS, DISABLING INJURY, MALIGNANT DISEASE
SOCIAL	-	RECENT LIFE EVENTS, EG THREAT OF REDUNDANCY, UNEMPLOYMENT, MAJOR ILLNESS IN THE FAMILY, A CHILD LEAVING HOME, SEPARATION OR DIVORCE, AND THE LOSS OF A SUPPORTIVE RELATIONSHIP.
PSYCHOLOGICAL	-	MALADAPTIVE FEELINGS OF HOPELESSNESS, HELPLESSNESS

321

Table 10
Causes of mental illness

MAINTAINING FACTORS

PHYSICAL   -   CHRONIC PAIN OR
                         DISABILITY, SIDE EFFECTS
                         OF MEDICATION, FAILURE
                         TO TAKE MEDICATION

SOCIAL   -   CHRONIC SOCIAL STRESS,
                         LACK OF SOCIAL SUPPORT

PSYCHOLOGICAL   -   LOW SELF ESTEEM, LACK
                         OF EXPECTATION OF
                         RECOVERY

1. factors intrinsic to the job
2. role in the organisation
3. career development
4. relationships at work
5. organisational structure and climate.

What are the consequences of mental illness?

For employers, this is generally an even more important consideration than the cause. (See table 11)

Firstly there are consequences for physical health

People with psychological disorders have an increased risk of physical illness, and indeed mortality which is not just from suicide. The risk of death from all causes is twice the norm in severe non-psychotic depression (Sims and Prior 1978) and the risk of death is four or five times the norm in schizophrenia and manic depressive psychosis, excluding suicide (Fox

Table 11
Consequences of mental illness

1. INCREASED RISK OF PHYSICAL ILLNESS AND DEATH

2. DOMESTIC CONSEQUENCES

    MARRIAGE

    FINANCE

    HOUSING

    FAMILY LIFE

    SOCIAL LIFE

3. OCCUPATIONAL CONSEQUENCES

    SICKNESS ABSENCE

    RELATIONS WITH COLLEAGUES

    WORK PERFORMANCE

    ACCIDENTS

    LABOUR TURNOVER

and Godblatt 1982). The risk of suicide for minor depression and anxiety is not so very great, but for very severe illness it is substantial: 10% schizophrenia; 15% manic depression; 10% alcoholics.

Secondly there are domestic consequences

Psychological illness may cause a variety of problems in the social domains of marriage, finance, housing, family life and social life. Thus those domains are not only the medium for stress and support, i.e., the causes of illness, they are also the medium for the consequences of illness. For example, continued depression or irritability may place a great strain on the understanding and tolerance of a spouse, eventually leading to marital problems. If prolonged, this may cause more serious disruption of the relationship, and may occasionally lead to divorce, with far reaching long term consequences for children and for the joint finance.

The depressed person may become unable to manage his financial affairs, bills may remain unpaid and letters unanswered. Essential house repairs may not be carried out, leading to further deterioration in the property which could easily have been prevented. Parental illness can lead to conduct disorders and emotional disturbances in the children. Children are usually affected if both parents are simultaneously depressed for any length of time, but usually remain unscathed as long as one parent is well and fully functional. There is a tendency to withdraw from friendships when depressed, thus losing opportunities for social support. All these social consequences form a vicious circle which in turn acts as further stress on the individual, maintaining the illness. On a more optimistic note, occasionally an illness can provide an opportunity to rethink one's life, reorder priorities, and that can be very positive.

Lastly but not least, there are:

The occupational consequences of psychological illness

and these include

    Sickness absence
    impaired relations with colleagues
    reduced work performance
    accidents
    labour turnover

All of these have measurable social and economic costs, and because these costs may be used in the decision as to whether it is cost effective to initiate preventive strategies in the workplace, I would like to take a closer look at one common consequence, sickness absence.

Assessing the contribution of mental illness to sickness absence

Three methods have been used to determine the contribution of psychological disorders to sickness absence. The first is based on the examination of the diagnoses given by GPs on sickness certificates. These figures are very helpful BUT although high are nonetheless considerable **under**estimates since, like all figures derived from rates of diagnosed or treated illness, they are affected by the individual's readiness to seek medical care for his symptoms, by the availability of medical services, and by the primary care doctor's ability to diagnose mental illness and treat it. And we know that on average GPs miss half the depression that presents to them (Goldberg & Huxley 1991). And even if the doctor does diagnose it, he may not label it as such on the certificate because he is aware of the stigmatisation that often occurs. And of course this method cannot include uncertified absence.

The second method, used by Fraser and his colleagues during the war, is based on retrospective attribution of spells of absence to depression and anxiety made by research doctors on the basis of lengthy personal interviews with the subjects, and access to their medical records. Using this method, Fraser and his colleagues found that depression and anxiety caused between a quarter and a third of all absence from work in the munitions factories. Such a method avoids the disadvantages associated with simply basing estimates on sickness absence certificates. However, the method is based on the notion that an episode of sickness absence may indeed be attributed to one particular cause, and it ignores the overwhelming evidence from Professor Warr's research unit that most absence is voluntary behaviour which is affected not only be demographic and environmental factors, but also buy the individual's attitude to his work, as well as by the presence of a physical or psychological disorder.

In order to overcome this latter problem, the third method makes no attempt to attribute one particular episode of absence to any one cause, but rather to make comparisons of the annual absence taken between individuals with identified minor psychological illness, and those without. Using this method, it is found that the presence of depression and anxiety, does make a huge contribution to sickness absence, and that this contribution is greater for certified absence than uncertified (even though the absence is usually certified as due to physical rather than psychological illness), and is greater for duration than frequency (Jenkins, Ferguson).

Labour turnover is another costly phenomenon. It is costly to the employer in terms of wasted training resources and work experience. It is costly to the individual in terms of disrupted career pattern, attendant social disruptions such as loss of colleagues, a break in income, insecurity for the family, and the risk of unemployment. Attempts to understand the causes of labour turnover have largely concentrated on the relation between occupational attitudes and labour turnover (Porter & Steers, Telaachi, Pettman), but there are a few studies suggesting that there is a link between mental health and labour turnover. My own study of civil servants showed that the psychological symptoms score was twice as high in men and women who subsequently left the organisation within the next twelve months than in those who stayed. Mental health was just as important as occupational attitudes in predicting labour turnover. So it would seem that there are definite advantages to treating psychological illness fast before it results in these costly consequences. So, what are the possibilities for preventing mental illness at work.

Primary prevention

i.e., preventing the illness from happening in the first place, this entails action to ensure that the workplace itself does not cause depression and anxiety. The major aetiological factors here are low job discretion, low use of skills, low or high work demands, low task variety, high uncertainty, poor working conditions and low interpersonal support. This entails consultation with employers and training of line management staff.

Secondary prevention

i.e., the early detection and prompt management of depression and anxiety so that they do not become chronic, and lead to excessive distress and knock on consequences to family and children, as well as sickness absence, reduce effectiveness and labour turnover. This can be achieved by general education of line managers to detect the early symptoms, and the establishment of an organisational policy of action, depending on the severity of the condition e.g., a simple exploratory and supportive discussion, referral to a welfare officer, or to the personnel department, referral to an occupational health department, referral to own GP, and in severe cases referral to the specialist services. It may be helpful for companies to form the requisite links with DHA occupational health departments if they don't have their own in house occupational health service, and also with a local department of psychiatry. It would also be worth considering, in addition, whether to set up a confidential counselling scheme, rather like the American Employee Assistance Programme.

Tertiary prevention

i.e., the rehabilitation back to work of people who have had a fairly severe illness with extensive time off work. They need to be 'titrated' back to work, and this requires careful dialogue and planning between the employee, their doctor and psychiatrist, line manager and personnel officer.

It is possible to target people in high risk situations for extra support e.g., those immediately pre-retirement, or undergoing job transition. This is reactive primary prevention as it is reacting to a particular stressor, either before or immediately after it. It is also possible to give everyone extra help with coping skills, self-assertion, exercise, stress management etc and this is proactive primary prevention.

In view of the considerable morbidity in the workplace, and its attendant consequences, it is initially important to encourage the dissemination of workplace policies on mental health.

Conclusion

I started this talk by identifying the paradox that we are all a little proud of pressure of stress but that we are ashamed of psychological illness. I would like to submit to you that both are inappropriate responses. **Taking pride** in the pressures or stress in our lives may prevent us from taking action to reduce it either for ourselves or our colleagues, and to increase our support, before the stress results in illness.

Similarly, **being ashamed** of depression and anxiety may also prevent us from seeking help to treat it as fast as possible. We will all experience it at some time or another. Rather, we need to take pride in our ability to minimise our stresses, mobilise our supports, and to seek help for ourselves or our colleagues if and when it is needed.

References

Bebbington, P., Hurry, J., Tennant, C., Sturt, E., & Wing, J. (1981). Epidemiology of mental disorders in Camberwell. *Psychological Medicine*, **11**, 561-581.

Brown, G. W., & Harris, T., (1978). *Social origins of depression. A study of psychiatric disorder in women*. London: Tavistock Press.

Cheng, T. A. (1988). A community study of minor psychiatric morbidity in Taiwan. *Psychological Medicine*, **18**, 953-968.

Cherniss, C. (1980). *Staff burnout: Job stress in human services*. Beverley Hills, California. Sage Publications.

Cobb, S. (1976). Social support as a moderator of life stress. *Psychosomatic Medicine*, **38**, 300-314.

Dilling, H. (1980). Psychiatry and primary health services: Results in a field survey. *Acta Psychiatrica Scandinavica Supplement* No. 285, **62**, 15-22.

Jones, D. P., & Henderson, P. (1978). The use of a two stage design in a prevalence survey. *Social Psychiatry*, **30**, 187-198.

Finlay-Jones, R. & Burvill, P. (1977). The prevalence of minor psychiatric morbidity in the community. *Psychological Medicine*, **7**, 474-489.

Fox, A. J., & Goldblatt, P. O. (1982). *Longitudinal study - sociodemographic mortality differential LS No. 1, 1971-1975*. London HMSO.

Jenkins, R. (1985a). *Sex differences in minor psychiatric morbidity*. Psychological medicine monograph No. 7, Cambridge University Press.

Jenkins, R. (1985b). Minor psychiatric morbidity in employed young men and women, and its contribution to sickness absence. *British Journal of Industrial Medicine*, **42**, 147-154.

Jenkins, R. (1985). Minor psychiatric morbidity and labour turnover. *British Journal of Industrial Medicine*, **42**, 534-539.

Jenkins, R. (1980). Preliminary communications: Minor psychiatric morbidity in employed men and women and its contribution to sickness absence. *Psychological Medicine*, **10**, 751-757.

Jenkins, R., MacDonald, A., Murray, J., & Strathdee, G. (1982). Minor psychiatric morbidity and the threat of redundancy in a professional group. *Psychological Medicine*, **12**, 799-807.

Jenkins, R., Mann, A. H., & Belsey, E. (1981). Design and use of a short interview to assess social stress and support in research and clinical settings. *Social Science and Medicine*, 15E, **3**, 195-203.

Johns, G. & Nicholson, N. (1982). The meanings of absence: New strategies for theory and research. In B. M. Slaur & L. L. Cummings (Eds.), *Research in organisational behaviour*. Greenwich: CTJAI Press.

MacBride, A., Lancee, W. & Freeman, S. (1981). The psychosocial impact of a labour dispute. *Journal of Occupational Psychology*, **54**, 125-133.

Mann, A. H., Jenkins, R. & Belsey, E. (1981). The twelve month outcome of patients with neurotic illness in general practice. *Psychological Medicine*, **11**, 535-550.

Mavreas, V., Beis, A., Mouijias, A., Rigeni, F., & Lyketsas, G. (1986). Prevalence of psychiatric disorders in Athens: A community study. *Social Psychiatry*, **21**, 172-181.

McDermott, D. (1984). Professional burnout and its relation to job characteristics, satisfaction and control. *Journal of Human Stress*, 79-85.

McGrath, A., Reid, N., & Boore, J. (1989). Occupational stress in nursing. *International Journal of Nursing Studies*, **25**, 343-358.

Myers, J. K., Weissman, M. M. Tischler, G. L. et al. (1984). Six month prevalence of psychiatric disorders in three communities. *Archives of General Psychiatry*, **41**, 959-67.

Orley, J., & Wing, J. (1979). Psychiatric disorder in two African villages. *Archives of General Psychiatry*, **36**, 513-520.

Regier, D., Boyd, J., Burke, J., Rae, D., Myders, J., Kramer, M., Robins, L., George, L., Karno, M., & Locke, B. (1988). One month prevalence of mental disorders in the United States. *Archives of General Psychiatry*, **45**, 977-985.

Sims, A., & Prior, P. (1978). The pattern of mortality in severe neuroses.

British Journal of Psychiatry, **133**, 299-305.

Stansfeld, S., & Marmot, M. (1991). (unpublished). Whitehall II study of civil servants.

Vazquez-Barquero, J., Munoz, P., & Madox, Jauregi, V. (1981). The interaction between physical illness and neurotic morbidity in the community. *British Journal of Psychiatry*, **139**, 328-355.

Vazquez-Barquero, J., Diez-Mannique, J. F., Pena, C., Aldama, J., Samaniego Roderiginez, C., Menandez Arango, J., & Mirapeix, C. (1987). A community mental health survey in Canbalima: A general description of morbidity. *Psychological Medicine*, **17**, 227-241.

Weissman, M., Myers, J. & Harding, P. (1978). Psychiatric disorders in a US urban community: 1975/76. *American Journal of Psychiatry*, **135**, 459-462.

27 Scotland wakes up to the idea of mental health

K. Keddie

The mental health movement in Scotland is in its infancy but, to my mind, there are significant changes occurring within the nation which I shall refer to shortly.

First, I would like to set the scene in its historical context and remind you that the treatment of people with mental health problems in Scotland goes back to 1781, when the hospital I work at - originally the Montrose Asylum, and now call Sunnyside Royal Hospital - was founded. Clinical records began there in 1818 with 'The Register of Lunatics'. The first entry for a patient was in relation to a Martha Wallace, a domestic servant who had been admitted at the age of 26 to the Asylum in 1784. Her malady had been caused by the 'conduct of a fellow servant, who stole some article and concealed this in Martha Wallace's trunk, thus escaping detection by directing suspicion to an innocent party'. That particular patient remained in the Asylum until her death at the age of seventy.

The careers of two Scottish asylum doctors, who worked in Montrose, reflect the high standards that were available for patients in our country last century. The first was William Alexander Francis Browne, who rose from provincial surgeon to the superintendencies at Montrose and then Dumfries before being appointed as the first Scottish Commissioner in Lunacy under the 1857 Scottish Lunacy Act.

In the autumn of 1836, at the age of 32, Browne broke new ground by giving a series of public lectures to the Asylum managers and local notables on the treatment of insanity. These lectures were published in 1837 in a book entitled 'What Asylums were, are and ought to be' (Browne, 1837).

The other influential doctor was Dr. James Howden who was appointed as Superintendent at Montrose in 1857. He had graduated from Edinburgh University and had spent some time at the Royal Edinburgh Hospital prior to moving North. His reign lasted for 40 years. Dr. Howden's strength, and one that was repeatedly acknowledged by the Commissioners in Lunacy on their six-monthly visits, was his ability to organise a programme of both work and recreation for all those patients well enough to be involved.

Like other such institutions in the latter half of the 19th century, Montrose Asylum functioned in the manner of a large, self-sufficient country household, where domestic concerns prevailed over medical matters. Moral management rather than therapeutic intervention was the order of the day. Among the hospital archives at Montrose is a collection of several hundred photographic plates - taken by William Orkney, the Clerk of Works - which capture the inmates as people and not patients. These plates, together with the Board Minutes and patient records, help to bring alive life at the Montrose Asylum at the turn of the century.

Treatment for those afflicted with serious mental illnesses - as opposed to neurotic disorders or the now seemingly widespread 'problems with everyday living' - has been until comparatively recent times ineffective, humiliating and cruel. There were however advances in the medical sciences after the Great War which began to have a major impact on the outlook for many of those with chronic mental illnesses. The Montrose Asylum took a lead in keeping up with contemporary developments. One reads that in 1926 at Montrose 'Malarial inoculation' was introduced for general paralysis of the insane (Presley, 1981). In 1938 the newly appointed physician superintendent noted that 'hypoglycaemic shock treatment', used in the treatment of schizophrenia, was 'still in its experimental stage'. A year later shock therapy - later to be known as ECT - was introduced for the first time within the hospital.

Moving on to more recent times I should like to emphasise the close collaboration there has been for the past 20 years between the Scottish Division of the Royal College of Psychiatrists and the Scottish Association for Mental Health, the voluntary organisation responsible for safeguarding standards of care for those with mental health problems. Currently there are within Scotland 24 psychiatric hospitals and 16 of these have more than 500 beds. The Association feels that psychiatric hospitals, being often large and remote, perpetuate the stigma that people with mental health problems experience and suggests that over the next 10 years there should be a gradual transfer of resources from institutions to the community.

For the past 5 years I have served on the management committee of the S.A.M.H. as the representative of the Royal College of Psychiatrists. As a result of this experience I have learned to examine my own feelings and ideas as a caring, professional person. I undertook my medical studies in the 1950s and my psychiatric training in the early 1960s. My attitudes to patient care have tended to reflect the orthodoxy of those decades. As a result of working with enthusiastic and energetic people from S.A.M.H. I have found myself less rigid in my approach to patients, relatives and colleagues. I prefer to be on first name terms with staff and I wonder if I have at last stepped off the pedestal marked 'Medical Professional: do not touch or even approach'?

A year or so ago S.A.M.H. laid down fundamental principles relating to the prevention and management of emotional disorders. The opening statement reads: 'In the pursuit of health, people should not be disadvantaged because of their ethnic group, age, gender, sexual orientation, religious beliefs or by reason of where they live, their economic or social conditions.' The first four principles are as follows:-

1. Health: our society must become aware of the positive need to promote mental health.
2. Dignity: the paramount consideration in planning mental health care must be recognition of the human dignity of those who need help.
3. Rights: the fundamental human rights of a person are not lost if he or she becomes ill.
4. Advocacy: people who use mental health services should be able to engage in self-advocacy and have representations made on their behalf.

Recently Robin Laing, Director of S.A.M.H., has been discussing with his colleagues the need to have a policy with respect to the promotion of mental health. The aims of such a policy would encompass the following:-

1. Allowing people to feel comfortable with themselves and with others.
2. Engendering feelings of confidence to deal with life's crises.
3. Ensuring that individuals have positive feelings about life.
4. Working to ensure that everyone fulfils as much of their potential as possible.

The Scots are well known for their strong objections to public expressions of affection. This in turn can lead to disquiet and even stress. S.A.M.H. think it would be in the interests of positive mental health to encourage the setting up of workshops in schools and within firms in order to encourage the idea that it is alright to discuss, and to share, feelings. S.A.M.H. hopes to issue some literature on these matters and see as a model the recent documents 'Promoting Mental Health at Work' produced by the C.B.I. and the Health and Safety leaflet 'Mental Health at Work'. S.A.M.H. encourages the setting up of local associations of mental health and there are now a total of 20 within Scotland, the most recent one being that of my own area, Angus. S.A.M.H. looks forward to working closely with local associations in the organising of local events which will promote public awareness of mental health.

Till now the associations have concentrated on providing facilities for ex-users of the psychiatric services such as day centres and counselling services. The angus Association has decided to concentrate on an educational role by having a series of public meetings in each of the towns within the county at which issues can be debated. The emphasis will be on helping individuals and groups in the community in ways of building up confidence and tackling stress.

Within Scotland in recent years there have been widespread changes in family patterns, social mobility and in the labour market. Some of the statistics make disturbing reading. The rising divorce rate means that 1 in 6 Scottish families is now headed by a lone parent, 9 out of 10 being women. Some of the most worrying statistics relate to nutrition with 40,640 families within a population of 5 million - according to a recent National Children's Homes survey - being reported as not having enough money for food (Duncan, 1992).

Women's Aid in Scotland is a network of locally based groups run by women, for women who have been abused, and any children they may have. The numbers of women in contact with Women's Aid has risen from 4651 in 1980/81 to 17257 in 1990/91.

Many of Scotland's current social problems relate to drinking habits. The use and abuse of alcohol is central to the question of the mental health of the Scottish population. This is not because the per capita consumption of alcohol is very high (there are many other countries in the drinking league table above us) but because the social pattern of consumption in Scotland is that of binge drinking.

This type of drinking is concentrated over a number of days or even hours and the resultant high levels of blood alcohol commonly result in social problems such as family discord and sexual abuse. It is a common mis-conception in Scotland, as elsewhere in the UK, that people drink because they are under stress. While stress may be the factor influencing heavy drinking in an individual at a time of crisis, drinking habits within a population are more to do with cultural norms and the availability of alcohol (Kendall, de Roumanie and Ritson, 1983). With respect to the

334

second factor, the availability of alcohol, alcohol is currently relatively cheap compared with the cost of living and there is little difficulty in obtaining alcohol when shopping in the supermarket. Increasingly women are experiencing social and medical problems from drinking. This is because women are drinking more as a result of a change in social attitudes which no longer stigmatize them if they are seen drinking in public or purchasing alcohol (Peter Rice, 1992).

There is within Scotland a growing realization that an effective way to bring about change is through community involvement. This has been particularly successful, for example, in Dundee district of Mid-Craigie and Linlathen, one of Scotland's five current Social Strategy Areas. With the collaboration of residents a health survey was published in 1988 which classified those factors which local people saw as having a bad effect on their health. Over 70% quoted as important factors poverty and the absence of a chemist. Subsequently a local health issues group was formed which campaigned for a chemist's shop which was in fact opened earlier this year. Another successful community project is that of the P.R.O.P. Stress Centre at Pilton in north Edinburgh. The basic philosophy of the team there is to encourage the members who attend to develop both social skills and practical know-how. People are encouraged to take increasing responsibility for their lives so as to increase confidence in their ability to cope.

There are other such projects throughout Scotland and I feel more public money should be made available to make these more accessible. It is, in my opinion, often only through the active participation of local residents that changes will come to areas of multiple deprivation. Such areas are beginning to learn how to successfully lobby both politicians and policy makers.

Having been involved in discussions during my visits to such community projects in Scotland, I have come to the sad conclusion that psychiatrists have a bad image problem. As a result of contact with members of this species, clients too often see psychiatrists as hostile and non-communicative. To offset this tendency it might be helpful for psychiatrists in Scotland to become more involved in what Manfred Bleuler regarded as 'the best type of psychiatry': 'humanistic, caring, thoughtful, empathic and oriented to the care of the whole person' (Mosher and Burti, 1989). On a positive note I can report that the membership of the Stress Centre at Pilton in Edinburgh have recently been asked to advise some of my colleagues about deficits in the training of psychiatrists. If this idea caught on, we could perhaps at last begin to see some progress and the beginning of the breakdown of the artificial barriers between psychiatrists and their clients.

I would like to say a few words about the mental health of the members of the caring professions. The doctors, nurses, psychologists, social workers and other therapists who care for members of the public, have emotional needs that are rarely addressed by employing authorities.

Many doctors, as a result of their training, see themselves as needing to be strong at all times. This in turn leads medical professionals, including psychiatrists, to the conviction that they shouldn't have personal problems and that, if they do, they don't need to share them. Psychiatrists are not an elite section of society - they have foibles, feelings and failings like everyone else. The Royal College of Psychiatrists earlier this year published a book in the Gaskell series entitled 'Management/Training for Psychiatrists'. In this there is a chapter 'Stress Management - Taking the Strain' by Dr. Helena Waters, a psychiatrist, who has been involved in the running of stress management courses for health care and social work professionals for some years. (Waters, 1992).

I attended such a workshop in 1991 run by the Life Foundation of Therapeutics (see References for address) and feel that my involvement in that has provided a catalyst for personal change and growth. The School is a non-religious, non-political and non-profit making organisation that aims to make available self-help techniques to improve health and generate self-awareness at all levels.

A recent B.M.A. report, 'Stress in the Medical profession' (B.M.A., 1992), argues that the high levels of alcohol and drug misuse and suicide among doctors typifies only those 'who may have reached the extremes of failure - the numbers of doctors suffering adversely from stress are likely to be much greater.' The authors of 'Community Mental Health: Principles and Practice' (Mosher and Burti, 1989) note that doctors and other professionals devote a considerable amount of time these days to the bureaucratic process. There is a danger that the emphasis of medical care will move from its proper focus - that of providing humane and individual approach to an ill person - to an overriding concern for providing reports on time. Another source of stress in psychiatric hospitals is whenever a suicide occurs. In the aftermath of such tragedies more and more I see myself as being somebody within the team who can help to comfort and console and communicate with those who often feel strained to the point of despair and I see this as an essential part of my job. This is often because there is no official, or even unofficial, system whereby individuals can seek support, succour and advice. The setting up of a counselling service, either within or outwith the health service, should be considered as a matter of urgency. In the meantime we should remember that the

336

Samaritans have recently extended their service - at least in England - into different areas such as hospitals. This is of course a completely confidential service and one that is available to *anyone* passing through a personal crisis or in imminent danger of taking their own life. Members of the caring professions carry no immunity to reacting to human problems and should be aware of this scheme in times of stress. We all need someone in whom we can trust. Surely this is a benefit that should be extended to Scotland.

You might be forgiven for believing that I have abandoned my original concept that Scotland is waking up to the idea of mental health and that I have allowed myself to drift in an elitist direction, but I remain deeply concerned for the welfare of professional carers in Scotland. An ill or disillusioned professional can cause untold damage. The mental health movement in Scotland, while basically a grass-roots one, still needs the involvement of doctors, nurses, psychologists and social workers who are energetic, enthusiastic and well integrated.

Some might argue that because of the conservative and allegedly stubborn nature of the Scots character, the waking up to the idea of mental health will take generations. I believe that, on the contrary, attitudes within the Scottish community are already changing. People are coming to accept that talking of feelings and sharing moments of deep emotion are essential for personal growth and self confidence. Educating the public in ways of achieving high standards of mental health must have a high priority in Scotland.

Problems resulting from social ills such as poverty, malnourishment and unemployment can result in feelings of despair and apathy and must be constantly addressed by our politicians and policy makers.

Despite the prevalence of such adverse social problems in Scotland, positive change at an individual level is nearly always possible.

Let me share with you a personal testimony. My own mental health has, for example been greatly influenced by the writings of the American psychologist Carl Rogers, known for his client centre therapy. Rogers wrote of his own philosophy, for the later decades in life, in his Paper 'Growing Old - or Older and Growing' (Rogers, 1990). He noted that for many the age of 65 marked the end of a productive life and the beginning of retirement - 'whatever that means'. He described his own 65 to 75 years as a time of embarking on many new adventures, involving psychological or even physical risk. He was willing to take chances because - so he said - in doing so, whether he succeeded or failed, he learned something new about life. In his words, 'All of this involved change and , for me, the process of change *is* life'.

The emerging lifestyle that younger people were, and are, helping to bring about fascinated him. He felt committed to 'a way of life that reflects certain inner convictions; first that it is better to have things on a human scale; secondly it is better to live frugally, to conserve, recycle, not waste; third that the **inner life**, rather than externals, is central'.

He was able to cast aside conventional thinking and unashamedly admit to being increasingly aware, at his age, of **his** capacity for love and **his** sensuality.

Like Rogers I find myself more in touch with my own feelings and as a result I am able to develop deeper relationships with men and women. I find myself able to share without holding back, trusting in security of friendship.

Finally it is the needs of individual people within any community - in this case Scotland - that have to be addressed. In this context I have been much impressed by the value of many self-help manuals. A little while spent reading these could be invaluable compared with the time often wasted by 'amusing ourselves to death' - in words of the american sociologist Neil Postman - in front of the television.

Susan Jeffers' 'Feel the Fear and Do it Anyway' has a whole Life Grid which I would commend to you (Jeffers, 1987). In order to have a balance within our lives, we need several areas of nourishment. These are:-

Friends
Partnership
Work
Leisure
Personal Growth
Alone Time
Family
Hobby
Contribution

The Contribution component refers to the area that allows us to make our own special difference to the world. It is not something in grand terms such as the visionary work of Gandhi or Albert Einstein, but simply those measures that we can adopt to affect some change, however small. Much of our self esteem and satisfaction in life comes from this.

Lord Boyd Orr was a Scot who was the first Director General of the Food and Agricultural Organisation of the United Nations. His motto was that 'You can't build peace on empty bellies' (Lubbock, 1992). Boyd Orr drew evidence from the past of the vital role of food supply for the flourishing of civilization and pointed the way that a New World Order could be started by the nations of the World agreeing to organise the World food supply to provide an adequacy for all.

Lesser mortals have to be content with something more basic and I would leave you with the inspiring words of the German writer Heinrich von Kleist.

These instructions if carried out conscientiously would, I contend, make a vast difference to the lives of many of us.

'One should at least every day read a good poem, look at a beautiful picture, listen to a gentle song or have a warm conversation with a friend in order to cultivate the finer and I would say the more human aspect of our essence.'

Acknowledgements

I would like to thank friends for sharing time with me to discuss the ideas in the Paper.

Christoph Correll, Florence Grote, Michael Hippisley
Ann Keddie, Robin Laing, David Lubbock
Peter Rice, Dorothy Robbie, June Schonfield
Claire Walker, Angus Whitson

References

B.M.A. (1992). *Stress and the Medical Profession.*

Browne, W.A.F. (1837). *What Asylums were, are and ought to be.* Edinburgh: Adam and Charles Black.

Duncan, G. (1992, June 25). *Scotsman,* p.3.

Jeffers, S. (1987). *Feel the Fear and Do it Anyway* (p.138). London: Arrow.

Kendall, R.E., de Roumanie, M. & Ritson, E.B. (1983). *The influence of economic factors on alcohol consumption.* British Medical Journal, **287**, 809-11.

Life Foundation School of Therapeutics, Maristowe House, Dover Street, Bilston, WW14 6AL.

Lubbock, D. (1992). *The Boyd Orr View: From the Old World to the New with proposal for action to banish hunger:* The late Lord Boyd Orr's Testament by his Collaborator David Lubbock. Rowatt Research Institute, Bucksburn, Aberdeen. ABZ 9SB.

Mosher, L.R. & Burti, L. (1989). *Community Mental Health: Principles and Practice.* New York: W.W. Norton & Company.

Postman, N. (1985). *Amusing Ourselves to Death.* London: Methuen.

Presley, A.S. (1981). *A Sunnyside Chronicle: 1781-1981.* Tayside Health Board, Dundee.

Rice, P. (1992). (Personal communication): Consultant in charge of Tayside Alcohol Problem Service, Sunnyside Royal Hospital, Montrose.

Rogers, C. (1990). Growing Old: or Older and Growing. Ian H. Kirschenbaum & V.L. Henderson (Eds.), *The Carl Rogers Reader* (37-42). London: Constable.

Waters, H. (1992). Stress management: Taking the Strain. In D. Bhugra & A. Burns (Eds.), *Management training for psychiatrists,* (pp. 200-224). London: Gaskell.

28 Establishing needs and allocating resources within the provider/ purchaser framework

Z. Kenyon

This paper attempts to describe a model for identifying the pattern of provision of mental health and mental illness services in South Kirklees of a population of 211,000. To date we have no fundholders in this area and so the picture has not been influenced by the fundholding initiative. Current services have been examined and pooled experience has gone some way to defining unmet need.

Our group, consisting of myself (Medical Adviser to the FHSA), the Head of Clinical Psychology Department, the Community Physician, Senior Social Worker, a representative of Community Psychiatric Nurses and the Business Manager from the Division of Psychiatry, has met regularly during the course of the last year. There was an obvious need for a mutually acceptable language and I would like to elaborate a little about the words and phrases used in this paper.

'Mental Health' is just that, not a euphemism for psychiatric illness. The medical model of disease seemed to exclude many who needed help and include some who were adequately contained within the community. For this reason we talk about maladaption, rather than mental illness. Winnicott, in his essay 'Concept of a Healthy Individual in 1971' said 'we use the words normal and healthy when we talk about people, so we usually know what we mean'. 20 years later can we so competently still identify the healthy and the normal? In the last 24 hours many people have told us what mental health is and what factors influence it but I am not so confident and think there is an intensely personal angle to this. I would like to ask when do individuals and society itself change constructs? A very simple culture-bound example is of our expectation of eye contact and vocal recognition on passing a stranger in the lane. Downcast eyes and no acknowledgement signals depression, withdrawal, or at least bad manners. In a different culture the converse would be true.

The implementation of the Community Care Act and the Purchaser/ Provider split influences the allocation of limited resources. The holistic approach is now widely accepted but talk and action do not always match up and we must be constantly aware of the frequently quoted phrase 'never mind the problem, here is the solution'. Territorial rights, a lack of clearly defined professional role, misunderstanding, power struggles, can compound the shared difficulties of underfunding. It seemed that we were stabbing at trying to clarify a four dimensional dynamic situation with infinite individual variations. Obviously an impossible task!

From all this discussion emerged the concept of using a triangular framework, divided into 5 bands, recognising that there is movement between the bands and that the degree of maladaption was one of the governing factors for placing any individual in a particular band.

Our task then has been to collect and collate current activities, to separate the well from the ill, to understand lay health beliefs, to identify social support networks (kind neighbours, the milkman, voluntary agencies). To do battle with the users of the phrase 'worried well' (who would not be worried if they were well, or well if they were worried).

There is variable interest, variable recognition and variable response from workers in primary care, and this is compounded by sparse resources, e.g. limited numbers of community psychiatric nurses and even fewer clinical psychologists. It is little wonder that we reached the conclusion that equity, if attainable at all, is beyond our horizon.

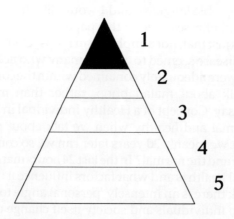

I have already mentioned the concept of maladaption and we will have to consider this when resources are allocated. For example, a patient may be clinically and functionally impaired but adapted to the environment in which they are living. The concept of maintenance (containment) or remedial (treatment) approaches were discussed.

Band 1 - The severely ill

That is those with a remedial but recurring condition, or severely ill but with no remedial input and so requiring containment (some psychopaths, manic-depressives, schizophrenics and those with organic psychosis or dementia may, at some stage, be in this band).

Band 2 - The moderately ill

Input could be at primary or secondary level. Those with irremedial conditions may, from time to time need containment somewhere other than their own homes.

Band 3 - Mildly ill

This group are, on the whole, suffering from remedial conditions and can be contained within primary health care. Other services outside the primary health care team can be incorporated into caring for these individuals. This group will contain, among others, patients who have problems with alcohol abuse, the bereaved, carers under stress, people having to cope with catastrophies, the effect of HIV/AIDS on the mental health, parasuicides, those with established irremedial physical illness (e.g. chronic disease, amputation etc.) sufferers from sexual abuse, tranquilliser misuse and drug dependency.

Band 4 - The potentially ill

Where known predisposing factors can be identified and early intervention can facilitate a rapid return to normality (major life events, lack of family or community support). This is where sensitivity of healthcare workers is essential if there is to be an early return to band 5.

Band 5

This last group at the bottom of our triangle is where maintenance of mental health depends on several factors outside the Health Service (employment or lack of it, environmental factors, housing, litter and even dog dirt, as referred to by other contributors to this symposium). The shift as we see it is away from the top of the triangle into the areas of prevention or remedial services and in this group we have included alcohol misuse, bereavement, the needs of carers, catastrophies, HIV/AIDS counselling, parasuicides, established physical illness, past sexual abuse, tranquilliser dependency and so on.

To avoid drifting up to the top of the triangle, a sensitivity and awareness is necessary in primary care. Consultation rates are high in those with a psychological need. In childhood this correlates with broken homes, separation of the child from either or both parents and a family history of psychiatric illness. Put another way, minor psychological disturbances doubles the consultation rate. Any GP who sees a pattern of frequent consultations for 'medical trivia' should speculate on the underlying cause. By early recognition and intervention the duration and severity of psychological disturbance can be minimised.

Rather than shrug and say 'it's their age', perhaps we should try to provide more empathic ears to listen to our adolescents (some 10% of whom have significant emotional problems).

'AGE' is also often blamed for dysmenorrhoea, dyspareunia, dysfunctional marriage etc. Organic reasons for pelvic pain are sought at great expense to the country and often great discomfort to the patient where again the empathic ear could have heard the underlying causes of prolonged and entrenched distress.

Try the 'AGE' excuse again. Of course we all know that 'AGE' causes forgetfulness, confusion, disturbed sleep patterns and so on, but what about the unresolved grief (a child dead 60 years but still clearly recalled), the inability to accept restricted physical activities, the mourning for the past and maybe fears about the future.

Earlier today Dorothy Rowe pointed out that professionals sometimes act like authoritarian parents and she asked us if individuals could release the empathy they had as newborn babies.

Thinking about mental health provision has focused our minds on several conflicts common to many areas of health needs assessment.

1. The first is the continuous danger of slipping back into service provision, rather than well researched assessment.
2. The second is the agonizing conflict of prioritising in an under-funded service.
3. Thirdly, society and professional pressures force us towards health prevention and disease promotion. (sic)
4. Health care workers are largely concerned about process but managers are understandably concerned with outcome.
5. Is the optimal site for mental health promotion and mental illness

care in the primary or secondary arena, or somewhere in between?

Finally, we have the conflict between our private empathy and involvement and our professional lives which some claim should be kept separate.

Having identified our task and recognised some of the obstacles we can now begin to move forward with missionary, rather than mercenary zeal.

29 Involving users in the planning of services

F. Ledwith

Abstract

This paper was originally planned to present the results of a process of collaborative planning, involving users, providers and purchasers of services for mental health. In fact it will be an account of the organisational blocks to that process, an outline of a tried and tested model and a description of what we have achieved so far with some suggestions on how to avoid the organisational blocks in the future.

Whence the organisational blocks

I would take it as a basic truism that those who have power wish to exercise it, and are not keen to give it away to others. Health Service professionals do have a good deal of power and prestige associated with their roles. It follows therefore that Health and Social Services, either as organisations or in the practice of their professional staff are likely not to give full value to the views of users, to give them any power to shape the pattern or style of services. In the case of mental health users, there is also the added burden that any critical views or wishes for improvements can be and often are taken as a symptom of their condition rather than as a legitimate concern. There is however the rhetoric of the Citizens' Charter, which NHS purchasers are insisting should be incorporated into contracts. Insofar as that Charter implies any sharing of power with users, it will not meet ready acceptance by professional provider staff within mental health services.

It is essential to make a distinction between consultation and collaboration in planning. Consultation means presenting already formulated plans for comment. Collaboration involves discussion of plans whilst they are still being formulated. Consultation has been around for a long time and is easily accepted. For example, the recent round of production of Community Care Plans, as required by the government, did have a process of consultation after the plan was produced. There were requests for comments and public meetings at which the weighty documents were discussed.

Any minor comments could be, and were, incorporated in the final version. On the other hand any issues of major substance, such as the pattern of service or its adequacy of delivery could only be noted. There was no power base, no sustained expertise with which to challenge the plan in its entirety. In those circumstances it is clear why Health and Social Services could live easily with consultation.

Collaboration would require that the public and particular interest groups were involved in the early stages of drawing up the principles for services, deciding on the allocation of resources available and then drafting the proposals for services to be developed, reduced or scrapped. Within such a process it is possible to avoid the presentation of a fait accompli, of constraints already set which determine the scope of any possible decisions. However collaboration requires a substantial change to methods of working. It is difficult enough to manage the processes of planning which involve all the relevant departments in an organisation, to consider the buildings and equipment needed so that they are available when needed, to ensure that the relevant staff are available and that the organisation can operate within its budget. (This difficulty is compounded when, as now, there are so many changes taking place in the structure of organisations with the purchaser provider split and now the move at great pace to Trust status for provider units.) To include voluntary bodies, advocacy groups and individual users into the round of meetings would add a massive degree of complexity to the process. The consequence is that to involve users would increase both the time taken to plan and the complexity of the task.

In addition, experience in a number of places has shown that to make a real contribution, users and outside bodies require the administrative and technical support and expertise which officers of Health and Social Services take for granted: at planning meetings we are looking for informed and considered inputs from those concerned with capital planning, personnel and finance. In the same way we want such high level of expert input from outside bodies. To achieve such expertise requires time to develop. It is for that reason that planning managers get paid comfortably large sums of money. In other words, effectively to involve users would cost no small amount of money.

To be fair, the NHS Management Executive paper on consulting users (NHSME, 1992) does seem to suggest a middle way whereby there are a series of consultation points in the planning process, from Purchasing Plan, through Service Specification to Contract Monitoring and Review of outcomes. In this way the public's views could in some ways be incorporated in the formulation of plans though there is no mention of how to support the development of any expertise for the process. In addition no mention is made of users' views, which presumably are thought to belong to the province of service providers.

The planning workshop model

There is a model for collaborative planning which has been used successfully for Learning Difficulty services in Bradford and Rochdale, having been developed originally for Manchester Housing Department. In outline the process is this:

1) Involve users and carers in initial discussions on the issues they wish to see tackled. This would lead to a public meeting involving users and carers at which the issues were raised and discussed, with delegates elected at the meeting to take part in the planning workshop.

2) The planning workshop would involve users and carers, providers of services and purchasers. It is very useful if the lead figures such as the Chair of the Health Authority and Chair of Social Services can be involved in the workshop. The workshop might involve from 50 to 100 people. The process consists of small groups of users and professionals discussing the main service issues as they see them. Then there would be small groups to brainstorm and then organise proposals for service developments. These proposals (typically on flip charts) would be put together into categories by the organising group. Each participant would then be given a sheet of 8-10 coloured stickers (coded by colour for the different constituencies of user, carer, provider and purchaser). Each person could examine all the options suggested (which might run to 50-100 proposals) and place a sticker against the 10 proposals they most favoured. After everyone had completed the task it would be possible to see what were the most favoured proposals and whether there were any systematic differences between different constituencies of interest.

The 5-8 most favoured proposals could then be looked at and volunteers sought for the person to lead the development of the proposal in the future. A timetable could then be worked out for the work to be carried forward for the year. If the planning workshop were held once a year, then a review could be made of progress on the previous year's work at the start. Experience in Bradford and Rochdale has suggested that where lay people take the lead, they do require administrative support that people within the organisation take for granted: access to phones, photocopying and specialist expertise and information. To achieve this there does require to be a support worker along the lines of the Federation in Derbyshire Social Services or the Liaison Officer as found in Blackburn.

This model was discussed in Preston by a subgroup including the Health provider, Social Services, the FHSA and the voluntary sector. When presented by the Health provider unit to the District Joint Planning Team (JPT) along with the cost implications of the workshop (around £1,000) and of a support worker, the proposal was rejected. The ostensible reasons for refusal were to do with cost and appropriateness. The Purchaser felt that they could and were obtaining the information they needed from consumer surveys and anyway doubted whether the provider should be involved in planning. Social Services felt that there could be other models (unspecified) which might be preferred. My own view is that a large part of the real reason for rejection lay in the quite explicit commitment to share some power with users.

A users' workshop

Whilst this proposal was being discussed I was having discussions with Preston Users Group (PUG) on the proposals for the planning workshop. Once the JPT rejected the proposals we decided to honour our commitments and hold a workshop to hear users' views and produce a report for our own use. That workshop was held, jointly organised by PUG and the Provider Division. Some 25 users attended, including a contingent of 6 men from a Night Shelter in Preston, all of whom had been users of mental health services. There was a wide spectrum of histories from people buying their own homes to those who were homeless whose most palatial home, if not a park bench, was the Night Shelter. The issue of homelessness featured very strongly. Apart from that, issues raised had to do with medication (severity of dosage and side effects), lack of information (on services available and on welfare benefits) and lack of understanding and courtesy from provider staff.

It was no easy matter to produce a summary report which properly represented users' views and yet was in a form which professionals would not reject out of hand: there were many blunt and critical comments. The next step will be to have a workshop with users, professionals and managers to discuss the report, look at the desired improvements and jointly select the 6-8 for most urgent action. In the meantime immediate action is being taken to assess the extent of our responsibility for ex patients who are homeless. All the indications are that the problem lies not with ex long stay patients but with 'revolving door' clients.

Lessons to be learned

The first and foremost lesson must be to expect that the process of collaboration with users will not be welcomed by most authorities. Expect stiff organisational resistance and plan to deal with it. It would seem to be wise to start small with the process of collaboration with users in planning, realising that it will be underfunded at first. After one or two years of struggling along it might be possible to get real logistic support. Once any collaboration is underway I would suggest that it would be important to involve our political masters in the process. A key person would be the Chair of Social Services (though this is much easier to do within a City or borough than in a large County authority). In this way it would be possible to avoid the trap of officers shielding politicians from meeting service users and thus from being presented with some quite blunt talking about service inadequacies.

A vital first step in the process is to build up a constituency of users. Without a Users Group it would be much harder to recruit a good cross section to any discussion or workshop. There is a real risk that a workshop would only involve the more articulate and less disadvantaged.

There is a good deal of organisational learning and change required to involve users in any meaningful way. We have found the first steps illuminating and a powerful reminder of some key priorities. On principle we intend to carry the process on though it will not be an easy road to pursue for the many reasons outlined above.

References

National Health Service Management Executive (1992) - *Local voices: The views of local people in purchasing for health*. London.

30 Mental health awareness training and the promotion of mental health

L. Lorenc. J. Hazell and J. Smith

Abstract

This paper describes an ongoing programme of mental health awareness training underway in Bromsgrove and Redditch Health Authority. The training aims to encourage participants to consider the way caring services affect the lives of people with mental health problems, and is offered to staff from Health Authority, Local Authority, Voluntary and Independent sectors involved in the support of people with mental health problems. The training is designed to help participants to clarify their own values and attitudes in relation to people with mental health problems; identify more closely with the lives and experiences of people who use mental health services; and to focus on possibilities for change in relation to their own practice, and in the services within which they work, to ensure that users have access to valued services. The training is of particular interest because it involves service users as paid co-trainers. We believe this has contributed significantly to the success of the training programme. The training has been evaluated and some brief evaluative data is provided. The implications of these findings are discussed.

Introduction

The following paper describes a series of workshops designed to promote mental health by altering potentially negative and unhelpful attitudes about people with mental health problems that prevail among service providers. These attitudes are believed to have an impact upon the individual self-esteem and self perceptions of people with mental health problems which can be detrimental to the restoration of mental health. In addition, these negative attitudes may contribute to the stress felt by service users and may, therefore, have an effect on relapse rates in those susceptible to such stresses (Ball et al. 1992). This is particularly crucial, given the current transition from hospital to community based mental health services. The opportunity of change is an ideal time to address these issues, particularly if we are to achieve the 'vision' of community care as set out in the strategic statements of 'Caring for People'. If these statements are to be meaningful, they have to be adopted at a personal as well as an organizational level. Professional workers from all agencies concerned with mental health care will need to review their values, attitudes and practice carefully, particularly in relation to users and carers. This is essential if we are to produce a service which, in being sensitive and responsible to the needs of individuals, will actively promote the mental health of users and carers.

To do this it is particularly crucial to confront the stereotypes that exist amongst professional workers about people with mental health problems and their capabilities: particularly in relation to their active involvement in planning, implementing and monitoring service provision. Negative attitudes can act as powerful obstacles to service change, particularly when those changes potentially threaten traditional professional (often paternalistic) practice.

Attitudes towards people with mental health problems in our society are generally negative. These perceptions develop from cultural and societal values to which we are all exposed. We need to recognise that although professional workers, we are also members of society and need to be aware that we are equally susceptible to these same attitudes and stereotypes. As there is often a close link between what we think and feel and how we subsequently behave and act the consequence of holding rigid and often negative attitudes about people with mental health problems is that users and carers are often in receipt of a devaluing and disempowering service.

The mental health awareness workshop was developed as an attempt to address these issues. The aim was to provide a non-threatening, non-judgemental climate where professionals could be helped to identify and challenge common views and attitudes about people with mental health problems: to develop some understanding about where those attitudes come from and to make explicit links between attitudes and behaviour. They would also be helped to understand the disabling effect that negative attitudes can have on practice and thus on the lives and experiences of users and carers. Through increased awareness of their own attitudes and personal power in positively influencing the service they deliver, participants would be encouraged to focus on possibilities for change in personal practice and the services within which they work.

Changes that specifically and directly benefitted users and carers in terms of promoting self-esteem and empowerment would be encouraged, given that these issues are fundamental to the maintenance and promotion of mental health.

It was felt to be important to involve local users and carers as paid co-trainers in the workshops as a powerful impetus to the process of attitude awareness and subsequent service change. This assisted in promoting a more positive and empowering image of users and carers in terms of their capabilities in articulating their needs and experiences clearly and dispassionately, and in withstanding the personal stress that might be engendered in talking to a large group of professional workers.

One feature of the mental health awareness workshops described was that they actively sought to bring together individuals from different professional backgrounds, different levels of training and experience and different agencies to provide a networking opportunity. In this way, individuals could collaborate and share a common commitment to realizing the values and aspirations embodied in 'Caring for People' as well as sharing good practice and ideas between agencies.

Method

Six workshops were run during an eighteen month period spanning from April 1991 to the present.

Workshop participants

A total of 109 people attended the workshops. The average number per workshop was 18. Staff who attended came from a range of agencies, e.g. Health Authority, Local Authority, Independent Sector and Voluntary Agencies. The type of professions represented included nurses, social workers, care assistants, police, psychologists, advice workers etc. Some of the staff who attended were professionally qualified and some unqualified, but all had regular contact in their work with people who experience mental health problems. The average duration of working with people with mental health problems was 9.9 years, with a range of 3 months to 33 years. The amount of contact with people with mental health problems varied from daily to monthly, with the vast majority having daily contact.

Workshop leaders

Each workshop was led by three clinical psychologists who introduced the topics under discussion and facilitated small group exercises and the large group discussions.

Workshop structure and content

Each workshop was run over two consecutive days. Each day started at 9.15 am and ended at 4.15 pm. The course content was split into four, half day sections. Each section focused on different topics but all built on the knowledge gained in the previous sections. The sections consisted of a mixture of talks, small and large group discussions and small group exercises.

The four sections were entitled; Images of Mental Health in the Media, How Beliefs and Labels Influence our Behaviour, How Attitudes affect service Delivery and the Service user's Perspective. These are described below:

Images of mental health in the media

This section consisted of a short introductory talk about service values, particularly in relation to the local joint mission statement and the implications for service delivery. The talk explored attitude formation and how attitudes in turn influence perceptions. Finally the talk briefly explored the attitudes held about people with mental health problems largely developed through parental messages, exchanges in the school playground and media reporting. The talk included examples of stories where the media presented only a selection of facts, which consequently distorted the truth. It was suggested that as a consequence negative and restrictive attitudes about people with mental health problems often develop in the general public. Participants then divided into three small groups to work on exercises relating to different aspects of the talk. The first group had to brainstorm words (both technical and slang) that are often used by the general public to describe people with mental health problems, for example lunatic, nutter, etc. The second group considered how people with mental health problems are portrayed in the media in terms of the kind of images of people with mental health problems that are put across in television, newspaper articles, films and books. The third group were asked to consider their own thoughts and ideas about people with mental health problems before they began working with them and since they have had experience of working with them. The feedback from the small group work was discussed and summarized in a large group forum at the end of the session.

How beliefs and labels influence our behaviour

This section started with a short talk about how our expectations and attitudes can influence our own behaviour and feelings, and the consequent impact it can have on the people we interact with. The group then divided into three small groups and completed an exercise which required them to give their opinion on a given topic. Examples of the topics used were 'Contraception in no circumstances should be available to girls under sixteen years old', 'Voluntary euthanasia should be offered to anyone over sixty-five years old', 'Violence in society is provoked by T.V. programmes, films and videos that glamorize violence, such as Rambo and Robo Cop'. While doing this, each participant was required to wear a 'label' on their forehead. Examples of the labels used were 'stupid', 'confused' and 'intelligent'. Participants were unaware of what their own label was but could clearly see labels worn by other group members. Group members were asked to respond to the comments made by each person in turn in a prejudicial way according to the label on that person's forehead and not in terms of what the person actually said. Discussion them followed, about how this felt in terms of being treated according to a label rather than based on what a person said or did, and how labelling often operates with people with mental health problems.

How attitudes affect service delivery

By means of introduction to this section of the workshop, participants were asked initially to identify several examples of good and bad services that they had personally received. Discussion abut what aspects of a service made it good or bad highlighted the fact that the experiences of a good service are more often based on the way the service is delivered, rather than on physical or practical aspects of that service. For example, individuals did not mind waiting for an appointment as long as they were kept informed as to why. Participants then divided into small groups to complete the 'Life-styles Package' (Brown and Alcoe, 1984). This exercise consists of participants making choices about aspects of services that they would value for themselves or a member of their family.

Discussion followed about these choices and whether these same choices were available to people with mental health problems that they worked with, and possible reasons for why they were not.

Service users' perspective

It was felt important for professional workers to see the services they work in from a user's and carer's viewpoint. To this end, a video recording an interview between one of the course leaders and a number of service users was prepared beforehand. The video lasted approximately 20 minutes and focused on user's experience of services and people's attitudes towards them. The video was shown at every workshop, with follow-up questions given to those service users who attended. This served to greatly reduce the level of stress of the service users and had the additional benefit of being able to be used alone should no service user be available to attend.

Assessment measures

All participants were asked to complete the following questionnaires:

Beliefs about mental health questionnaire

This questionnaire consisted of eight statements about people with mental health problems and the services they receive. Each statement was rated on a five point scale ranging from 'disagree strongly' through 'not sure' to 'agree strongly'. (See Appendix 1). Participants were asked to indicate the extent to which they agreed or disagreed with each statement. This questionnaire was given at the beginning and the end of the workshop.

Course evaluation and feedback form

Participants were asked a series of questions about the content, presentation, relevance and time allowed for discussion. Participants were also asked to identify the most and least useful aspects of the workshop, and to make any additional comments or suggestions. (See Appendix 2). This questionnaire was given at the end of the workshop.

Pledge form

At the end of each workshop participants were asked to state a personal 'pledge', i.e. to decide on one service improvement or change that they could personally make in an aspect of their work during the next week. This pledge had to be an easily managed change of behaviour which would in some way provide an improved service for clients. This was recorded on a pledge form (see Appendix 3). These pledges were followed up by telephone within two weeks of completing the workshop.

As far as participants were concerned, this was the end of contact with the workshop organizers. However, a follow-up survey was conducted on those who had attended the first four workshops (that is, between 7 and 14 months following completion of the workshop). Those who were contacted were asked whether they remembered the workshop, and their pledge, whether they were still carrying it out and whether they had made any other changes to their work practice as a result of having attended the workshop. Everyone was asked to say what their pledge had been, and those who were unable to do so were reminded of the details. If people said that they had changed their work practice, they were asked to give details of changes made.

Results

Beliefs about mental health questionnaire

The results of this questionnaire were considered in terms of apparent attitude change. That is, we were looking at the numbers of people who shifted their views in relation to the eight statements given, in the desired direction. Table 1 shows the number of people who apparently altered their responses, plus the number of people who remained at ceiling level (ceiling being the response to each statement which we considered to be most desirable).

Table 1
Table showing results of beliefs questionnaire
(N = 76, data from 4 workshops only)

Question	No. moving in expected direction	%	No. moving in opposite direction	%	No. at ceiling point	%
1	10	15	0	0	57	85
2	20	30	28	42	19	28
3	3	4	1	1	63	94
4	12	18	11	16	44	66
5	5	7	5	7	57	85
6	8	12	0	0	59	88
7	20	30	20	30	27	40
8	21	31	18	27	28	42

Note: Percentages may not add up to 100% due to rounding off.

For most statements, the majority of people were at ceiling point. It is to be noted that questions 2, 7 and 8 engendered a large variance in response.

Course evaluation and feedback

Table 2 provides the figures for those responding to questions concerning course content, presentation, relevance and time allowed for discussion.

Table 2
Satisfaction with workshop
(N = 88, Combined figures from five workshops)

		Nos. Responding	%
1.	**Content**		
	Was the course content:-		
	Over Familiar	6	7%
	Useful	72	82%
	Overspecialized	1	1%
	Did we Cover:-		
	Too little	6	7%
	About right	72	82%
	Too much	2	2%
2.	**Presentation**		
	Were the presentations:-		
	Boring	0	0%
	Fairly interesting	12	14%
	Interesting	64	73%
	Were they:-		
	Confusing	0	0%
	Fairly clear	19	22%
	Clear	63	72%
3.	**Relavance to your work**		
	How relevant was the workshop:-		
	Irrelevant	1	1%
	Fairly relevant	33	38%
	Relevant	49	56%
4.	**Time allowed for discussion**		
	Was there:-		
	Too much	5	6%
	About right	65	74%
	Too little	12	14%

The vast majority of participants were satisfied with the workshop in all four areas assessed. It is important to note that not everyone provided an answer for every question so, therefore, figures do not add up to 100%.

Tables 3 and 4 show those aspects highlighted as being 'most' and 'least useful' respectively:

Table 3
Table showing sections highlighted as 'most useful'

	Nos. responding	%
- Involvement of service users	41	47
- Labelling exercise	10	11
- All of it!	10	11
- Meeting different professionals	7	8
- Lifestyles exercise	4	5
- Images of mental health exercise	4	5
- Small group discussion	4	5
- Practical exercises	3	3
- Being made to think	2	2
- Second day of workshop (sections 3 and 4)	1	1

Table 4
Table showing sections highlighted as 'least useful'

	Nos. responding	%
- Labelling exercise	11	12
- Images of mental health exercise	8	9
- None of it!	3	3
- Lifestyles exercise	2	2
- Number of people working full-time in mental health	1	1
- Staying in the same small group	1	1
- Involvement of service users	1	1
- Lunch/coffee breaks	1	1
- Completing questionnaires	1	1
- Everything	1	1

Pledge form

The pledges made by individuals were idiosyncratic and related to an individual's specific contact with people with mental health problems. Some examples of pledges made were as follows:-

- 'I will restart keep fit class on a Thursday, even if only one or two clients are interested. (Day centre worker).
- 'I will take a resident who rarely gets a chance to go out, for a walk'. (Residential care assistant).
- 'I will check daily that there is toilet paper in the client's toilet'. (Social Worker).

Initial Follow-up

The results of the initial pledge follow-up are given in Table 5.

Table 5
Table showing results of initial pledge follow-up
(N= 103, data from all 6 workshops)

Category	Numbers	%
Completed pledge	79	77
Failed to complete pledge	16	16
Unable to contact	2	2
No available record	6	6

Note: Percentages may not add up to 100% due to rounding off

The vast majority of participants reported that they had completed their pledge.

Extended follow-up

68 people were identified to be contacted by telephone and asked about their pledge. At the time of writing, contact had been made with 33 people. A further 10 were not contactable (mainly because they had moved to a new job). Table 6 shows the results of this follow-up.

Some people were no longer carrying out their pledge because it had involved a one-off action on their part. Example of further changes in

Table 6
Table showing results of extended follow-up pledges (N=33)

Question	Yes		No	
	No.	%	No.	%
Do you remember the workshop?	33	100	0	0
Do you remember your pledge?	31	94	2	6
Are you still carrying our your pledge?	22	66	11	33
Have you made any further changes?	18	54	15	45

work practice tended to be fairly general. For example:-

- 'more considerate'
- 'more aware'
- 'different approach - spending more time with difficult residents - more patience'
- 'more aware of clients' social needs'
- 'take residents to Bingo and the Social Club'
- 'try to be more aware of residents needs generally'.

Discussion

Overall, we have studied three aspects of the workshop: attitude change, satisfaction with the workshop, and subsequent behaviour change.

The results show that, despite an apparent failure to effect the desired attitude change, participants did accomplish a self-reported behavioural change in at least one aspect of their usual work practice. Overall, participants expressed a high degree of satisfaction with the workshop and claimed in particular to have benefitted from the involvement of service users.

Attitude change was measured using the beliefs questionnaire. Unfortunately, it would seem that this was an insufficient discriminator of attitude change, given that the majority of responses to the statements reached ceiling level at the first administration of the questionnaire. Most people attending the workshop were already giving desired responses at the beginning of the workshop and there was no possibility to measure even subtle attitude changes as a consequence of attending the workshop. One possible reason for this may be that a Mental Health Awareness workshop attracts people who are already quite 'aware' in terms of mental health issues. If this is the case, then we need to find a way of picking up small or subtle changes in attitudes. Also, we need to consider how to attract to a Mental Health Awareness Workshop of this kind, those people who are not appropriately 'aware'.

It is interesting to note, that questions 2, 7 and 8 generated a very mixed response, with an equal number of respondents moving in the desired direction as moving in the opposite direction. Two possible explanations present themselves. Firstly it may be that people are identifying unintended subtleties in the questions. For example, it may be that people have learned, during the workshop, that it is wrong to make assumptions regarding all people with mental health problems. They are perhaps discriminating against questions which suggest that 'all people with a mental health problem' should be treated in a certain way, even if the statement actually suggests introducing choice for mental health users: for example ' people with mental health problems should have a right to refuse a service that is offered to them'. Secondly, some participants on the initial day of such a workshop may have given 'expected' rather than truthful answers. It may be that the workshop then gives them pause for thought, particularly the non-judgemental approach which gives them permission to express their true opinions. This could then lead to apparent changes of opinion in the opposite direction when participants respond more closely to their true point of view and move away from the desired response originally given. Without knowledge of their true opinion at the beginning of the workshop it is difficult to assess any change in attitude.

Levels of satisfaction with the workshop in general were measured using the post workshop evaluation form. In general the responses to this questionnaire were largely positive, although it must be pointed out that the responses to most satisfaction questionnaires are generally positive. Clearly on the issue of the areas which people find either least or most useful there is a wide divergence of opinion. This can probably be best explained by the knowledge, different levels of experience, and different degrees of contact with people with mental health problems. It may be, therefore, that this background affects what aspects of the workshop are found particularly useful or relevant. Of particular interest was the inconsistency of response in regard to the usefulness of the labelling exercise. This exercise was designed to be particularly powerful in that people were expected to gain insight into the feelings which arise from being labelled, in a very short space of time. Some people in some of the workshops clearly found this exercise very threatening and were unwilling to get involved. It seems likely that those people later reported this exercise as least useful. Those who did get involved were often quite shocked at the depth of feelings that could be evoked during the exercise.

The third area of assessment concerned consequent behavioural change, assessed using the pledge forms which were subsequently followed up by telephone calls to check whether the change had taken place. These pledges, because they must relate to the person's work practice, are clearly idiosyncratic. Some people chose one-off actions as opposed to continued ongoing change, and this was reflected in the second follow up at a later date. Some people had continued with the behaviour change whereas those who had chosen a one-off action clearly could not continue. Obviously, there are problems with the telephone follow up of behaviour change, in that we rely on self reported activity. We have no means of testing out whether behaviour has actually changed in practice.

A further difficulty lies in the fact that we cannot be sure that the pledges that people have chosen to make are actually the sort of pledges that would make a difference to the lives and experiences of people with mental health problems. Clearly it would be useful to have some measure of whether there is a positive outcome for users and carers, either in terms of their experiences, or the attitudes of staff that they come into contact with.

The data that we have collected, therefore, seem very promising. It would appear that some people are making attitude, and consequently behaviour, changes. Generally people claim to be satisfied with the workshops, although we have pointed out that it could be that we are attracting onto such workshops people who have an interest in improving their practice rather than those people who might benefit most from questioning their current attitudes and practice.

One spin-off from the workshop involves the improved self-esteem of the service users who participated in the training. This in turn had an immediate impact on those attending the workshop, who then see people with a mental health problem in the role of 'expert', rather than in the role of service recipient. Clearly it is of value to professionals to hear directly from users concerning their experiences about the services that they receive.

Finally, the potential limitations of a two-day workshop in maintaining attitude and behaviour change need to be recognized. The probability is high that people will return to old attitudes and old habits of practice without continued support and supervision. How to provide this is a difficult issue. One possibility is to provide a further advanced workshop to build on this basic introduction, but as yet, this is very much in the pipeline and could at best only provide further intermittent support. It can only be hoped that, given that enough service providers attend the workshops sufficient numbers of people will have had their attitudes and practices challenged to ensure that a changed ethos pervades in the provision of care to people with mental health problems.

Acknowledgements

We would like to acknowledge and thank the following people for their contribution to the workshops, particularly to the process of data collection and analysis: Helen Close and Lesley Price, Assistant Psychologists, Barnsley Hall Hospital, Bromsgrove; Paul Chadwick, Clinical Psychologist, All Saints Hospital, Winson Green, Birmingham; Christine Heaven, Redditch Social Services, Redditch. We would also like to thank Lesley Clarke and Dorothy Richardson, Secretaries, Psychology Department,

Barnsley Hall Hospital, for their support in word processing many drafts of this manuscript.

References

Ball, R., Moore, E., & Kuipers, L. (1992). Expressed Emotion in Community Care Staff. A comparison of patient outcome in a nine month follow up of two hostels. *Social Psychiatry and Psychiatric Epidemiology,* 27, 35-39.

Brown, J., & Alcoe, J. (1984). *Lifestyles for people who use mental health services: A quality care training exercise for staff and service users.* Brighton: Pavilion Publishing.

Appendix 1

Beliefs about Mental Health Questionnaire

Listed below are 8 statements. Please read each statement and indicate whether you strongly agree (1), agree slightly (2), are not sure (3), disagree slightly (4) or strongly disagree (5).

In order to keep the questionnaire anonymous please do not put your name on the sheet. However, it would be useful for us to know whether you are male or female, you date of birth, and the extent of your contact with people with mental health problems.

Sex Male/Female   Date of Birth: / /19

□   □

For how many years have you been in contact with people with mental health problems?

(years)

How often do you come into contact with people with mental health problems?

Daily   Weekly   Monthly   Less often

□   □   □   □

Now please rate the following 8 statements as honestly as possible.

	1 Disagree Strongly	2 Disagree Slightly	3 Not Sure	4 Agree Slightly	5 Agree Strongly
1. It is a waste of money to provide plush surroundings and furniture for people with dementia.					
2. I feel it is appropriate that there should be separate staff toilets in facilities for people with mental health problems.					
3. It is too late to help people over 65 with their emotional problems					
4. Informal carers should make an equal contribution to discussions about care and treatment of their relatives, as professionals.					
5. It is okay for people with mental health problems to stop taking their medication because of side effects even when no alternative treatment is available.					
6. It is okay to talk about confused older adults when you are standing nearby.					
7. People with a mental health problem should have the right to refuse a service that is offered to them.					
8. People with a mental health problem should receive payment when asked to talk about their experiences at a staff training workshop.					

Appendix 2

Course Evaluation and Feedback Form

We would like to know how you felt about the workshop so that we can make appropriate changes to future workshops. Would you please complete the following questionnaire. Please tick the appropriate box.

1. CONTENT
Was the course content: Over familiar[ ] Useful[ ] Over specialized[ ]
What did you find most useful?

_____

What did you find leat useful?

_____

2. COVERAGE
Did we cover: Too little [ ] About right [ ] too much [ ]
Is there anything we did not cover that you would have like included?

_____

3. PRESENTATION
Overall were the presentations: Boring[ ] Fairly interesting[ ]
                                                    Interesting[ ]
How might we have improved the presentations?

_____

4. CLARITY
Were the presentations: Confusing [ ] Fairly clear [ ] Clear[ ]

5. RELEVANCE TO YOUR WORK
How relevant was the workshop: Irrelevant[ ]Fairly relevant[ ]
                                                    Relevant[ ]

How might we have made the workshop more relevant to your work?

_____

6. TIME ALLOWED FOR DISCUSSION

Was there: Too much [ ] About right [ ] Too little[ ]

7. Any further comments or suggestions for change

_____

_____

Appendix 3

PLEDGE FORM

- Think about the exercise you have just taken part in and consider one thing you could do differently or alter at work which would help to provide a better service.

- When deciding on this, consider the following points:

1. Will I have the opportunity to do this over the next week?
2. How much control do I have over the change?
3. Is it small, discrete and possible?

EXAMPLES OF PLEDGES FROM PREVIOUS WORKSHOPS

- Next week I will take someone shopping that I don't normally take who rarely gets the chance to go out.

- To restart 'keep-fit' class even though only one or two people were interested

- To knock on the door and make sure the resident replies before I walk into a room.

'NEXT WEEK I WILL — — — — — — — — — — — — — —

— —

— —

— —

— —

— —

— —

31 Defining the goals and raising the issues in mental health promotion

G. MacDonald

'Psychology contains experimental methods and conceptual confusions.'
Wittgenstein quoted in Ingleby (1981) p 24

'Operational definition is an obstacle in front of which whole armies of theoreticians have blunted their weapons because, blinkered by their natural-istic assumptions, they have failed to take account of the distinctive problem of characterising human behaviour and experience.' Ingleby (1981) p 30

'The norms of mental 'health' and 'illness' are essentially matters of cultural judgement, although positivism misrepresents them as matters of empirical fact.' Ingleby (1981) p 43

Introduction

This paper began its life as an attempt to make progress in understanding how goals for mental health promotion can or should be set, and how mental health issues to do with patients / clients / people / colleagues can or should be raised. What at first seemed a very large task would, I thought be simplified because these two issues are related in that the sort of statements that are made about goals will have certain consequences for what sort of issues get raised and in what sorts of ways. To put it another way, I thought it was important to get our ideas about goals for mental health promotion sorted out before we decide - or slip into -ideas about methods.

In the event, the paper neither defines goals nor specifies issues for mental health promotion. Instead it questions the assumptions people make when they try to define goals for mental health promotion. One of these assumptions is that it is possible to define mental health. Another, is that it is justifiable to define mental health and in doing so, set the agenda for which mental health issues should be raised. The paper argues that these assumptions rest on philosophical confusions as well as ethical inconsiderations.

Clearly, in thinking about what sort of goals are appropriate or acceptable for promoting mental health, people will inevitably have a view about the nature of the thing they are trying to promote. Being clear about goals depends on being clear about what sort of thing mental health is. Is it the absence of mental illness? Or if more than this, what else should be included in a description of mental health? Can there be a mental component to health? And does mental illness exist and if so, how is it decided where illness stops and health starts? As Ingleby (1981) points out, these are as much **political** issues as anything else, and depend on our views of what society should be like.

'...is it sufficient, for example, to define health merely in terms of availability for work, or readiness to fulfil whatever role society has laid down for one? Is our society such, indeed, that 'normality' could ever be equated with 'sanity'?' (Ingleby, 1981).

These are theoretical questions which are being grappled with by practical people wanting to be clear, honest and rigorous about their plans for promoting mental health.

But in trying to find answers, there seems to be a cultural leaning towards wanting a definition, as if it is possible to complete a sentence which starts 'mental health is...'. I think there are problems, not only about how agreements can be reached about the sort of things that go into a definition - and the things that get left out - but also about the sort of activity you are doing - and the sort of assumptions you are making - in trying to define mental health.

What I want to argue is that it is not appropriate - both philosophically and ethically - to define mental health. This does not mean that the concept of mental health passes in to relativistic chaos - it just means that definitions are not what are required to make any sense of the issues. Similarly, I do not think it is appropriate to define goals for mental health promotion. This does not mean that there cannot be goals for the promotion of mental health - it just means that none of us are in any philosophical or ethical position to dictate what these are.

In putting forward this argument, I want to show that it is possible to talk about mental health in ways that make sense and in which agreements can be reached. But these agreements can only be reached when we have cleared away the conceptual confusions that building definitions places in our way.

The main part of the paper compares the goals for mental health promotion as they are viewed from four fundamentally different perspectives or paradigms. To compare the goals, we must necessarily compare the other features of these paradigms. Having done this, I look at the strengths and weaknesses of each paradigm - view before going on to expound more detailed criticism of one of these in particular - namely the functionalist view. In doing so, I think I point up some of the important issues about mental health that can be promoted. Finally, I point out some of the implications of my arguments, particularly for the sorts of things people who want to promote mental health need to be doing. **Goals for promoting mental health**.

Behind all our efforts to promote mental health will lie a personal construction about what it is we are trying to promote. I believe it is not only the detail of this construction - what we say mental health is or isn't - that needs our attention. Also, it is assumptions about the processes we go through, and the **sort of answer** we are looking for that are often left unattended and need prior scrutiny. So if it is possible to draw together a list of abilities and attributes that characterise what it is to be mentally healthy, then do we take this list as a definition - as a kind of check list - or do we take it as a menu - as a tool to help open up negotiation?

To define is to assume that what is needed as an answer to the question 'what is mental health?' is a definition, something to set a standard by, something to judge against, something achievable, an end to be reached. The implication set by this approach is that it is possible to answer the question 'what is mental health?' objectively.

To negotiate is to believe that what is mental health depends upon the individual, recognising that we are all individuals and that for example one person's stress is another person's driving force. Here, mental health is seen perhaps more as a journey than as an arrival. The implication is that it is only possible to answer the question subjectively.

I think a lot hangs on whether we are defining or negotiating when we try to characterise what is mental health. Not least of which concerns the sorts of things that are done to people if their personal abilities and attributes do not match the definition, the 'ideal'.

My own feeling - like others' I guess - is that there is something to hold onto **and** something to reject from both of these positions.

Regarding objectivity, I would like to hold onto the view that there is something objective about mental health in the sense that it is an idea or concept that there can be some agreement abut. What I would like to reject is that there is or can be an unequivocal standard of what counts as mental health which can be prescriptive of what counts as mentally healthy behaviour, and which can draw a line and categorise us as mentally healthy or ill.

Regarding subjectivity, I would like to hold onto the view that any agreement about what is mental health needs some flexibility, some variation to allow for the fact that people are different, as are their circumstances, their aspirations and their experiences of life. But also, I want to reject the idea that what counts as being mentally healthy is entirely relative to each individual.

How strongly you agree or disagree with me about holding on to or rejecting these points depends on where you are on the subjective - objective dimension. In part this is a matter of ideological persuasion. In part, it will depend on practical considerations on how effective you believe various promotional strategies to be, which arise out of these ideologically differing viewpoints. Also, there is something about feeling comfortable with certain strategies, perhaps to the point of defending established professional positions.

Of a more fundamental nature though, there are certain philosophical considerations which argue, not against the **desirability**, but the **appropriateness or legitimacy** of trying to define a concept like mental health.

Against 'the act of definition'

The point here is that it is not necessary to have a definition of something for it to have intelligible, credible meaning. You can try to invent a definition - draw a line - for the concept but this is for your own use. You cannot expect other people to necessarily agree with you, and you must be very careful about what **status** you hold their objections.

What you cannot do is deny that anything outside the line is meaningless. This is what Ayer (1956) and other positivists wanted to do - anything that could not be proved as true (this was his line) was meaningless. And for Popper (1959), anything that in principle could not be falsified was meaningless. I think that something like this sweeping disregard for what falls outside your definition still exists in debates about mental health. But I think we are unwise to disregard as irrelevant or meaningless ideas that are different to our own, just on the basis that they are different. One way to avoid disregarding the views of others is to avoid the temptation to make a definition in the first place. But as well as this pragmatic argument against definitions of mental health, there is a more fundamental problem which I now want to explore.

374

Wittgenstein (1953) used the notion of a game which will serve as a parallel to our thoughts about mental health. His reasoning is that we don't get our understanding of the word 'game' from a definition - even if what you mean by 'game' and what I mean by 'game' are different. But there are **limits** to how different these understandings of the word 'game' can be for us to have a sensible (meaningful) conversation. These limits are set by the way the word 'game' functions in language. Neither of us needed a definition of the word 'game' to learn these limits. Further, there is no definition which encompasses all the variety of activities which it makes sense to call games. In particular, there is no single feature common to all games which can act as the defining feature of what a game is - though there may be certain resemblances between one game and others. So any attempt to think up a definition - however convincing, all-embracing or credible it sounds - may appear to have a usefulness but we must remember that we knew how to use the word 'game' sensibly before the definition came along, and that there are going to be cases, either now or in the future, when people will use the word 'game' quite meaningfully, to which the definition will not apply.

This for me is where objectivity comes from - the meaning that comes from words being used intelligibly in language (this is what **language** is.) Or rather, it is because words are already used in language that the possibility of objectivity can arise. As Hamlyn (1970) puts it,

'We can raise the question of what is objective or otherwise only within the conceptual scheme that we have, given our form of life.......we cannot get outside these concepts to raise questions about objectivity independent of them.'

This is why subjectivity does not equate with relativism.

The parallel with mental health depends on whether 'mental health' functions descriptively in the same way as 'game' does (see Fogelin 1976). My own view is that the parallel is sound, and runs as follows.

We don't get our understanding of the words 'mental health' from a definition, especially if your understanding and my understanding are different. The fact that they are different does not mean only one of us understands and the other is wrong. What this difference in understanding depends on is there being a concept which we both use in language in a way in which communication happens and sense can be made. Again - we neither of us needed a definition to learn how to use the words 'mental health' in ways that made sense. Further, there is no definition which encompasses all the variety of features which it makes sense to describe as mental health. In particular, I do not see any single feature common to all meaningful uses of the words 'mental health' which can act as the defining feature of what mental health is - though there may be certain resemblances between one use of the words and another. So any attempt to think up a definition - however convincing, all-embracing or credible it sounds - may appear to have a usefulness but we must remember that we knew how to use the words 'mental health' sensibly before the definition came along, and that there are going to be cases, either now or in the future, when people will use these words quite meaningfully, to which the definition will not apply.

This may seem an over-technical argument, but I think its relevance is as follows. I think that what is important in setting goals and raising issues about mental health and its promotion is being able to discuss these things in meaningful ways with all those involved. What is not important is needing a definition before we can start discussion, for as Wittgenstein shows, any definition **depends** for its sense on the ordinary and everyday meanings that words have when we use them in language. Far from adding clarity, 'the act of definition' adds conceptual confusion because a definition will never cover everything that anyone will want to say about mental health, and will cloud the real issues which I think are about the assumptions being made - either in an unattended or intentional way - about the criteria for what goes in and what is left out.

So why do we search for a definition?

It is worth considering why definitions are sought for a concept like mental health. In the main, I think this is because there is a temptation to work in ways analogous to the physical sciences in which concepts are given definitions which do not correspond to everyday usage. The person wanting a definition is acting rather like a scientist who needs to define a new phenomenon. But we ought to note that we are not dealing with a **new** phenomenon - people have been engaging this question for as long as there have been people.

Science is often seen in this way as the paradigm model of human thought. If a method such as definition works in science, the argument goes, then it will work just as well in other areas.

This temptation is based on the assumptions.
* that methods used in the physical sciences 'work', and
* that these methods are translatable to human questions like 'what is mental health?'

I think there are many problems with this Popperian / Skinnerian view that cannot be gone into in this paper. My view is that in discussing mental health, we should not be scientists -our methodology is quite different. (Winch, 1964, Rhees 1970, Graham 1986). And as Ingleby points out,

'The physicist's definition......is justified by its meaningfulness and utility within a well-established theory, and the theory itself translates readily back into the language of everyday experience. None of this is true of the 'operational definitions proposed in psychology.' (1981).

There is also a further problem about trying to find scientific answers to fundamentally human questions. As Ingleby also points out,

'...increasing public mistrust about scientists' aims has complicated the notion of 'objectivity' and opened up a new discourse about the social and political roots of science.' (ibid).

And as Graham has noted,

'Nietzche....regarded the scientific search for absolute truth as a reflection of a desperate need for certainty in an uncertain world, and the outcome of fear' (1986)

So far from being a model of discourse independent and free from human perspectives, science might best be seen as itself a dependant and tied to the emotional, social and political under-currents of our lives.

So if we cannot be said to be acting scientifically in wanting a definition, are we acting philosophically? I do not think so. For as Wittgenstein says, 'when philosophers use a word ..... and try to grasp the **essence** of the thing, one must always ask oneself: is the word ever actually used in this way in the language-game which is its original home?' What philosophers should do is not to invent new homes (new meanings) for words, but to 'bring words back from their metaphysical to their everyday use.' Wittgenstein (1953)

A second attraction of searching for a definition of mental health is that it is assumed that a definition provides objectivity. But as I have shown, objectivity does not depend on definitions - rather, it is the other way round. So, if an **objective** definition is what you were after, then are you happy with the possibility that it will not include all cases?

A third point as to why people feel that definitions are appropriate is that they assume that their experiences, training, education, profession, job, status, social position, etc., give them the **entitlement** to define what counts as mental health. But what gives anyone the right to make a definition which excludes what other people might want to include? This is no longer a discussion about philosophy but about power. Whatever the profession or social position, there are clearly ethical as well as philosophical problems about 'the act of definition' which I feel we should do well to avoid.

377

Objectivity, society and our view of mental health

As we have seen above, there are problems about asking for an 'objective' description of mental health. Objectivity is already there if we look for it in the language we use. Trying to **add** objectivity through 'the act of definition' merely muddies the discussion because a range of unfounded assumptions about pragmatism, philosophy and power are being employed.

But as well as these difficulties, I believe there are other assumptions at work in many statements made about what is mental health. These concern how we see other people and ourselves, and the roles and positions we occupy in the society in which we live. This introduces another dimension which has an influence on the sort of mental health we feel we should be aiming for - a dimension about society. For as Caplan and Holland (1990) point out,

'If mental health is about how we experience ourselves in the world, then it is important to have a well thought out view of society.'

Burrell and Morgan (1979), in their sociological analysis of organisations (their arguments pertain to far wider issues in society than mental health alone) characterise this dimension. Society is seen

'in terms of structural and other social conflicts such as that between capital and labour, the fight against racism and other forms of discrimination. It is these contradictions and tensions reflected in various modes of domination of some classes and groups which lead to various forms of social, economic, political and cultural deprivation.....' (ibid)

As Caplan and Holland have pointed out, how each of us sees mental health depends on our position along this dimension. In the social control view,

'mental health or illness would have more to do with the make up of the individual, or the faulty functioning of particular primary institutions in which the individual develops, such as the family. The idea conveyed here is one of regulating individuals or institutions so as to fit them into an otherwise harmonious and integrated social whole.' (ibid).

In the social change view, mental health or illness has more to do with the make up of society in general.

Burrell and Morgan (1985) have provided a framework which enables the discussion to be taken further by crossing the two dimensions we have so far discussed, i.e.

* theories about knowledge, objective vs. subjective
* theories about society, social control vs. social change

This produces a four quadrant or paradigm metatheory which has been used to good effect by Caplan (1986) and Taylor (1990) in helping to illuminate various aspects of health education and promotion, including mental health promotion Caplan and Holland (1990) and Tudor (1991).

Burrell and Morgan use the labels 'Functionalist', Radical Humanist' etc to characterise each paradigm. I think that these terms may be misleading, especially as regards the two 'humanist' paradigms. For as Helen Graham

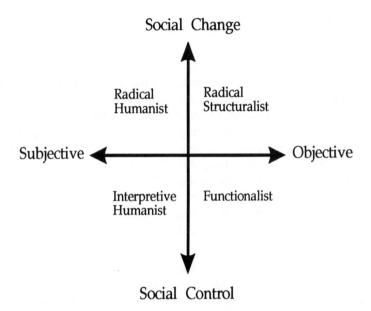

has pointed out, any humanist worthy of the name is holistic in orientation and is thus concerned with the total entity, and not with abstracting certain features (e.g. cognition, emotionality) from the whole.

On the other hand, I do think the four paradigm analysis is helpful in pointing out how approaches to mental health have typically been made. In particular, I think it helps us see the strengths and weaknesses of each paradigm view so that we gain insight into a more unified, holistic way forward.

Four paradigms of mental health

What I would like to do now is take the present discussion further by seeing how mental health has been variously described under each paradigm, and in doing so, begin to draw out the implications of each of the four paradigm positions for the raising of mental health issues in practice.

Functionalist

The functionalist definition of mental health is based, as we have said above, on the assumption that there is or can be an unequivocal condition called mental health. As Tudor (1992) has pointed out, Wooton (1959) and Preston (1943) describe their vision of mental health in terms of 'mental hygiene' and the idea of a 'good productive worker' as if there is a clearly 'correct', 'good', or 'wholesome' way of behaving mentally which, if followed will no doubt lead us to fulfil our destiny and place in society.

Words that have been used to describe mental health in this paradigm are: *autonomous, self governing, in touch with reality, being in control, being credible, being useful, being rational, making rational choices, being purposeful, being consistent, having direction in life, recognising boundaries, sustaining effort despite frustration, acceptance, independence, respect for others.....*

The focus of the functionalist paradigm seems to me to be changes in an individual's behaviour or presenting symptoms - these changes brought about by whatever methods and means the 'expert' consultant or therapist deems appropriate because (and there have been many examples in the history of mental health) to the functionalist view, the end will justify the means. Or perhaps some 'higher principle' is brought in to justify the end, as when Szasz insists that psychiatrists should

'return to a contractual relationship with the patient, aimed simply at promoting individual liberty' (in Ingleby, 1981).

The strength of this view is perhaps its clarity, and that in many cases, it is the behaviour or symptom that first presents itself as the block to mental health. The weakness is that I think that blocks to mental health often go a lot deeper, and into other dimensions than behaviour or physical symptoms, and that the latter will be concentrated upon in disproportionate and ethically worrying ways.

Interpretive humanist

Kakar (1984) has written about mental health in terms of an 'integration of psychological functioning' and 'conduct of personal and social life' which could be taken to highlight the importance - at least for Kakar - of maximising the effectiveness and autonomous power of the individual **within** the confines of a fairly static social whole. Phrases like 'overcoming negative thought patterns' are common in this area (Beck, 1976). It is also about helping people move their concentration away from certain limited features of the problem in order that they may see other possibilities for its solution.

'although people believe themselves to be looking for the solution, they are actually hanging onto the problem.' (Graham, 1992).

For me, interpretive humanism is about helping to free the thinking of individuals via processes (and by people) which are defined socially e.g., maintaining a professional - client control and distance; middle class - defined notions such as assertion training, stress management and relaxation. It's almost as if these are the new prescriptions. This sort of control of the process seems to me to be very predominant in a lot of contemporary work done in the name of mental health promotion.

Words that have been used to describe mental health in this paradigm are: *autonomous, able to make decisions, relating to others, being able to say no, having self worth, being calm, being relaxed, being assertive, recognising boundaries, ability to communicate, ability to make relationships, ability to seek help, having coping strategies, being intelligent, dealing with life, being calm, clarity of thought, making choices, capacity to learn, capacity to develop and change one's characteristics....*

It seems to me that the main focus of the interpretive humanist paradigm is the self - awareness and development of an individual's cognitive processes. The strength of this is that it takes into account the phenomenology of mental health problems - that is, that we all see them so we are both the source and the solution of the problems we create. As Hay (1988) asserts.

'The only thing we are ever dealing with is a thought and a thought can be changed.'

The weakness may be placing too little emphasis on how the individual feels, and too much on what s/he thinks. There may also be too much emphasis on the role of assertiveness training and other personal development technologies as a prescription for mental health problems, and on the assumption that these problems can **in principle** be solved by the way an individual thinks and reacts. As Ingleby argues.

'Postulating variables like 'stress' is no substitute for a properly interpretive account of the way people's situations, as they perceive them, give them grounds for their conduct.' (Ingleby 1981)

Radical humanist

The writings of radical humanism often appear similar to the previous paradigm. For Kittleson (1989).

'mental health should deal with communication skills, decision making skills, values awareness and self esteem.'

Berne (1968) talks of 'autonomy, awareness, spontaneity, intimacy'. Both of these could come from either the Interpretive or Radical Humanist camps. Tudor (1992) places them in the latter, but does not give much indication as to why. For me, the difference is about the role of the worker and her relation to the individual. Often the difference is about assessment or accessing needs - about prescription or negotiation of processes aimed at fulfilling such need.

Words that have been used to describe mental health in this paradigm are: *expressing positive and negative emotions, being happy with yourself, relating to others, having a feeling of self worth, having self worth, being calm and relaxed when I want to be, feeling I have a purpose, recognising I have rights, ability to make and develop relationships, finding simplicity, letting go, having a positive self image, having an internal locus of control, being genuine, being able to love and play, feeling empathy for others, having respect for self and others, clarity of feelings, spontaneity, intimacy.....*

The main focus of the radical humanist paradigm seems to me that issues are dealt with at an emotional level. The feelings of the people involved are the substance of the promotional work with outcomes such as change in behaviour being incidental. The strength of this is that for me at least, a really important and often ignored aspect of what mental health is - the affective domain - is put firmly to the fore. The weakness may be that even if people feel better about situations they are in, by placing the main emphasis on the individual's emotional perception and response, certain injustices in the situation may be condoned, ignored and perpetuated, where a degree of social action may be at least as appropriate.

Radical structuralist

Fromm (1956) defines mental health as

'the ability to love and to create, by the emergence from incestuous ties to clan and soil, by a sense of identity based on one's experience of self as the subject and agent of one's powers, by the grasp of reality inside and outside of ourselves, that is, by the development of objectivity and reason.'

These last three words remind us which end of the subjective - objective dimension we have returned to. Fromm argues that mental health

'cannot be defined in terms of the adjustment of the individual to his society, but, on the contrary....must be defined in terms of the adjustment of society to the needs of man.'

As Ingleby (1991) points out, under this view,

'to achieve mental health and the way in which one does so, depends to a small extent on individual factors, but is largely a question of what society makes possible.'

An example of this approach is the work of Basaglia (1981) and his staff at a provincial psychiatric hospital in Gorizia, Italy. Their aim

'was not seeking simply to make the asylum 'work better', but to lay the groundwork for its total destruction.'

This is because Basaglia believes that as long as there is such an institution as an asylum, there will be a spurious reality given to the notion of mental illness. For him, mental illness

'is not what the mental hospital cures but what it creates; from this source emanate both the categories of disorder and the fundamental meaning of mental illness as something to be segregated and contained.'

Words that have been used to describe mental health in this paradigm are: *expressing emotions, relating to others, being able to say no, being able to lobby, being able to make demands, ability to react against oppressive forces, identifying with a social purpose, ability to articulate, purposive social behaviour.....*

The focus of the radical structuralist paradigm is the change of society and its systems by collective social action. The strength of this approach seems to me, that it does seek to address and rectify injustices, intolerances and inequalities which many people believe - with a good deal of justification in my view - to be at the root of a range of the mental health problems people have. The weakness would be that this approach somehow undervalues how an individual characterises and interacts with these social issues, and how individual growth and learning can often flow from focusing on this interaction.

The following diagram is an attempt to summarise the discussion so far by listing what I see as the characterising goals, beliefs and focus in each paradigm, together with implications for subsequent promotional activity:

Paradigms and practice

Depending on your paradigm, you will have varying empathy with the different focuses described above. And you will minimise or maximise the various strengths and weaknesses as I have described them. Or, following Evans - Pritchard, you may be so closely wedded to your own paradigm view that 'you cannot think that your thought is wrong' (1973). This illustrates an important point about paradigms,

'they conform to different **mentalities**.....(and) to this extent, adherence to one or other paradigm is equivalent to membership of a sort of community.' (Ingleby, 1981)

And of course, various professional groupings are in many cases the physical embodiment of paradigm mentalities.

Radical Humanist	**Radical Structuralist**
mental health: subjective goals: personal re-orientaton relationship: person-person focus: feelings methods: negotiated counselling, groupwork "what would be of help to you to be what you want to be"	mental health: objective goals: social change relationship: advocate-activist focus: social behaviour methods: collective action "what do we need to change in society to redefine the norm"
Interpretive Humanist	**Functionalist**
mental health: subjective goals: personal coping skills relationship: professional-client focus: thinking skills, self talk methods: interpreting, counselling, groupwork "you need me and my skills/technologies to help you be what you want to be"	mental health: objective goals: curing individuals relationship: expert patient focus: individual behaviour or symptoms methods: experimentation, organic treatment "this is what you need to do to start being normal"

Choosing paradigms

The four paradigm analysis of mental health issues is offered as a view of current practice -a description not a prescription. The question now is, what are the implications of the four paradigm analysis for the practice of mental health promotion?

The first implication for all of us, professionals especially, is that there are, as I have indicated, a number of assumptions that we make - perhaps in a very unattended way - which will guide our perception of the mental health issues we come across. These assumptions will also guide **what we see and accept as** a mental health issue, as well as the actions we make in response.

The second point is that each paradigm has its strengths. This is not the same as saying that each has equal merit so it's just a matter of taking your pick and choosing the one you are most comfortable with. Rather, it is to recognise that there are certain mental health issues that will benefit from being seen in particular cases and by particular people from one particular paradigm. It is worth noting that if you accept this view, then you are already rejecting the functionalist mono - view.

To say that each paradigm has its strengths is not the same as saying that once we begin to see a mental health issue from one paradigm that this is where it should end. Rather, as Sue Holland (1990) has pointed out, there is enormous scope for **moving through the paradigms** - perhaps beginning with the paradigm that meets the specifics of the circumstance, but following through to help develop the thoughts, feelings or social activity of people as is appropriate to the needs and aspirations they identify. As Holland says,

'through all the shifts and diversions I keep in my head the notion of moving people through the different spaces (paradigms). They all seem to start off as functionalists, that is, they see themselves as machines that need a bit of adjusting; they need a tonic, or they need some tablets for their 'nerves'. Working class people, in contrast to those from the middle class have been taught to think like this.' (Holland 1990).

So it is not so much a decision for all time about which paradigm we fit into, but about which features of a particular individual's circumstances and experience are best addressed by which paradigm. And it may well be that for many, their experiences and circumstances cannot be made sense of or helped from only one paradigm view. The task may well be to **move away** from the paradigms to a much more holistic view.

As I have pointed out above, belonging to a paradigm view corresponds to a **mentality** - a certain ideology or weltanschauung from which it can be very difficult to see another point of view. But what I want to argue is that although each paradigm might have its strengths, and although the people whose mental health we are trying to promote may begin the interaction in one paradigm or another, there **are** arguments which point to the need for movement.

These arguments are not simply pro-humanist or anti-functionalist - although I admit to **an emphasis** in this direction. Rather they are arguments which are relative to situations. They are arguments which I hope begin to map out where one paradigm should be abandoned for the strengths afforded by another. In the main, I am following Habermas, whose view is that

'These fundamental questions of paradigm choice are to be settled by **moral** reasoning, which is not a matter of brute force and emotion, but of negotiation and a common search for ideals.' (in Ingleby, 1981)

Thoughts about functionalism

As will be gathered from earlier comments, I think that the scope for a functionalist approach to mental health promotion has severe limits. Not least of these are difficulties in 'the act of defining' a concept like 'mental health'. But as well as objecting to this **activity**, I also have some objections to its results. But in raising these, it ought to be borne in mind that the starting point for functionalists embodies the same views and assumptions about objectivity that are shared by structuralists. So it is not surprising that some of these thoughts about functionalism apply to radical structuralism as well.

The first point to make is that the functionalist, believing in the possibility of an objective definition, will come up with a closed and unnecessarily **narrow** list of words to describe mental health. The list cannot be extended and varied depending on changes in society and the perceptions and aspirations of the people you are working with. I think that given both of these variables - society and its people as individuals - we need to keep the lists open and under review both from time to time and from situation to situation. But sometimes, our professional specialism leads us to view mental health in this narrow, functionalist way. For example,

'Psychiatry takes on itself the responsibility for people's pain and frustration; it confiscates their problems, redefines them as 'illnesses', and (with luck) exterminates the symptoms.' (Ingleby, 1981)

So for me, functionalism tries to limit the scope of mental health to something it can deal with on its own terms - not on the terms of the people concerned. By rejecting the subjective, functionalism leaves too much out and inaccurately translates what goes in. It denies what for Ingleby is undeniable.

'...that events affect us not for what they are, but for what they mean to us.' (ibid)

This brings us to a second point about functionalism that I think is wrong: this is about 'reality' and how we see the world. For the functionalist, there is a reality which is 'out there', waiting to be discovered by the rigours of scientific method. It's as if the world has 'its own story' and that science 'describes the world in the same way that the world would describe itself if it could.' (Luntley, 1992)

but this assumes that the language science has used to describe the world actually works in this 'naming' way - as if scientific language has simply found names to talk about the various bits of the universe that we can see. As Wittgenstein showed however, this is not how language works. Naming is not the end in itself, indeed

'naming and description do not stand on the same level: naming is a preparation for description. Naming is so far not a move in a language-game - any more than putting a piece in its place on the board is a move in chess. We may say **nothing** has so far been done when a thing is named. It has not even got a name except in the language game. This is what Frege meant too, when he said that a word had meaning only as part of a sentence.' (1953)

What this means is that naming can only happen **within** a language. As Fogelin puts it

'if we take ostensive definition (naming) as the **fundamental** method of assigning meanings to words, we have failed to notice that the activity of giving an ostensive definition makes sense only within the context of a previously established linguistic framework.' (1976)

So what we call reality depends on the language game we have available to describe it. And it is the culture we live in in which that language game will be based. As Luntley observes,

'the language of science is just as culturally determined a way of looking at the world as religion.' (1992)

- or as any other language game. So how we see things in the world - how we characterise our experience - depends on a culturally determined language. But **which words we choose**

'involves a subjective selection, categorisation and interpretation and is ultimately a matter of choice...and as the concepts thus selected are chosen to suit personal purposes, values necessarily enter into even the most mundane description.' (Graham, 1986)

All this argues against functionalism in favour of a **phenomenological** approach -

'the study of the appearance of things as they appear in consciousness, rather than the study of things in themselves.' (Graham, 1986).

In terms of mental health, this does not mean accepting that any person's perception of events is without difficulty - indeed the perception of a problem is in many cases the **source** of the problem. The functionalist response to problem - causing perceptions has been to treat them as 'deviations' from the 'norm', requiring treatment. But this takes from the person both the essence of the reality they are experiencing, and the possibility of finding their own solutions. It amounts to an inadmissible denial of our affective life - our feelings. The structuralist too can make a similar mistake by 'blaming it all on society'. On the other hand, humanism can go too far if it denies that meaning is a social variable, and that how a person perceives a situation will depend on the social conditioning s/he has received thus far (i.e., perception depends upon the moves we have learnt to make in the language games which create our reality.)

A third point is the way functionalism often goes hand in hand with Cartesian thinking, To mix Ingleby and Ryle, they think that the human machine has both faults and ghosts. But is mental health something that can be viewed and dealt with in isolation from what is happening in the rest of the individual's physical, emotional and spiritual experience? I would argue that it cannot. Indeed, Graham has pointed out that 'mental health' is a contradiction in terms. As Perls has argued, health

> 'Can only be achieved through the integration of all the parts of the self, because it is only in this way that the self emerges as unified or 'whole' in relation to its environment, and is able to assert or express its needs and satisfy them.' (Graham, 1992)

This brings us to the fourth point: a consideration of people's needs. As has been mentioned above, what you will do to promote mental health depends in part on whether you see it as your role to define or to negotiate the health needs of the people you are working with. Maslow

> 'conceived of a hierarchy of needs, basic to which are physical needs.....
> (and) that health must be viewed as the fulfilment of physical, psychological and spiritual needs.' (Graham, 1992)

If you believe Maslow, then like me, I think you will want to avoid defining an individual's need, but work through negotiation to help both you and the people you are working with to identify what these needs are. This argues for a more interpretive view than functionalism allows.

This may involve finding a balance between different and often competing mental health needs. e.g. being genuine **and** relating to others; being consistent **and** being calm and relaxed when I want to be. Graham asserts that

> 'the satisfaction of one's needs is something of a balancing act, maintained by a self - regulatory process of constant awareness of self and its situation.' (ibid)

I would want to add that it is in terms of what the individual sees as **important, significant or fulfilling** about herself and her situation that fuels this self-regulatory process. Again, for me, this points to the need for negotiation and creating the conditions for a kind of comfortable reflection in order for this adjustment or balance to take place. Also, I would want to allow for flexibility in the **degree** to which any one aspect of mental health is taken on board. Again, I think talk about negotiation and flexibility are more interpretive / humanistic than functionalism would allow. And structuralism too can be very dogmatic in its assumptions about the needs of people. I think we need to allow for the fact that no matter how strongly our conviction may be that mental health should include a certain aspect, the people we are dealing with may not share this view, may not **ever** share this view, or may only see what you judge as the relevance of this view after other needs and aspirations have been met. Even then, this relevance may be seen as less important to them than it does to you, and I would hope that if we are genuine and respectful of the people we work with, that we allow for the possibility of changing our minds.

Finally, if mental health can be thought of as adjustment or balance, then as Perls argued, 'much of the difficulty in maintaining this balance can be attributed to the way individuals are required to conform to one central, enduring social role, and the expectations that are attached to it.' (ibid).

For example, the patriarchal pressures in society can mean that finding a balance between stereotypical gender roles is difficult. As Graham points out,

'...males characteristically suppress the more sensitive side of their natures, and thus certain emotions and their expression, intuition and aesthetic qualities, whereas females typically fail to assert their independence, aggression, sexuality and intellect. Consequently, individuals experience confusion as to where they end and others begin, and cannot satisfy their needs as they are not aware of what they are.' (ibid)

Functionalism has nothing to say about these social pressures. But structuralism can be in danger of saying too much, by leaving out the interaction between social objectivity and the person. As Ingleby points out, the capitalist system, pay and legislation

'are sustained by the individual psyche.' (1981)

Regardless of social conditions and deprivations, people often **do** recognise and meet their needs. They may have similarities with those who have survived illness, war and other deprivations and who, as Siegel (1990) has noted, have in common a **flexibility** which tight stereotyping is not going to allow. This flexibility shows itself as characteristic traits which are biphasic, that is

'they are both serious **and** playful, logical **and** intuitive, rational **and** emotional, hardworking **and** lazy.....' (Graham, 1992).

Another aspect of the need for flexibility concerns our western cultural preoccupation with verbal expression. This is perhaps saying the same thing as the criticism of being too tightly defined in gender stereotypes.

Again, functionalism with its emphasis on a correct, ordered and ordained view of how society should be is often the source of the mental health pressures people face, and offers solutions which only look at the symptoms whilst carefully ignoring the cause. As Ingleby observes,

'As this apparatus perfects itself, so the goal of a society fit for human habitation recedes further and further into the future.' (1981)

To conclude thus far, functionalists

'bamboozled by their own scientific self-image, have accepted the servile position of functionaries in the modern state; emancipated from that role, hopefully they may be in a position to be critical of society itself.' (ibid)

Some implications for mental health promotion

There is something that for me threads through the points I have just made. If we are to be flexible about how we describe mental health, tolerant of how others describe it, serious about the real needs that people have, accepting the likelihood of conflicts and opposition between different needs and willing to work with people to help them find balance and resolution, then mental health is perhaps much more like a journey than an arrival. It is much more like developing and growing than a finished product. What are the implications of this view for the promotion of mental health? In essence, this must mean doing whatever we can to help people on their journey.

Firstly, this must mean helping people find where they are and identify where they would like to go. It means finding ways in which the people you are working with can be helped to identify their own area of concern, in language that they generate, and in ways that do not prescribe, set standards or goals other than those that the individuals have negotiated and are happy with. In some cases, this will start from judgements made by people by themselves or on their behalf at the functionalist stage. This is a starting point, but someone needs to work through with the individuals where it is they would like to go. I guess this sometimes means doing a lot of unpacking of all of the issues that are tied into the original presenting problem.

In other cases, there may be no presenting problem - at least, none that any of the people concerned are willing or able to identify or admit to.

Working to promote mental health in these cases needs to begin by establishing a dialogue abut people's lives, their needs, their aspirations and the cognitive, emotional and social obstacles that people see as standing in their way. It may mean looking outside the obvious - it may mean looking outside of the 'normal' focus imposed by your job and your worldview. It means taking the whole person seriously, starting with people and their concerns, not with your ideology. It means not using technical and medical language but it may mean helping people develop a language in which to explore their experiences and make progress in getting to where they want to go.

This language may not be verbal, and making progress may involve using imagery and visualisation, art or drama to help find ways of saying when words and thoughts fail.

So promoting mental health may mean finding new ways of working. It will certainly mean answering difficult questions of yourself as a worker about the degree of professionalisation that you have invested in and may have to leave behind. It will involve addressing your own personal needs and aspirations, your own personal journey and growth. It will require honesty about goals, about methods and effectiveness, and collaboration with other workers who can take over where your skills leave off.

In consequence, promoting mental health needs to be about open debate and interagency collaboration across agency and professional boundaries. For some, if not all of us, this means letting go of rigid rules. But as Hay (1988) points out, this ability to 'let go' is itself a very humanistic view of what it is to be mentally healthy. By their own definition therefore, it will be functionalists who may find it most difficult to get involved in this debate. So perhaps it will be functionalists who will need the most help. This is paradoxical, as often functionalists are the people with the most power.

What you do in response to these thoughts is a bit like what we expect our patients / clients / people to do when dealing with a mental health issue. Do we use it as an opportunity to examine our thoughts, develop our competencies, explore our feelings or move to change the system if this is the real block to progress? Or should we do all of these things?

Acknowledgements

I should like to thank the following people for their help and ideas which have helped me to write this papers.

Tracey Austin, Fiona Mooniaruch, Robert Davies, Craig Newns, Keith Tudor.

References

Ayer, A. J. (1965). *The problem of knowledge*. Penguin.

Basaglia, F. (1981). Breaking the circuit of control. In D. Ingleby *Critical Psychiatry*. Penguin.

Beck, A. T. (1976). *Cognitive therapy of depression*. International Universities Press.

Berne, E. (1964). *Games people play*. Penguin.

Burrell, G., & Morgan, G. (1985). *Sociological paradigms and organisational analysis*. Gower.

Caplan, R., & Holland, R. (1990). Rethinking Health Education Theory. *Journal of Health Education*, **49** (1) 10-12.

Evans-Pritchard, E. E. (1937). *Witchcraft, oracles and magic among the Azande*. Oxford University Press.

Fogelin, R. J. (1976). *Wittgenstein*. Routledge & Kegan Paul.

Fontana, D. (1992). *Know who you are, be what you want*. Fontana.

Fromm, E. (1956). *The sane society*. Routledge.

Graham, H. (1986). *The human face of psychology*. Open University.

Graham, H. (1992). *The magic shop*. Rider

Hamlyn, D. (1970). *The theory of knowledge*. MacMillan.

Hay, L. (1988). *You can heal your life*. Eden Grove.

Holland, S. (1990). Psychotherapy, oppression and social action: Gender, race and class in black women's depression. In Perlberg & Miller (Eds.) *Gender and power in families*. Routledge.

Ingleby, D. (Ed.) (1981). *Critical Psychiatry*. Penguin.

Kakar, S. (1984). *Shamans, mystics and doctors*. Unwin.

Kittleson, M. J. (1989). Mental health vs. mental illness: A philosophical discussion. *Health Education*. April/May 40-42.

Luntley, M. (1992). *The real thing*. Channel 4 Television.

Popper, K. (1959). *The logic of scientific discovery*. Hutchinson

Rhees, R. (1970). *Without answers*. Routledge and Kegan Paul.

Ryle, G. (1949). *The concept of mind*. Hutchinson.

Taylor, V. (1990). Health education - a theoretical mapping. *Health*

Education Journal. **49**(2) 13-14.

Tudor, K. & Holroyd, G. (1992). Psyche and society. *The promotion of mental health, vol. 1.* Avebury.

Tudor, K. (1992). Unpublished paper to the Howard Morton Symposium on psychological approaches to the promotion of mental health. University of Sheffield.

Winch, P. (1964). *The idea of a social science and its relation to philosophy.* Routledge and Kegan Paul.

Wittgenstein, L. (1953). *Philosophical investigations.* Basil Blackwell.

Wittgenstein, L. (1974). *Philosophical grammar.* Basil Blackwell.

32 A report on a study of views and attitudes of people in contact with former patients discharged from a Northern Ireland hospital

R. Manktelow

Introduction to the study

i) The researcher

I was employed as a social worker at a Northern Ireland hospital for over twelve years. During that time I have worked in the acute admission wards, the intensive nursing wards, the continuing-care wards and from 1987 in rehabilitation. Three years ago the Community Rehabilitation Team was formed to provide long-term follow-up and support to former long-stay patients and to those people chronically disabled by their mental illness living outside hospital. I am a founder member of this multi-disciplinary team and continue to be centrally involved in providing services to this client group.

This research developed out of my professional experience. Whilst a considerable amount of work is being undertaken to find out what the individual leaving hospital feels about the changes he is experiencing, it is also important to prepare the communities in which former patients will reside. The project is therefore action research which sought both to educate and change attitudes as well as investigate what people think.

The paper is a merger of my views as a social worker in rehabilitation and a report on research findings, which are inevitably interpreted through the eyes of a practitioner.

ii) The study

The aim of this preliminary project was to investigate the response of the local community to the discharge of long-stay patients from the county Psychiatric Hospital. Since the policy of reducing the number of long-stay patients began in Northern Ireland in 1987, the extent to which former patients have integrated with the wider community has depended on the attitudes of the people amongst whom they live. Also community attitudes influence the quality of life which may be experienced by resettled long term psychiatric patients.

Only 102 long-stay patients were discharged from the hospital over the five years, 1987-1992. The majority of the general population are unlikely to have experienced direct contact with this group. The project focused, therefore, on the attitudes, behaviour and reactions of those members of the local community who had had contact with former patients.

Usually these interactions took place in the neighbourhoods in which they lived. Contact also occurred between former patients and their families and between former patients and those individuals who made up their informal social networks.

The study explored the possibility that groups in contact with former patients had sympathetic and tolerant attitudes towards people with mental illness. Associations between certain characteristics of these 'host' communities or groups and positive attitudes were explored with a view to identifying the types of communities which might be most receptive to former patients. The Researcher also included an investigation of neighbourhood views of the local sheltered care scheme. A question of particular interest for future projects was how far familiarity with former patients had increased tolerance towards people with mental illness. Information describing former patient/community interaction was collected in order to illuminate the social process of 'community care'.

The aims of the study are summarised in the following research questions:-

1. What is the nature and extent of knowledge about the policy of community care and local services for people with mental illness or those in some degree of contact with them?
2. How do residents in neighbourhoods containing a Community Mental Health Facility view its impact?
3. What are the attitudes of those in contact with former patients towards people with mental illness?
4. What is the amount and type of contact between former patients and people in the community?
5. What is the nature of interaction between these members of 'The community' and former patients? Specifically, how does interaction occur and what form does it take?

The geographical location of the study was a town in Northern Ireland, although some families lived elsewhere. The research was built around interviews with 114 people. The study sample consisted of a number of sub-groups distinguished by the manner of their contact with former long-stay patients. These forms of contact were living in a neighbourhood containing a community mental health facility, being a befriender of a former patient and being a relative of a former patient. Also included were a group of pupils from a local secondary school.

iii) The broad themes of the study: The community response

There is a considerable body of literature (Goffman, 1961) which holds that institutional care has involved the removal, isolation and stigmatisation of the mentally ill. Furthermore, it has been argued that this process has encouraged a public reaction of ignorance, prejudice and rejection (Busfield, 1986).

The current policy of community care in Northern Ireland (DHSS, 1986) holds that long-stay patients should be resettled in smaller home-like settings in the community. If such stigmatised individuals are to live outside hospitals then public attitudes towards the care and treatment of people with mental illness become crucially important as they determine the nature of the community response.

This community response to people with mental illness may be viewed from a number of perspectives: sociological, psychological and geographical. Each of these outlooks on community response highlights certain issues about the social integration of former patients. These are: the concept of deinstitutionalisation and the concept of destigmatisation (associated with the sociologist and the social-psychologist); and the concept of decentralisation (associated with the social geographer).

The sociological perspective (Becker, 1967) emphasises the labelling of mental illness by others as the crucial event in becoming mentally ill. Being mentally ill becomes a 'master status' (Scheff, 1966) by which acts of the individual, inside and outside hospital are defined by others. Labelling theory (Lemert, 1972) suggests that outside hospital the individuals will still be perceived negatively in terms of former psychiatric patient status. The potential for reintegrating may be severely limited as others continue to interpret actions according to past history as a psychiatric patient.

The social-psychological perspective (Rabkin, 1974) emphasises the importance of public attitudes in influencing the community response towards people with mental illness. Attitudes are related to social behaviour, although the precise nature of this association is unclear. For instance, a person may hold very definite attitudes but may not act on them. Alternatively, a person may profess to hold different attitudes from real ones because the individual is concerned to give a socially acceptable response. Bearing these caveats in mind, the measurement of attitudes may be an important indicator of the community response to the resettlement of ex-patients. In this investigation the Community Attitudes towards Mental Illness Scale (Taylor & Dear, 1981) was used to assess attitudes.

The third perspective is that of social geographer (Smith & Giggs, 1988). Such a perspective links tangible factors like proximity, location and neighbourhood to the more intangible factors already mentioned, such as societal reaction and public attitudes. Public facility location theory (Dear & Taylor 1982) deals with the spillover effects of public facilities on the surrounding communities. These external effects may be negative or positive and are important factors in shaping local attitudes. Facility characteristics like size, design, visibility and level of supervision are one set of external variables. Neighbourhood characteristics like household composition, home ownership and beliefs about property prices are another.

iv) Summary of findings

The main findings of the research are summarised below:-

1. All the groups studied held positive attitudes to people with mental illness. These were three neighbourhoods containing a sheltered care accommodation for discharged long-stay patients, family and volunteers who made up the key social networks of ex-patients, and a group of school pupils with no direct contact with former patients.

2. All three neighbourhoods reported a positive level of acceptance of the sheltered accommodation located on their estate. The three types of accommodation were statutory mental health hostel, group home and sheltered flatlets.

3. The knowledge amongst respondents about local services was not high and the policy of community care, as conceptualised within the caring professions, was not familiar to many people. However, their responses indicated a basic understanding of its principles, a respect for individual freedom and a rejection of long-term institutional care.

4. Although it was not possible to make any statistically significant comparisons between sub-groups it was clear that the responses of relatives of people suffering mental illness were rather differ-

ent. They were less critical of institutional care and more cautious about the ability of ex-patients to lead normal lives.

5. Contact was highest between former patients and their immediate families with whom they were most likely to stay overnight. However, because of the ageing of relatives this contact is likely to decline over the years.

6. The study described the everyday interaction between ex-patients and the community as represented by neighbours, befrienders and relatives. It appeared that when former patients lived in facilities which encouraged independent living there was more potential for social integration. When they were shopping, paying bills, using public transport and other activities ex-patients were accepted as normal residents within their community.

Methods of research

The study sample was made up of a total of 114 individuals. This total consisted of a number of sub-groups as follows -

1) Three sub-groups drawn from neighbourhoods where residential facilities for people with mental illness were concerned. These were a Statutory Mental Health Hostel, two Group Homes and a Sheltered Flatlets Scheme.

2) A sub-group composed of relatives of former long-stay patients.

3) A sub-group made up of befrienders who provided social and recreational activities for ex-patients.

4) A sub-group of Secondary School pupils who had been taught on mental illness.

A questionnaire was administered by the researcher to the respondents. The interview schedule comprised of three parts: Part I contained structured questions about the policy of community care and local psychiatric services. Part II consisted of the 40 Item Likert Attitude Scale. This was the 'Community Attitues Towards the Mentally Ill (CAMI) Scale (De Taylor & Dear 1981). Part III included a semi-structured interview with those respondents who had experienced contact with former patients, about the nature and circumstances of that contact.

Data was collected over a three month period from December 1990 to February 1991 by the researcher.

Discussion of results

This study aimed to document the community response to the discharge of former patients from a Northern Ireland hospital, by assessing the

attitudes towards ex-patients of sub-groups of the local population likely
to know former patients, and by investigating the relationships between
familiarity with policy and knowing ex-patients, individual and neighbourhood characteristics and levels of tolerance. The results of the study
are discussed in relation to the objectives as set out in the five research
questions posed in the introductory section.

It is important that the implications of the study's findings be interpreted
with caution, for a number of reasons. In the first place, the study is very
much an exploratory piece of research within an area not previously
investigated. The importance of such work is as much in the delineation
of areas and the identification of questions requiring detailed research. In
the second place, the size and selection of the sample necessarily restricts
the impact of the study's findings. Bearing these caveats in mind, the
study has produced some important findings.

What is the amount and type of contact between former patients and people in the community?

The research study was based on the assumption that, given the relatively
small number of long-stay patients discharged from psychiatric hospital,
the majority of the population were unlikely to have direct contact with
them. The attitudes of the general population towards people with mental
illness have been widely investigated and it has been found that the public
are not familiar with the behaviour associated with mental illness (Rabkin,
1974). This study, therefore, concentrated on investigating those groups
in some form of contact with ex-patients, although the level of contact
varied between sub-groups.

Overall, the sample was predominantly female, young to middle-aged,
married with children and drawn from Social Classes III to V. This was
not a representative sample in terms of the general population, but it was
these 'stay at home' housewives who were most likely to have contact with
ex-patients living in their locality, and whose attitudes were, therefore, of
paramount interest.

The sub-groups experienced a number of forms of contact with discharged long-stay patients in a number of places and at varying levels of
contact. The sub-groups included family, neighbour, befriender and a
school group. Form, place and level of contact are both likely to be
influences on attitudes. For example, it has been found that befrienders
visiting patients in mental hospitals have developed more positive attitudes towards mental illness (Kulick et al, 1969). Befrienders were likely
to be positively motivated individuals who have chosen to become
involved with people with mental illness. This is in contrast to families

400

who were bound by the obligations of kin to their mentally ill relative.

Neighbours exercised some control over their contact with ex-patients, although to avoid all contact they would have had to take the drastic solution of moving home. It may be that the public is more likely to accept such individuals in their locality because the stigma of mental illness is attached to being a patient in a mental hospital, rather than to the illness itself (Johannsen, 1969). As community care brings ex-patients into contact with the public it is hoped they will become more familiar with their behaviour and develop more sympathetic attitudes.

Contact between the school group and people with mental illness was limited to visits to the hospital and the statutory hostel. Pupils had also learnt about mental illness in their studies and a small number of them had had some direct contact with ex-patients at the Social Club which had originally been located at the school. The school group, therefore, were more similar to the general population in their amount of contact with discharged long-stay patients.

When overall levels of contact with people with mental illness were investigated, it was found that they were higher than anticipated on the basis of sample selection. For instance, over half of respondents had had contact with a person with mental illness as a carer or befriender, and a third of respondents as a friend. This is similar to the figure of 50% reported in a survey of the general population in Magherafelt (O'Brien & Normand, 1991). However, frequency of contact varied enormously with under a third having contact with a person with mental illness more than once a week.

Relatives were likely to be in most frequent contact despite the fact that family ties often unravelled during hospitalisation (Fisher & Tessler, 1986). Individuals living in community mental health facilities, because of the disabling effects of their mental illness, were most likely to depend on their families for social support, although the amount of family contact varied enormously. A study of the social networks of residents of the sheltered accommodation scheme found that only five out of eleven residents saw relatives every week (Doherty et al, 1992).

What is the nature and extent of knowledge about the policy of community care, local services for people with mental illness, gaps in the services and views of the hospital?

Questions about the respondents' knowledge about community care and local services were a starting point in the interviewing and as well as

401

collecting information, served to clarify the subject. Probe statements were used to define terms but respondents had to name local services and were not given a check-list, unlike two other recent surveys of public awareness in Magherafelt and Bangor (O'Brien & Normand, 1991; Magee, 1992).

Comparisons between the three surveys should bear in mind this difference in methods.

The fact that respondents were unfamiliar with the term 'community care' may be an indication of the gap between social planners and the community in question. After all, public awareness is a crucial issue in the development of community care schemes. Only one of the sheltered-care schemes investigated had been preceded by a consultative exercise between service providers and the local community. They were met by a positive response from locals which should encourage others to avoid a 'fly by night' approach. Some researchers have identified the 'not in my backyard' response from communities with concerns such as falling property values (Moon, 1988). In contrast, the results of the present study showed a public that understood the basic principles of community care, rejected institutional provision and was committed to the values of individual freedom.

It was found that respondents' knowledge of local psychiatric services was patchy. As in Bangor, the most well-known facility was the Day Centre. This may be because it serves people with a range of problems and is not restricted to people with mental illness. Local services are dominated by the psychiatric hospital so it is difficult to make comparisons with Bangor and Magherafelt where half the sample identified psychiatric day hospitals as a local service. Neither was the voluntary sector as well known, with only a quarter of respondents naming one of the voluntary group as compared with 80% knowledge of the Northern Ireland Association for Mental Health in the other two towns. Of course, any survey of this type is in the nature of action research which aims to increase public knowledge of local services.

Consumer involvement is now one of the principles of service delivery and the questionnaire gave an opportunity for respondents to make suggestions for future developments. The scope of their replies demonstrated the real contribution which ordinary individuals can make given the opportunity. Half of those who had been inside a psychiatric hospital condemned it as 'institutional' or 'custodial'. This is striking evidence of how far the psychiatric hospital must still change if it is no longer to be seen as a 'last resort', to be avoided at all costs.

How do residents in neighbourhoods containing a community mental health facility view its impact?

The policy of community care involves a process of decentralisation from the isolated mental hospitals to redistribution of resources in numerous locations. It is often one of urbanisation, from the countryside asylum to the inner city locations of hostel and sheltered care. In the present case, this movement has involved short distances from the edge of town into local housing estates. Local reaction to community based schemes for people with mental illness can now be measured. When neighbours of the three sheltered care schemes were asked their opinion of these local schemes they were overwhelmingly positive.

Rothbar (1973) has identified the Liberal Distance Function to describe the social phenomenon that favourable support for a social reform increases as the distance between subject and the locus of reform increases. However, studies of attitudes towards local psychiatric facilities and proximity in Toronto (Taylor et al., 1979), New York (Rabkin et al., 1984) and Portsmouth (Moon, 1988) show no clear association. This finding is supported in the present study. A lady who lived next to the hostel for five years had only discovered its identity when she was persistently questioned as to its whereabouts!

The three neighbourhoods which contain C.M.H facilities are similar in their demographic composition, consisting of families drawn from Social Classes III to V, living predominantly in public housing. Studies of sheltered-care schemes in Canada and California reveal that the most supportive communities are where there exists neither strong social cohesion, as in a suburban area, nor severe disorganisation, as in a slum area (Segal & Averim, 1978). In the present study, as no facilities had been located in private housing estates, it was not possible to compare the reaction of two different socio-economic groups.

The strongest level of acceptance amongst the three schemes was found for the Sheltered Flatlets. At the time of interviewing, the scheme had only been opened eight months and it may well have been in a honeymoon period. Nevertheless, it was clear that there existed a fund of goodwill for the scheme which involved a significant investment in the locality. Respondents explained their positive views in terns of normalisation and integration i.e. 'it helps them to be among ordinary people and treated normally'. Segal and Averim (1978) suggest that the facility regime is a crucial factor in encouraging positive integration of residents in the local community. The authors reported that a facility which encouraged social dependence was likely to limit the possibilities of integration, whereas a facility in which residents were more independent meant better external integration. The regime of the sheltered flatlets fitted this second category of social independence. Residents were responsible for their own cooking, shopping, payment of bills, transport etc. In these activities, on an individual basis, they interacted with their neighbours in a normal way, at the shop, the bus-stop, the post-office, etc.

The level of support from respondents for their local C.M.H facilities was compared with the support given for a hypothetical facility by those who had no neighbourhood experience of an existing facility. The results showed a higher level of acceptance for an existing than a hypothetical facility. This may suggest that acceptance of such schemes and their residents increases with familiarity as respondents were able to build up their own positive experience of the ex-patient as a 'good neighbour'. In support, Segal and Averim (1978) suggest that the most important variable influencing integration is a positive response from neighbours.

It was beyond the scope of the present study to compare the acceptability of facilities for the mentally ill with those for other disadvantaged groups. Research in this area has unearthed some rather negative views: that the mentally ill were less acceptable than the mentally retarded and physically disabled (Tringo, 1970); that group homes were viewed less favourably than facilities for the elderly (Wilmoth et al, 1987); and that C.M.H facilities emerged as only marginally less unpleasant than sewage plants in one study of public evaluations (Smith & Hanham, 1981).

The fact that the local response to sheltered care schemes for discharged long-stay patients is overwhelmingly positive is very encouraging. However, planners should not take such results as 'carte-blanche' for the wholesale location of further projects in local communities. Researchers have documented the American experience in which community based projects have been over-concentrated to the point where a new type of urban ghetto has developed. They are termed 'service-dependent ghettos', where welfare populations and the facilities to assist them are concentrated (Dear & Wolch, 1987).

What are the attitudes of those in contact with former patients towards people with mental illness?

Attitudes are seen as a crucial factor in the acceptance of discharged long-stay patients living in the community. In the present study, such attitudes were investigated by the Community Attitudes Towards the Mentally Ill (C.A.M.I) Scale first developed to study community attitudes in Toronto, Canada (Dear & Taylor, 1982).

Public attitudes and beliefs about mental illness have been extensively investigated over the last forty years. In a comprehensive review of the literature, Rabkin concluded that people are now better informed and hold more enlightened attitudes (Rabkin, 1974). Research in Dublin has revealed a public which discriminated between different mental illness labels (O'Mahoney, 1981), and a general agreement between public knowledge and psychiatric symptomatology over one particular category of mental illness, namely schizophrenia, has been reported from an English study (Jones & Cochrane, 1981).

The present study found that those in contact with former patients held positive attitudes towards people with mental illness on all four dimensions of the C.A.M.I Scale. This is a very encouraging response for the policy of community care although how far positive attitudes translate into a sympathetic and welcoming response remains in question. When the results were analysed on each dimension it was seen that there were some interesting differences in the responses.

Respondents were most positive on the benevolence scale which tapped into liberal sentiments and aspirations towards people with mental illness. On the social restrictiveness scale, respondents were required to report on how they would act in situations involving people with mental illness. Their responses were more cautious with a sizeable number avoiding offering an opinion on a number of items about the suitability of such individuals for positions of responsibility as babysitters, spouses and authority figures. It can be seen that the sample had reservations about the inclusion of people with mental illness in their personal and family life.

The desire of respondents to maintain social distance is contrasted by their wholesale endorsement of C.M.H facilities being located in residential neighbourhoods, as expressed in their positive responses on the Community Mental Health Ideology Scale. The Authoritarianism Scale might have been more sensitive in picking up on how respondents would behave in reality. Although the sample expressed their rejection of institutional care, a substantial minority, numbering a quarter of respondents, supported a moral approach towards the care of people with mental illness. However, it may well have been that such respondents were confused between mental illness and mental handicap. In this study, the sample was not asked to differentiate the two conditions, unlike the Bangor and Magherafelt surveys. In both those towns, between 15 to 40% of those interviewed did not know or gave incorrect answers when asked the differences between mental illness and mental handicap (O'Brien & Normand, 1991; Magee, 1992).

When the responses of the different sub-groups to the C.A.M.I Scale were examined separately, some interesting differences were apparent.

Relatives stood out as a distinctive group, being more in favour of early hospitalisation, recognising differences between people with mental illness and others, and being reluctant about marriage for such individuals. Relatives had experienced all the disruptions of mentally ill behaviour within their families and this experience was likely to harden attitudes as shown in these results.

The other distinctive group was the school group who were significantly less positive about the location of mental health facilities in residential neighbourhoods. This result may be indicative of a more cautious attitude amongst the general population from which the school group were drawn. One American study has revealed that whilst the better educated hold more enlightened views of mental illness, 'host' communities of lower social status had a more positive response to local community care schemes (Trute & Segal, 1976).

All three neighbourhoods studied held positive attitudes towards people with mental illness as measured on the C.A.M.I Scale. This is a very encouraging response to the location and operation of local sheltered-care schemes. However, because all three areas were similar in their socio-demographic composition, it was not possible to compare attitudes between different types of communities. The administration of the C.A.M.I Scale to a higher socio-economic sample drawn from private housing would make this possible. The results would help to resolve the dilemma between quality of environment as found in private estates and social integration which is better achieved in mixed housing areas.

The Canadian study found that public attitudes towards people with mental illness were significantly related with life-cycle stage (Taylor & Dear, 1981). The authors reported that six demographic variables showed relatively strong relationships with scores on the C.A.M.I Scale. Respondents with less sympathetic attitudes were likely to be older, male, married and widowed with children, and of lower socio-economic status. However, in order to make these comparisons the authors used parametric tests to relate attitudes, as measured on an ordinal scale, to socio-demographic variables, measured on a nominal scale. Such tests should only be used when all variables are on a continuous dimension and are normally distributed. In the present study, when non-parametric tests were used to investigate the relationship between attitudes and socio-demographic variables the results were not statistically significant.

What is the nature of interaction between members of 'contact groups' and former patients?

Much sociological effort has been concerned with finding the ideal form of social organisation. One such idealisation of life has been the village community characterised by mutual support based on close personal ties of friendship and kinship. In their study of urban society, sociologists have identified urban villages, usually working class, containing extended families and situated alongside heavy industry which provided local employment. Today, however, individuals usually live in one area, work in a different location, socialise elsewhere and have limited contact with their widespread extended family. The focus of attention has, therefore, changed to the links and contacts of people within and between their social worlds.

The present study describes the social worlds of former patients based on family, befriender and neighbourhood. These groups are identified as providing the non-psychiatric social worlds as opposed to the psychiatric ones to which the former patient often remains attached (Prior, 1991). They represent the interface between discharged patients and the community, providing the context in which their behaviour is experienced and judged.

There are a number of crucial determinants of the quality of this interaction. Interaction which takes place in ordinary settings involving everyday activities is normal and normalising. This social process offers the ex-patient the opportunity to act as a normal member of, and be accepted by, the community. A greater degree of social integration will be achieved by facilities which maximise the opportunities for residents to be in frequent contact with their locality.

However, contacts between discharged patients and the wider community have been described as 'few and fleeting' (Prior, 1991). Befriending relationships represent increased opportunities for interaction within the wider community. Various strategies might be employed by ex-patients in these interactions and this is a second crucial determinant of their quality. These might include 'covering' their mental illness, 'passing' as ordinary people until they have gained enough confidence in their companions to reveal their past biography, or being 'up-front' with their psychiatric condition and making a positive identity of it.

It may well be easier for discharged psychiatric patients to 'cover' than people with physical disabilities for a number of reasons. They do not usually have visible signs of their conditions apart from the side-effects of medication such as restlessness and tremors. Of course, their ability to 'cover' will depend on their social skills as it is precisely in social interaction that the disabling effects of mental illness become apparent. Research has discovered that the public are most reluctant to label mental illness and will only do so as a last resort (Lemkau & Crocetti, 1962). If, as has been suggested (Johannsen, 1969), the public use the fact of being a patient as a definition of mental illness, then ex-patients are more likely to avoid labelling. Evidence from New Zealand has shown that the status of ex-mental patient carries a number of positive ratings as compared with the persistently negative stereotype of the mental patient (Green et al, 1987).

This draws attention to the possibility that the stigma of mental illness is as much a stigma of place as of behaviour. Once discharged, the individual is no longer attached to hospital, but, in order to manage in the community, is required to live in sheltered accommodation supported by regular visiting from mental health professionals. Whilst former patients may go about their daily business anonymously, their residence in sheltered care with supportive visiting will give them a separate identity. The extent to which this makes them in 'a place apart' is determined by public attitudes towards people with mental illness, the local reaction to the C.M.H facility and the nature of interaction between former patients and the community as discussed.

The part played by the family of the discharged patient is rather different and evidence of this difference has been shown in the results from the C.A.M.I Scale. Families may be pulled in opposite directions in their effort to do what they feel is best for their relative. Prior to hospitalisation, they may endeavour to cope with the disruptions of disturbed behaviour for as long as possible. But the legacy of this behaviour may end up destroying family ties in

the future. During hospitalisation, family contact lessens, ageing parents cannot maintain their level of support and siblings are unlikely to maintain as close involvement. By the time the former patient is returned to the community, family contact is sporadic, or likely to become so. It is for these reasons that the sponsorship of social activity for former patients is so important.

Conclusions and recommendations

The findings of the research study, 'The Attitudes of People in contact with Long-stay Patients Discharged from a Northern Ireland Hospital', are summarised in the Introduction to the study. A number of recommendations are proposed based on the main findings.

1. The level of knowledge about local services was not high and the policy of community care, as conceptualised within the caring professions, was not familiar to many respondents. However, there existed a basic understanding of its principles and a commitment to the values of individual freedom.

A programme of public mental health education is recommended to build on public goodwill towards people with mental illness. Such a programme would seek to impart an understanding of mental illness which recognised and explained the importance of social and environmental factors. More information about local services is required. The question of access, availability and take-up of existing services should be examined.

2. There was evidence of a rejection of institutional care, as shown in the respondents' views of the psychiatric hospital and the results on the C.A.M.I Scale.

The hospital needs to examine its role in a new integrated model of care, working towards removing the boundary between hospital and the outside world. If the hospital is unable to adapt to helping people with social and interpersonal problems who end up as its patients then alternative models of care, such as Crisis Intervention Centres or Community Mental Health Centres, should be developed.

3. When respondents were asked about gaps in services, they showed good practical reasoning about people with mental illness, the nature of their disability and unmet needs.

The resources of ordinary people should be capitalised upon by the development of locally based friendship schemes, informal support networks and social activities.

4. Families are in the most frequent contact with people with mental illness. However, because of the ageing of relatives, they are a declining source of long-tern support.

Systems of informal care need to be fostered by statutory services in partnership with the voluntary sector. The Mental Health Support Workers (run by the National Schizophrenia Fellowship) are an example of such a scheme. These informal carers need suitable training in relating to and working with people with mental illness.

5. The sample held generally positive attitudes towards people with mental illness as measured on the C.A.M.I. Scale.

This is an encouraging response for community care planners and suggests that the policy has been implemented successfully to date. Respondents placed a clear duty on professionals that their community should not be put at risk through their discharge policy. Standards of assessment and preparation of potential dischargees in hospital and their care in the community must be fully maintained in the long-term.

6. The three neighbourhoods investigated all expressed positive opinions of their local sheltered care accommodation for discharged patients.

Further research is required to measure attitudes in areas of private housing with a higher social class composition to make possible direct comparisons between levels of tolerance in public and private housing estates. The positive response locally should not necessarily be taken to signal further developments in these areas as care must be taken to avoid geographical over-concentration and the creation of 'service-dependent ghettos'.

7. The response from the relative group on the C.A.M.I Scale was rather different than the other groups investigated. This suggests that there were other mechanisms at work.

The family care and management of people with mental illness is likely to become an area of increasing importance with the growth of community care. As discharged patients are returned to the community and as patients are maintained at home with professional support without resorting to hospitalisation, the burden on the family is likely to increase. Families as carers will need their own support from statutory services. In order to develop the most appropriate interventions, further research is required into the family management of relatives suffering mental illness.

8. The importance of normal, everyday activities, such as shopping, paying bills and using public transport was emphasised as a means towards effective social integration for former patients.

Hospital social skills programmes in rehabilitation need to be directed towards teaching competence in these areas of activity. Facility regimes should not encourage social dependence and residents should be given as many opportunities as possible to interact with their local community.

References

Becker, H. (1967). *The other side: Perspectives on deviance*, New York: Free Press.

Busfield, J. (1986). *Managing madness: Changing ideas and practices*, London: Unwin & Hyman.

Dear, M. & Taylor, S. (1982). *Not on our streets: Community attitudes to mental health care*, London:Pion.

Dear, M. & Wolch, J. (1987). *Landscapes of despair.* Oxford: Polity.

DHSS (NI) (1986). A regional strategy for the Northern Ireland Health and Social Services: 1987 - 1992 DHSS (NI).

Doherty, H., Graham, C., McCrum, B., Manktelow, R., & Rauch, R. (1992). Antrim - one year on: An evaluation of the first year of operation of the flat cluster accommodation and support scheme in Antrim, PRAXIS, Belfast.

Fisher, G. & Tessler, R. (1986). Family bonding of the mentally ill: An analysis of family visits with residents of Board Care Homes. *Journal of Health and Social Behaviour*, **27**, 236-49.

Goffman, E. (1961). *Asylums: Essays on the social situation of mental patients and other inmates*. Harmondsworth: Penguin.

Green, D., McCormack, I., Walkley, F. & Taylor, J. (1987). Community attitudes towards mental illness twenty two years on. *Social Science and Medicine*. **24**, 417-22.

Johannsen, W. J. (1969). Attitudes towards mental patients: A review of empirical research. *Mental Hygiene*. **53**, 218-228.

Jones, L. & Cochrane, R. (1981). Stereotypes of mental illness: A test of labelling hypothesis. *International Journal of Social Psychiatry*, **27**, 99-107.

Kulik, J., Martin, R. & Scheibe, K. (1969). Effects of mental hospital voluntary work on student's conceptions of mental illness. *Journal of Clinical Psychology*, **25**, 326-329.

Lemert, E. (1972). Human deviance, social problems and social control. Englewood Cliffs: Prentice Hall.

Lemkau, P. & Crocetti, G. (1962). An urban population's knowledge and opinions about mental illness. *American Journal of Psychiatry*, **118**, 692-700.

Magee, M. (1992). A mental health promotion and public awareness strategy - The Bangor Report. Northern Ireland Association for Mental Health, Bangor.

Moon, G. (1988). Is there one around here? - Investigating reaction to small scale mental health provision in Portsmouth, England. In C. Smith, & J. Giggs, (Eds.), *Location and Stigma*. London: Unwin & Hyman.

Nunnally, J. (1981). *Public conceptions of mental health*. New York.

O'Brien, M. & Normand, C. (1991). Public awareness and attitudes towards mental illness -A survey of Magherafelt. Health & Health

Care Research Unit, Queen's University of Belfast.

O'Mahoney, P. (1981). *Public, professional and patient perceptions of the mentally ill*. Unpublished Doctoral Thesis, Trinity College, Dublin.

Prior, L. (1991). The social worlds of psychiatric and ex-psychiatric patients in Northern Ireland. Health and Health Care Research Unit, Queens' University, Belfast.

Rabkin, J. (1974). Public attitudes towards mental illness: A review of the literature. *Schizophrenia Bulletin*, **10**, (Fall), 9-33.

Rabkin, J., Muhlin, G, & Cohen, P. (1984). What the neighbours think: Community attitudes to local psychiatric facilities. *Community Mental Health Journal*, **20** (winter), 304-12.

Rothbar, M. (1973). Perceiving social injustice: Observations on the relationship between liberal attitudes and proximity to social problems. *Journal of Applied Social Psychology*, **3**, 291 - 302.

Scheff, T. (1966). *Being mentally ill*. (London).

Segal, S & Averim, U. (1978). *The mentally ill in community based sheltered care*. New York: Wiley.

Smith, C. & Giggs, J. (1988). *Location and stigma*. London: Allen & Unwin.

Smith, C. & Hanham, R. (1981). Any place here: Mental health facilities as noxious neighbours. *Professional Geographer*, **33**, 326-30.

Taylor, S., Dear, M. & Hall, G. (1979). Attitudes towards the mentally ill and reactions to mental health facilities. *Social Science and Medicine*. **13D**, 281-90.

Taylor, S. & Dear, M, (1981). Scaling community attitudes towards the mentally ill. *Schizophrenia Bulletin*, **7**, 225-39.

Tringo, J. (1970). The hierarchy of preference to ward disability groups. *Journal of Special Education*, **4**, 295-306.

Trute, B. & Segal, S. (1976). Census tract predictors and the social integration of sheltered care residents. *Social Psychiatry*, **11**, 153-61.

Wilmoth, G., Silver, S. & Severy, L. (1987). Receptivity and planned change: Community attitudes and de-institutionalisation. *Journal of Applied Psychology*, **72**, 138-45.

33 Women and violence: A local authority response

L. McDougall

Introduction

We know from many sources that men experience more criminal violence than women and yet women's fear of violence is greater than men's. While for many years the focus of Home Office activity was crime reduction, recently a significant shift of focus has taken place. Tackling fear of crime has now become so significant that, in June this year, the Home Office announced that it would only be publishing the British Crime Survey biannually and national statistics six monthly because of the impact their publication has in increasing fear of crime amongst the public.

Women's fear of crime was often seen as irrational because women's experiences of crime were not reflected in national crime statistics. Researchers have struggled over the years to illustrate that women's fear of crime is justified and that the problem has been in the way in which these experiences have been reported, monitored and addressed. As a result, the relationship between women's experiences of violence, their likelihood to report these experiences, the response they get from statutory agencies when they do report and how these incidents have been monitored have been the subject of much discourse over the last 10-15 years. Much of this has tested the legitimacy of women's fear of violence.

The focus of this paper is the role of a local authority as an agent in responding to such issues. Does it have a role in addressing violence against women and if so what should that role be? How does it fit in with a local authority's other major responsibilities, particularly in times of financial stringency? And if it decides to act, what can it actually do?

In attempting to answer those questions, I want to briefly refer to some of the work which identifies women's experiences of and responses to aggression; to look at the question of whether, if and how, local authorities can devise responses to violence against women; and lastly, to use as a case study, some recent work in one local authority.

Living with violence

In the Violence Against Women - Women Speak Out survey carried out in Wandsworth in 1983-84, the 314 women interviewed reported 1046 incidents of men's violence which they had experienced or witnessed or which had happened to women they knew well during the preceding year (Radford, 1987). These included 280 reports of sexual and racial assaults or harassment, 137 of violent attack, 41 of being threatened in a public place, 32 of being threatened or attached by a stranger in their home, 35 reports of obscene telephone calls, 121 of sexual harassment at work and 39 of being threatened and/or attacked by men they were living with. In addition, 64 of the women had seen another woman being threatened or attacked and 206 knew other women who had been attacked.

A study in Manchester in 1985 produced similar evidence of the extent of women's daily, regular or recurrent experiences of male aggression towards them (Manchester Police Monitoring Unit, 1986).

A recent sample of 100 women in Coventry had experienced 256 sexual offenses, yet only 15 of these had been reported (Leda Group, 1992). Within this group of women, 2 out of 5 had experienced domestic violence and the average length of time they had endured this violence was eight years.

Such information gives rise to two questions. How serious are these incidents and how seriously should they be taken? What impact do such incidents have on women's lives?

The seriousness of incidents can be measured in a number of ways. Traditionally, seriousness had been determined by historical, legal and socio-cultural factors which identify what is crime and how it should be punished. Using those measures, rape, for example, has been treated more seriously than domestic violence. Sexual harassment or incidents that are not criminal offenses have been dismissed as trivial or outside the scope of action. But as Kelly shows, other criteria can be used to determine the seriousness of incidents, for example, the degree of violence and the frequency of occurrence (Kelly, 1987).

Using the degree of violence inflicted as the standard for measurement, then domestic violence and incest could be seen as more serious because of the physical and emotional brutality and injury they inflict. Using

414

frequency of occurrence, then sexual harassment and threat of rape could be viewed as more serious because of the extent to which fear of rape and the expectation of harassment limited many women's lives and their access to public activity. The seriousness with which any incident is treated also depends on subjective criteria. This has led to substantial discrepancies between the viewpoint of victims and the response from professionals from whom they have sought help.

Liz Kelly talks about a 'continuum of sexual violence' to illustrate that many women have a series of encounters with sexual violence throughout their lives and that these experiences underpin women's reactions to any given incident (Kelly, 1987). This cumulative experience reflects a range of occasional, regular or recurrent incidents of male violence, of differing levels and severity, from strangers, acquaintances and family.

Women's reactions to experiences of aggression, both at the time they occur and over a long period, differ, but are the result of a complex range of factors. The familiarity and expectation of harassment is one of the most important of these factors and also affects whether and to whom women report incidents.

A 1989 survey by 'Living' Magazine of 1,000 women found that nearly half had received obscene telephone calls, been flashed at or groped by a stranger in the last 5 years. Nearly 9 out of 10 of those who had received an obscene phone call and 3 out of 5 of those who had been flashed at had not reported the incidents. Nearly half of those interviewed thought it inevitable that they would fall victim to a flasher, a groper or an obscene caller at some time, and it was to this feeling of inevitability that the magazine attributed the low levels of reporting.

Establishing the relationship for women between casual non-violent incidents and other more physically and emotionally violent occurrences has taken time. For example, women's reactions to flashing have often been seen as excessive. Mohr (1964) suggests that the main influence on a woman's reaction is her psychological state of health. But McNeill (1987), in a study of 100 women covering 233 incidents, finds that women's reactions to flashing frequently reflect a realistic personal assessment of the possible danger they might be in at the time.

Furthermore, for many women, flashing is not only, as might be expected, a fear of rape but also a fear of death. Women's fear of rape is very high and exceeds women's fears of all other crimes (Warr, 1985). However, research by Stanko concludes that women's fear of rape reflects a greater fear of the likelihood of rape resulting in mutilation and death (Stanko, 1985). Women's fear of death is one of the reasons why many women, once attacked, do not resist rape. This association of incidents in the minds of women mean that, what are often seen by men as relatively minor incidents such as harassment, flashing or obscene telephone calls, to women are reminders of much greater threats. Fear leads to changes in women's patterns of behaviour which are not necessarily responses to incidents they have encountered but to the possible implications of those incidents.

Not only are women's responses to incidents a result of their lifetime experiences of violence but also of their experience of other people's reactions to them. Stanko says, 'In effect, women's feelings of fear may relate to their tacit understanding of the likelihood of experiencing male violence and the lack of protection they receive from those around them, and in particular, from those in positions of authority, to protect them from abusive situations' (Stanko, 1987). Non-reporting of incidents results from a realistic assessment based on personal and second-hand experience of the likely benefits, dis-benefits and outcomes attached to reporting.

The policing of male violence is too large a subject to discuss here. However, how male violence should be tackled within the workplace is an issue which needs addressing. Is an employer or service provider, in this case a local authority, responsible for making women staff, users and residents safe or for policing the male violence which makes them unsafe? Where should the priority lie? What are the parameters of local authority responsibility?

Local Authority responses

Local Authorities have a statutory obligation to provide key services. But how an authority delivers those services and how it prioritises work on non-statutory functions will depend on local circumstances. Many factors will shape the process by which decisions are made. One is the level of commitment to any particular issue and whether the existing political circumstances can or should accommodate work on that issue. A change of political control, for example, can result in a complete reversal of current priorities and work programmes.

Another factor is the legitimacy of the local authority to act, in other words, does the local authority have a responsibility on this issue? In areas of statutory obligation this question becomes easier to answer although much debate may then ensue about how the responsibility should be delivered. Gaining support for non-statutory functions is much harder.

Which issues receive attention and support is affected by a range of factors including:

     i)   the political expediency of raising a given issue and the need to reflect local political circumstances and histories,

ii) the resource implication,

iii) the level of public support,

iv) the level of importance attributed to any given issue compared to the many others simultaneously competing for support and resources,

v) the starting place for each particular authority on that issue and how much work it may have already done,

vi) the likelihood of achieving the objective.

Work on responses to violence against women has to be located within this context. Whether individual local authorities have chosen to work in this area, how support has been manifest and the extent of resources committed to it has varied around the country. The National Association of Local Government Women's Committee's report 'Responding with Authority' (1990) chronicles much of the recent work undertaken by local authorities. This shows that support has successfully been won and that responding to violence against women has been identified as a legitimate area of local authority concern. How has this been achieved?

Dobash and Dobash (1992) have identified the relationship between socialist politics and the emerging women's movement in the 1970's and particularly the influence of the Labour left in the style and direction of the battered women's movement. In the late 1970's and early 1980's, the establishment of women's units and women's committees, usually by Labour-controlled metropolitan councils, gave a voice to women's issues within local government that has not previously been possible. This meant that, in addition to work on homelessness and with refuges already being undertaken in some Social Services and Housing Departments, the whole issue of women and violence began to be discussed corporately and with Elected Members of the Council. This fusion of interests substantially raised the profile of violence against women in the 1980's and identified the possibility of a role for local government.

Enhanced media coverage facilitated the process. Public discussion, particularly about domestic violence, has been escalated by a series of controversial sentencing decisions which have led to a high degree of interest in the issue. Widespread dissatisfaction with police responses has led to Home Office intervention and the establishment of a number of local Police Domestic Violence Units. Aggression at work received media attention following the murder of a Birmingham social worker and the disappearance of Suzy Lamplugh in 1986. Subsequent work has usually focused on the responsibility of employers under the Health and Safety at Work Act to provide a safe work environment and for employees to use safe work practice. As a consequence, the need to provide support to victims of violence became more recognised and more accepted.

During the 1980's many statutory agencies and organisations began to review their practice, reassess their priorities and change their structure or focus in dealing with violence. Voluntary and community organisations, who had been the major source of support to survivors of violence, lobbied for and, in some cases received, greater financial support. Sympathetic local authorities took stock and reviewed their own policies, practices and responsibilities (NALGWC, 1990), fuelled by partnership arrangements with other statutory and voluntary agencies for developing work on community safety.

Local authorities carry many different responsibilities for responding to violence, depending on local circumstances and their relationship to the provision of Policing. However, four areas of responsibility can be clearly identified which accrue to a local authority in the delivery of its own functions:

a) as an employer,

b) in providing and delivering services to customers and residents,

c) in the provision of grant aid to voluntary and community organisations which provide support to victims of violence,

d) in the development and maintenance of the built environment.

Responses to violence against women can be made in any or all of these areas. However, within each of these areas most local authorities have pursued strategies which provide support for women in avoiding, minimising or dealing with the results of men's violence. Tackling men's violence remains outside the scope of local authority provision.

Making a response

Local authorities have developed work programmes responding to violence in many different ways, but they have typically arisen from equal opportunities initiatives on women's issues or, more recently, under the umbrella of community safety. The impetus and shape of this work often differs from that already undertaken with local authority service departments. Taking a corporate focus means identifying and developing responses across all areas of local authority activity, not only those which carry statutory responsibilities.

This section will describe some of the work undertaken in two local authorities, Wolverhampton since 1989 and initiatives now underway in Coventry.

In November 1989, Wolverhampton Council held a conference on responding to violence against women (Conference Report 1990). Although work with women had been ongoing in Wolverhampton for a number of years, this was the first time that the agencies involved had come together with individual women who lived and worked in the town to discuss their experiences and concerns. The issues raised by participants formed the basis for an action plan which was taken forward by agencies working both individually and jointly.

The objectives underpinning the work were:

i) to provide a voice for women to describe their experiences of violence and aggression,

ii) to respond to those issues identified by women as most relevant,

iii) to encourage joint working between organisations,

iv) to ensure that the concerns of black and disabled women were acknowledged and addressed,

v) to maximise the limited resources available to women survivors,

vi) to effect change to policy and practice in order to provide better services for women and children in need of support.

Inter-agency working in Wolverhampton has been fundamental in the development of a number of important initiatives to which the local authority has been a contributor. However, these are issues for which the local authority carries sole responsibility and for which it must take the lead. As outlined above, these are employment, service provision, voluntary agency support and changes to the built environment.

Employment issues

Local authorities, as the major employer in many of the geographical areas where they are based, are in a strong position to: i) minimise the incidence of some kinds of violence against women and, ii) to affect the quality of the response which women receive following any violent incident.

Although studies from elsewhere (Company magazine, 1989; Living magazine, 1989; Phillips, Stockdale and Loeman, 1989; Harris Research Centre, 1988) had identified the type and extent of women's experiences of and concerns about violence, there was little information available about women's experiences in Wolverhampton. In order to gain more understanding of local issues, a survey of women staff of the Council was undertaken, which asked women about their experiences of violence at work, on the streets and at home. The questionnaire was unusual in that it recognised that women staff were also users of services and that many of them are residents of the borough in which they work. This was the first time the Council had acknowledged the role of its own staff as customers with experience of issues that were not job related.

The survey, conducted as an anonymous and confidential postal questionnaire, provided 218 respondents - a response rate of 72.6%.

It found that at work, 1 in 2 had been on the receiving end of verbal abuse, 1 in 5 had suffered threatening behaviour, 1 in 6 had been sexually harassed and 1 in 18 had been physically assaulted. 1 in 5 of black women respondents had been racially harassed.

On the streets, half the respondents had been threatened or attacked outside their homes. 1 in 5 had suffered verbal abuse, 1 in 6 had been followed, 1 in 8 had been flashed at, 1 in 10 had been sexually or physically assaulted or harassed, and 1 in 15 had been mugged or had suffered theft.

At home half had suffered obscene phone calls, 1 in 7 said that they avoided being alone at home and 1 in 6 had experienced violence from a partner.

The survey's findings illustrated the need for urgent action and the Council subsequently adopted new corporate policies on aggression against staff and domestic violence. This second policy was unusual in that it recognised the Council's responsibilities as an employer of women who were subject to violence. The policy committed the Council to a programme of training for managers and staff to increase awareness of domestic violence as both an employment and service issue and to the introduction of an anonymous and confidential counselling service for women staff who had been subject to violence. The policy also contained procedures for staff on providing an appropriate response to women customers who might be victims of violence and these procedures were subsequently produced as leaflets for use by all front line staff.

The survey results became very important in developing initiatives in Wolverhampton. Although many of the findings mirrored national statistics, it was useful to be able to provide a local perspective on the issues raised. Some points, for example domestic violence, which had not previously been seen as employment issues, suddenly came into focus. And because there was no reason to suppose that women Council staff were any more likely to be subject to violence at home or on the streets than any other women, that information became useful to other agencies who were working in the field.

In June 1992, the survey, slightly amended to fit local circumstances, was used by Coventry City Council. 750 questionnaires were distributed and 392 returned, a response rate of 53%. The results show very similar patterns of experience and concern.

Although further work needs to be done to clarify some issues, the findings of the surveys are important. Both surveys show the extent to which many women suffer abuse, harassment and violence in all areas of their lives. These experiences interlink. Women in both surveys report discussing their experiences of domestic violence with their work colleagues and, in some cases, their line manager, trade union representative or welfare officer. (In the Coventry survey, 2 out of 5 of those women reporting domestic violence had discussed it with someone at work).

The survey findings also substantiate the view of violence as a continuum. Women do not compartmentalise their experiences and so information about violence is often shared with individuals or agencies where it is not monitored. How women share information needs further exploration.

An acceptance of the role of managers in
    i)   preventing, handling and responding to violence,
    ii) developing and implementing safe working procedures,
    iii) monitoring the safety of the workplace,
    iv) minimising potential danger to both staff and customers, can have
        a substantial impact on the lives of many women.

However, encouraging managers to see violence as an issue for which they carry responsibility is sometimes difficult, particularly when managers are dealing with so many other issues which they, and/or their employers may see as more important or urgent.

Service provision

Local authorities can use their position and influence to affect the way services are designed and delivered to women living with violence.

One key area where local authorities make direct provision to women who are experiencing violence is in housing. Indeed local authorities have a statutory obligation to provide housing for women who may become homeless as a result of leaving violent relationships. Many authorities have revised their allocations policies to facilitate the needs of women and children who are fleeing violence (NALGWC, 1990). Social Services will also be in regular contact with women survivors.

Less evident and less acknowledged, is the extent to which teachers are encountering violence. Teachers will often be aware of violence within a family home and may sometimes be subject to violence from a parent in search of a child who has fled, usually with her/his mother, from a violent home. Similarly, education welfare officers will have to deal with cases arising from violence within the family. Again, the issues interlink because violence within the home may result in aggression against a local authority employee who is involved, via their work capacity, with a member of that family. The same or related issues may also arise for youth and community service staff.

In Wolverhampton, these concerns have led to staff training within

Social Services, Education, Housing, Finance and Leisure Services for staff whose role may involve them in working with families characterised by violence.

Much of the progress of this work in Wolverhampton resulted from a highly successful collaboration between agencies with similar concerns, most notably the Council, Wolverhampton Safer Cities Project and Wolverhampton Domestic Violence Initiative. This inter-agency working also produced conferences in 1989 and 1991 on Women and Violence; leaflets on sources of help to women who are experiencing violence, aggression at work and sexual harassment; research on prostitution; and the establishment of multi-agency fora on Domestic Violence and Prostitution. The Council also organised a workshop with both national and local representation on black women and domestic violence (November, 1991).

In Coventry a Safer Cities funded conference on domestic violence resulted in a piece of research funded by Coventry City Council and Safer Cities, which looks at women's experiences of violence in one area of the City. Its findings show a high level of dissatisfaction with all statutory services by women who have suffered violence. Amongst a range of responses under development, an inter-agency focus group on domestic violence has been established under the Community Care Plan to look at how responses to domestic violence can be improved in the City.

Voluntary agency support

Work in both Wolverhampton and Coventry has depended on inter-agency working, particularly between the statutory and voluntary sectors. The work in Wolverhampton has relied on good working relationships between the Council, the women's refuge, victim support organisations and local women's resource centres, most of which are funded by the local authority.

Collaboration is also a key issue in Coventry. Much of the work in Coventry over recent years has been driven by funding from Safer Cities, working with local agencies, including a refuge for Asian women, a black women's centre, and the anti racial harassment and attacks network. A network, Workers for Change, has been established to help information exchange and co-working between agencies dealing with violence against women.

As financial constraints have become an increasing problem for local authorities, a key issue around continuing support for work on women and violence is the availability of funds to keep the voluntary and community organisations going at existing or even reduced levels of funding. Violence against women is an issue which, as a non-statutory function for local authorities, becomes increasingly difficult to prioritise.

Voluntary sector agencies providing support services to women who have experienced violence are finding themselves increasingly beleaguered. Demand for their services does not diminish; to the contrary, in many cases, it is steadily growing. Over recent years media attention has further served to increase demand. But this increased demand for services coincides now with a cut in the available grant provision.

Built environment

One of the questions within the survey asks if there are occasions when women feel less safe. In the Wolverhampton survey, 4 out of 5 said they felt vulnerable in subways, two thirds expressed serious concern about car parks, in empty buildings and when their car breaks down and a third said they felt uncomfortable in taxis, waiting for buses and on trains.

Wolverhampton followed up the original survey with another which explored use of subways by 100 men and women (July, 1991). This found that over half (equal numbers of men and women) never use subways after 7pm.

As a result, the Council commissioned a study of the problems experienced by pedestrians using subways to cross the town's Ring Road. Over 1,000 interviews were conducted with local people (March, 1992).

The main priorities identified by the public were, firstly the requirement to choose the way in which the Road is crossed rather than being forced to use a subway, and secondly the need for greatly improved lighting. The Council has subsequently agreed a programme of improvements to subways, including lighting and graffiti removal, and to review the situation with regard to providing surface level crossings in place of subways.

In addition, a Women's Safety Forum has been established, made up of representatives from statutory and community organisation, to look at the issues for women in using public places and to make recommendations for improvement and change.

Coventry has undertaken considerable work, particularly on the design and improvement of car parks and lighting, much of which has been led and funded by Safer Cities. Also with Safer Cities support, a women only taxi service, Feline Cars, was successfully introduced which has subsequently been taken over by a major taxi operator. In the survey carried out by the Council of its own staff, 9 out of 10 women indicated a preference for a woman driver and a quarter had actually used the women only service.

Conclusion

The future for this work in local authorities is unclear. The demand for services within the statutory sector and the voluntary sector it funds is growing. The exposure of the extent of regular violence requires all responsible agencies to respond. Individual women are clear about the need for more services, more choice, more understanding and more support. But how can this be met?

Local authorities are labouring under ever increasing financial constraints. If direct and indirect provision from local authorities stands still or ceases, there are no obvious contenders to take it over. Health authorities and charitable trusts are equally beleaguered.

Furthermore, the expansion of compulsory competitive tendering in local government undermines a local authority's ability to act corporately, either as an employer or as a service provider. As more services go out to contract, fulfilling a commitment to standardise provision across all sectors becomes harder and harder to achieve.

However, both community safety and community care are issues which continue to grow in importance. As the necessity for inter-agency working increases in order to develop responses to the NHS and Community Care Act, Children Act and other central government initiatives, maybe the only future lies in pursuing violence against women as a health, community safety and community care issue.

References

Dobash, R.E., & bash, R.P. (1992). *Women, violence and social change.* London: Routledge.

Kelly, L. (1987). The continuum of sexual violence. In J. Hanmer & M. Maynard, (Eds.), *Women, violence and social control.* London: The Macmillian Press.

McNeill, S. (1987). Flashing: Its effect on Women. In J. Hanmer & M. Maynard (Eds.), *Women, violence and social control,* London: The Macmillian Press.

Radford, J. (1987). Policing male violence - policing women. In J. Hanmer, & M. Maynard, (Eds.), *Women, violence and social control.* London: The Macmillian Press.

Stanko, E.A. (1987). Typical violence, normal precaution: Men, women and interpersonal violence in England, Wales, Scotland and the USA. In J. Hanmer, & M. Maynard, (Eds.), *Women, violence and social control.* London: The Macmillian Press.

Phillips, C.M., Stockdale, J.E., & Loeman, L.M. (1989). *The risks in going to work: The nature of people's work, the risks they encounter and the incidence of sexual harassment, physical attack and threatening behaviour.* London School of Economics.

Responding with authority: Local authority initiatives to counter violence against women (1990). National Association of Local Government Women's Committees.

Violence against women - whose concern? Leda Group (1992). Coventry City Council and Coventry Safer Cities Project.

Women and safety: Responding to violence against women (1990). Wolverhampton Borough Council and Wolverhampton Safer Cities Project.

Women and violence: Responses to aggression against women. (1990). Wolverhampton Borough Council and Wolverhampton Safer Cities Project.

34 Making a panorama out of a crisis: A Crisis Centre and its evaluation

A. McGuire

Introduction

Crisis Intervention has become a useful way of responding to the acute distress of individuals. This paper outlines the philosophy of Crisis Intervention, describes the work of Leeds Crisis Centre, and reports the results of a programme of evaluation of the service.

The crisis model

The word 'crisis' is by most people used loosely to indicate an acute state of affairs or a personal emergency of some type. A number of words and phrases whose use commonly overlaps with 'crisis' is given below.

Breakdown	Disturbance	Acute Situation	Disaster
Accident	Out of Control	Dysfunction	
Chaos	Shock	Problem	Emergency
Injury	Trauma	Failure	
Tense Situation	Major Stress	Immediate Need	Casualty

This list, obtained by asking a group of people on a training course 'What does a crisis mean to you?', indicates that the term 'crisis is employed imprecisely in normal speech. In the theory and practice of Crisis Intervention, the word is used as a term of art with a definite and specific meaning.

Lindemann's paper (1944), describing the after-effects on those involved, of a fire in a night club, is usually regarded as marking the beginning of Crisis Intervention theory. Lindemann described the symptoms of shock and bereavement seen in those affected by the fire, and outlined some of the ways in which the needs of the people concerned might be responded to.

Caplan (1964) defined crisis as 'an upset in a steady state, when an individual faced with an obstacle to important life goals, finds that it is for the time being insurmountable through the utilisation of customary problem solving methods'.

All individuals acquire and maintain a repertoire of *normal coping skills* and strategies to enable them to deal with the stresses of everyday life. A challenge to the individual which is dealt with successfully by the use of those coping skills is, no matter how severe, not a crisis. A crisis involves a diminution of coping ability.

The model identifies the possibility of factors that operate over an extended period of time and which increase the risk of a person not being able to cope with stressful challenges. Such *vulnerability factors* include e.g. problems with the use of alcohol or drugs and previous mental health problems.

It is also usually accepted that specific *life events*, even if successfully negotiated, can increase the risk of later crises. (Tyrhurst, 1957). Examples of this would include domestic difficulties, debt, problems at work, bereavements, and, indeed, most, if not all, stressful life events.

The crisis process proper begins with a *precipitating event*, a challenge to the individual, which requires the use of coping strategies to be dealt with. If the person's normal coping abilities fail to meet the needs of the moment, then the person tends to try new ways, usually starting with modifications of previous ways of responding to stress, but then becoming increasingly haphazard. This stage of *trial and error* response may, through serendipity, lead to a solution. But if, as is often the case, it does not, then the person has the experience of repeatedly failing to cope.

The trial and error state commonly leads on to psychic *exhaustion*: attempts to solve the difficulties diminish in number and degree and are replaced as a primary concern by that of having the pain or discomfort relieved.

The crisis reaches a natural *turning point* in that external or internal events will bring the state of acute distress to an end. If this outcome was accompanied by, say the gaining of relief through medication but also by the development of a sense of failure, then it is likely that the person's coping skills will be significantly diminished in the long-term. Future crises will be more likely, and accelerated seeking of distress-relief will then further damage the person's self-efficiency and self-esteem.

It is, however, possible to provide an intervention which will assist the person to return to more useful attempts to resolve the crisis. If this is done successfully, then the person has the positive experience of gaining mastery over a previously insurmountable problem and of increasing their repertoire of coping strategies. Such an outcome will mean that future crises will be less likely to develop, but that if they do, then the person will have a much-improved chance of there being beneficial outcome. Figure 1 shows the stages of the crisis process graphically.

Consideration of how Crisis Intervention is best delivered leads to a distinct style of working.

1. The support offered should be *normalising*. By emphasising that people commonly react to crises in particular ways, and that what the client is experiencing is not abnormal, the damage to the person's self-esteem is minimised.
2. The work done should be *intensive, brief, flexible and rooted in the here-and- now*. The person's distress is a powerful motivant for change. Given that crises tend to be self-limiting in time, there is a 'window of opportunity' which needs to be utilised.
3. The intervention should be *confronting*, in the sense of encouraging the person to focus their attention on the unresolved problems of the crisis, and in seeking to counteract the person's desire to make distress-relief the focus.

Farewell (1976) has used the term 'furore' to describe a process where repeated apparent crises are in fact ritualised re-enactments of earlier events, where the discharge of emotion enables the person to continue in an unsatisfactory but nonetheless relatively stable mental state. In furore, the person is likely to want any professional helpers who are involved to witness how bad things are, rather than actually use them to try to change things.

Leeds Crisis Centre

There is a wide range of services that respond, in different ways, to crisis. Jacobson (1979) has described a hierarchy of crisis-orientated interventions, and Ratna (1978) has identified different types of crisis service. Among services in the UK that identify themselves as specifically crisis - focused, the Huddersfield Crisis Intervention Team, Lewisham Mental Health Advice Centre, Napsbury Hospital's Team, and the, sadly now-defunct, Coventry Crisis Centre, may be mentioned.

Leeds Crisis Centre opened in 1989. The idea for the Centre had been developed by a multi-disciplinary group of interested individuals looking for ways of responding to the mental health needs of people in Leeds; the process of clarifying ideas and, especially, of gaining funding was lengthy, the group first having met in 1982. Funding was insufficient to enable the desired 24-hour service to be achieved, and a partial service operated until early 1992.

The Centre is directly managed by Leeds City Council's Department of Social Service. Staffing consists of a Co-ordinator, Deputy Co-ordinator, twelve full-time Crisis Centre Workers (two of whom have particular responsibilities for work with Afro-Caribbean and Asian people), two Community Service Volunteers, plus administrative and domestic support. The workers include RMNs, Social Workers, and Counsellors & Therapists. The Centre opens from 10.00 am to 10.30 pm, and has limited overnight facilities including a helpline, and crisis beds. A creche is available.

Referrals are accepted from any relevant person, and an initial contact with the client is offered for the same day if possible, or for the following day. At an assessment that usually lasts between two and three hours, the worker explores with the client the difficulties and a contract for work, normally for a maximum of twelve weeks, is formed. There are no upper or lower age limits for referrals.

The service is designed to be user-friendly: there is a high level of confidentiality, formalities are kept to a minimum, and clients have access to their files.

An Advisory Committee oversees the Centre's work; it includes a range of representatives from Social Services, the Health Authority, GPs, Voluntary Agencies and others. Clients and carers are both represented on the Committee.

A few types of referral are not accepted. These are referrals where the person is homeless and the homelessness is the main or sole reason for the referral; referrals where the reason for the referral is the problematic use by the person of alcohol or substances; persons who are so floridly psychotic that counselling or similar methods are unlikely to be of use; and persons who are likely to be violent. Referrals where the presenting needs of the person clearly will not benefit from short-term work are normally not accepted. In all cases where a referral is not accepted, attempts are made to suggest or refer to other sources of help. It will be seen from the data below that 88% of referrals are accepted.

From the outset, it was intended that research would be an integral part of the Centre's functioning. A small research group, comprising the Co-Ordinator, a Social Services Development Officer, a Lecturer in General

Practice from the University of Leeds, and a representative from MIND, meets regularly to review the research protocols and to monitor results.

A process of on-going monitoring, research and evaluation needs to be seen as an integral part of the overall management style of the Centre. As the process identifies the degree to which the Centre is meeting its stated aims, then modifications occur to work practice and, sometimes, to the aims themselves in consequence. That changed practice is then itself evaluated by the process. It is important that research is not an 'add-on' extra item, but an essential part of the Centre's activity. Good research reflects what we believe in and our commitment to delivering the best service possible.

The research

A. monitoring and demographical data

Because some clients are very distressed when first seen, it is not always possible to obtain full information, and a small number of clients choose for whatever reason not to give information. In all following statistics, people for whom the relevant information was not available have been excluded from the calculation of percentages, etc, and the value of n varies accordingly. Except where otherwise specified, all data refer to the period of three years from 25th June 1989 to 24th June 1992 inclusive.

(i) Presenting problems

The following table shows the numbers and percentages of clients

	Main		Main or Secondary	
Relationship problems	270	43.1%	610	97.4%
Mental Illness or Disturbance*	58	9.3%	279	44.6%
Isolation	18	2.9%	215	34.3%
Other difficulties	80	12.8%	211	33.7%
Sequelae of Abuse	45	7.2%	184	29.4%
Financial Difficulties	11	1.8%	154	24.6%
Workplace/school problems	24	3.8%	144	23.0%
Violence	27	4.3%	143	22.8%
Bereavement	53	8.5%	131	20.9%
Consequences of pregnancy	6	1.0%	77	12.3%
Physical Illness	14	2.2%	62	9.9%
Effects of Discrimination	2	0.3%	36	5.8%
Gaining Access to Children	1	0.2%	13	2.1%
Stress of Caring for Adult Dependant	1	0.2%	9	1.4%
Committing an offence	1	0.2%	7	1.1%

*: Mental Disturbance includes: Schizophrenia, Manic-Depressive Psychosis, and other Psychoses, Personality Disturbance, Obsessions and Compulsions, Severe Anxiety State, Phobias, Panic Attacks, non-psychotic Depression, and addiction-related disorder.

whose main presenting problem fell into the category shown, and who presented a problem in the category as a primary or secondary difficulty.

It is notable that the frequency of presentation as the main problem does not indicate the overall occurrence of that problem; thus while 7.2% of persons presented with the sequelae of childhood abuse as their main problem, it was a focus of work for 29.4% of people. This feature is of particular importance in the case of mental disturbance (as defined above); only 9.3% of people presented their mental disturbance as the main reason for contacting the Centre, but 44.6% of people overall presented it as a focus of concern.

(ii) Referrers

The following table shows the sources of referrals for the first three years

	All	Accepted		Became Cases	
General Practice	237	232	(97.9%)	197	(83.1%)
Psychiatry	87	78	(89.7%)	56	(64.4%)
Casualty	52	47	(90.4%)	35	(67.3%)
Sub-total, Medical Sector	376	357	(94.9%)	274	76/6%)
Educational Agencies	13	12	(92.3%)	10	(76.9%)
Official Agencies (eg DSS, Police)	14	12	(85.7%)	8	(57.1%)
Other Sources	69	58	(84.1%)	38	(55.1%)
Sub-totals, Other Sources	96	82	(85.4%)	56	(58.3%)
Friends	96	92	(95.8%)	76	(79.2%)
Relatives (inc partners)	48	44	(91.7%)	33	(68.8%)
Sub-total, Personal Referrals	144	136	(94.4%)	109	(75.7%)
Social Workers	163	137	(84.0%)	85	(52.1%)
Other Social Service	29	23	(79.3%)	16	(55.2%)
Sub-total, Social Work Sector	192	160	(83.3%)	101	(52.6%)
Self-Referrals	108	82	(75.9%)	36	(33.3%)
Advice Agencies	32	23	(71.9%)	21	(65.6%)
Counselling Agencies	132	112	(84.8%)	86	(65.2%)
Housing Agencies	10	6	(60.0%)	6	(60.0%)
Self-Help Agencies	20	18	(90.0%)	13	(65.0%)
Other Voluntary Agencies	16	13	(81.3%)	11	(68.8%)
Sub-total, Voluntary Sector	210	172	(81.9%)	137	(65.2%)
Totals	1126	989	(87.8%)	727	(64.6%)

of activity, with the numbers and percentages of referrals accepted and of accepted referrals becoming cases. Instances where the referrer was not recorded or identifiable (15) have been excluded.

Figure 2 shows the sub-totals in graphic form. It will be seen that medical referrals are the biggest single group, amounting to one-third of all referrals; about two-thirds of these are GPs, who value the speed with which their patients can be seen, and the fact that there is an extra option available to them. The pattern shown established itself fairly early on in the Centre's life; since then the most significant change has been former clients referring friends and relatives.

(iii) Demographic data

The gender of persons referred to the Centre was:

	All		Accepted		Became Cases	
Male	430	(37.7%)	372	(37.1%)	271	(37.2%)
Female	711	(62.3%)	630	(62.8%)	458	(62.8%)
	1141		1002		729	

These ratios of women to men are typical of mental health work generally. The constancy of the ratio from referral to acceptance to commencement of work is remarkable, and, since it indicates that the Centre is successfully avoiding gender bias in its acceptance of referral, gratifying.

The ages of clients at assessment were:

0-15	16-19	20-29	30-39	40-49
2.8%	5.6%	38.6%	30.5%	14.9%

50-59	60-65	>65
5.3%	1.2%	1.2%

(n=729, see Figure 3)

The mean age of clients was 33.47 years. The virtual absence of clients over 60 might reflect a lessening of crisis occurrence with age; it might also, and perhaps more probably, arise because referrers refer older people for counselling less frequently.

The marital status of clients at assessment was:

Single	241	39.2%
Married	139	22.6%
Widowed	11	1.8%
Divorced	73	11.9%
Separated	54	8.8%
Cohabiting	63	10.2%
Other	34	5.5%

(n=615,see Figure 4)

The preponderance of single people is in part related to the location of the Centre in an area used for student accommodation. But that is only part of the picture; it is well known that the isolated single person is more at risk of mental health problems.

The accommodation had by clients at assessment was:

None - homeless	6	1.0%
Owner/occupied	182	30.2%
Privately rented	105	17.4%
Council	123	20.4%
Housing Association	55	9.1%
Living with relatives, parents or friends	85	14.1%
Other	47	7.8%

(n=603,see Figure 5)

The employment status of clients at assessment was:

Employed(inc self)	289	47.7%
Unemployed	137	22.6%
Student	55	9.1%
Sick or Disabled	45	7.4%
Manages home	42	6.9%
Other	38	6.3%

The percentage of clients who are unemployed is substantially higher than the local rate.

(iv) Psychiatric morbidity

Of 675 clients, 105 (15.6%) were in the care of a psychiatrist at the time of assessment. Of 660 clients, 111 (16.8%) had been psychiatric in-patients at some time. Of 674 clients, 221 (32.8%) had received psychiatric out-patient care at some time. Of 585 clients, 244 (41.7%) had either been psychiatric in-patients at some time or psychiatric out-patients at some time or both. Of 675 clients, 341 (50.5%) had consulted their General Practitioner for some reason in the six months prior to assessment. It is important to note that the majority of people with mental disturbance were not currently in the care of a psychiatrist: 44.6% of clients showed mental disturbance of some kind, but only 15.6% were in the care of a psychiatrist.

Of 675 clients, 212 (31.4%) had taken a deliberate overdose at some time in their lives before assessment, and 87 (12.9%) had taken more than one. 157 (23.3%) had harmed themselves deliberately in other ways at some time. Of 171 clients assessed in the period 1.1.92-24.6.92, 73 (42.7%) had either taken an overdose at some time or harmed themselves deliberately at some time or both. The percentage of clients who either had a psychiatric history or a history of overdose/self-harm was 61%.

B. Equal opportunities

As part of the process of evaluation of the Centre, we began from 1st January 1992 a programme of monitoring for equal opportunities purposes. Each person is asked, during their first attendance at the Centre, if they will complete an anonymous questionnaire. They then 'post' the completed form, in an envelope, into a box which is emptied periodically. In this way, the person is assured confidentiality.

In the period 1.1.92 to 16.6.92 (24 weeks), 209 forms were returned, a return rate close to 100%. One form was returned blank and has been excluded from the percentages calculated below; all others were fully or partly completed.

Ethnic Origin

WHAT WOULD YOU DESCRIBE AS YOUR ETHNIC ORIGIN? - AFRO-CARIBBEAN; ASIAN; BRITISH AFRO-CARIBBEAN; BRITISH ASIAN; BRITISH WHITE; OTHER (PLEASE SPECIFY).

206 people answered this question:

Afro-Caribbean/British Afro-Caribbean	8	3.8%
Asian/British Asian	5	2.4%
British White	180	87.4%
Other	13	6.3%

The 1981 Census gives, for the relevant area, 82.3% of the population as of UK or Irish birth, 13.3% of New Commonwealth & Pakistan origin, and 4.4% from the rest of the world.

Disability

WOULD YOU DESCRIBE YOURSELF AS PHYSICALLY DISABLED? IF SO, ARE YOU A REGISTERED DISABLED PERSON?

208 people answered this question, of whom 13 (6.2%) described themselves as disabled. Of these 13, 4 (30.8%) were registered disabled, while 9 (69.2%) were not.

Sexuality
WHAT IS YOUR SEXUALITY? - HETEROSEXUAL; LESBIAN/GAY;
BISEXUAL
199 people answered this question:

	All	Male	Female
Bisexual	13 (6.5%)	5 (6.9%)	8 (6.3%)
Heterosexual	164 (82.4%)	61 (84.7%)	102 (80.1%)
Lesbian/Gay	22 (11.1%)	6 (8.3%)	16 (12.7%)
Totals	199	72	126

Slightly more men than women did not answer this question:
Question not answered 9 (4.3%)   4 (5.2%)   5 (3.8%)

The fact that 17% of clients (15% of males, 20% of females) do not describe
themselves as heterosexual is significant in evaluating the assumptions
which underlie service provision. As many people are non-heterosexual
as are non-white, yet in how many services are the needs of non-
heterosexual people taken as seriously as those of non-white people? This
question becomes more significant when the numbers of persons reporting discrimination are considered; as shown below, 37% of lesbians and
gay men report feeling discriminated against.

Childhood Abuse
WERE YOU ABUSED OR NEGLECTED AS A CHILD? IF SO, PLEASE
TICK ANY OF THE FOLLOWING WHICH APPLY: SEXUAL ABUSE,
PHYSICAL ABUSE, EMOTIONAL ABUSE, NEGLECT.
206 people answered this question.

	All	Male	Female
Sexual Abuse	35 (16.7%)	9 (11.8%)	26 (19.9%)
Physical Abuse	41 (19.6%)	16 (21.1%)	25 (19.1%)
Emotional Abuse	67 (32.1%)	24 (31.5%)	42 (32.1%)
Neglect	31 (14.8%)	11 (14.5%)	20 (15.3%)
Sexual or Physical Ab.	51 (24.8%)	19 (25.0%)	32 (24.4%)

Discrimination
DO YOU FEEL DISCRIMINATED AGAINST IN ANY WAY? IF SO,
PLEASE SAY HOW.....

66 persons (31.58%) indicated that they felt discriminated against in
society in some way. This table shows the types of discrimination they
reported, together with , where appropriate, the percentage of the relevant group that this represents (e.g.: 26.9% of non-white people felt
discriminated against because of their race).

436

Age	4	
Class/lifestyle	6	
Disability	4	23.1%
Domestic responsibility	5	
Ethnic Origin or Race	7	26.9%
Gender	28	21.4%
Mental Health	4	
Not specified	5	
Other	10	
Sexuality	13	37.14%

It is notable that the percentage in the case of discrimination on grounds of sexuality is considerably higher than that for any other group.

C. Evaluation

In the period 25.6.89 to 31.12.92, clients were asked to complete the General Health Questionnaire, 60 question version (GHQ-60), at assessment and again at closure. The General Health Questionnaire is a widely-used self-administered psychometric test used to measure levels of psychic distress. The more commonly used of the scoring methods (CHQ as against Likert) gives a single score out of 60. The threshold scores are 11/12. (Goldberg & Williams, 1988). 390 clients completed GHQ-60 at assessment. Because a proportion of clients drop out, the number of clients completing GHQ-60 at closure was 257.

The following table shows the number of clients whose score fell within each decile at assessment.

Decile	Score Range	Number of Clients	Percent
1	0-6	16	4.1%
2	7-12	10	2.6%
3	13-18	23	5.9%
4	19-24	23	5.9%
5	25-30	38	9.7%
6	31-36	51	31.1%
7	37-42	71	18.2%
8	43-48	66	16.9%
9	49-54	59	15.1%
10	55-60	33	8.5%

n=390; mean = 37.2 ± 13.9

At closure the number of clients whose scores fell within each decile were:

Decile	Score Range	Number of Clients	Percent
1	0-6	119	46.3%
2	7-12	38	14.8%
3	13-18	22	8.6%
4	19-24	16	6.2%
5	25-30	19	7.4%
6	31-36	11	4.3%
7	37-42	19	7.4%
8	43-48	8	3.1%
9	49-54	5	1.9%
10	55-60	0	0.0%

n=257; mean = 13.9 ± 14.7%

Figures 7 to 10 show the shift graphically.

The difference between the two means is 23.3 points, and, using the Wilcoxon Signed Rank Test, is significant with $p < .00001$.

The Crown-Crisp Experiential Index (CCEI) is a 48-question, self-administered test, which provides both an overall score and scores for six sub-scales of Free-Floating Anxiety (FFA), Phobic Anxiety (PHO), Obsessional Anxiety (OBS), Somaticisation (SOM), Depression (DEP), and Hysteria (HYS).

CCEI was administered in the same way as GHQ60. The following table shows the number of clients whose total score fell within each decile at assessment.

Decile	Score Range	Number of Clients	Percent
1	0-10	4	1.1%
2	11-19	7	1.9%
3	20-29	22	6.1%
4	30-38	48	13.3%
5	39-48	80	22.1%
6	49-58	104	28.7%
7	59-67	68	18.8%
8	68-77	27	7.5%
9	78-86	2	0.6%
10	87-96	0	0.0%

n=362; mean=48.6 ± 14.1

The following table shows the number of clients whose scores fell within each decile at closure.

Decile	Score Range	Number of Clients	Percent
1	0-10	7	2.9%
2	11-19	9	3.8%
3	20-29	35	14.7%
4	30-38	74	31.1%
5	39-48	66	27.7%
6	49-58	35	14.7%
7	59-67	13	5.5%
8	68-77	0	0.0%
9	78-86	0	0.0%
10	87-96	0	0.0%

n=238; mean=38.1 ± 12.1
The difference between means of 10.5 is significant with p<0.00001.

Figures 11 to 14 show these results in graphic form.

Sub-scale results for CCEI at assessment and at closure are shown in figure 15. Figure 16 shows these results with data for normal subjects (Crisp et al, 1978) and for in-patients with psychoneurotic illness (Crown, 1974).

The results that we have obtained show to a very high degree of significance that clients' mental distress markedly declines between assessment and closure. For GHQ60, at assessment only 6.7% of clients score below the threshold score, while at closure this has risen to 61.2%.

Because of the fact that there is a significant drop-out rate, it is not possible to be certain that these results give a completely fair indication of the efficiency of the Centre. The clients who drop out might be significantly different in mental state when they finish than those who do not drop out. For this reason, from 1st January 1992, we have been using the Global Assessment of Functioning as a comparison, which since it is worker-ascribed avoids this difficulty. It rates persons on a single rating scale of 1 to 100 (psychological sickness to health) according to objective criteria covering psychological, social and occupational functioning. (Burbach, 1991) Figures 17 to 21 show preliminary results from this, and demonstrate that there is a significant (p<.00001) shift in mean GAF between assessment and closure. (Since the GAF scale scores health higher than sickness as opposed to GHQ-60 and CCEI, the GAF deciles have been reversed).

Comparison with psychiatric out-patients

O'Dwyer (1991) has undertaken a survey comparing morbidity and demographic data for clients at Leeds Crisis Centre with patients referred to two Leeds consultant psychiatrists. She reports finding virtually no differences between the two groups demographically. Administration of GHQ-60 and CCEI to the outpatient cohort produced scores which were almost identical (Figure 22). The differences she found were in terms of presenting symptoms. The out-patient group presented as 'ill' and had significantly more history of psychiatric disorder than did the Crisis Centre clients, who presented with specific difficulties. Her work reproduces results found by Caccia (1987) who conducted a similar comparison between clients of the Westminster Pastoral Foundation and out-patients at Guy's Hospital Department of Psychiatry and found analogous results.

Conclusion

Two independent methods of measuring change in mental distress have shown that clients at the Crisis Centre who completed their contracts experienced substantial benefit during the time that they were receiving Crisis Intervention support. Preliminary results from a third method appear to show that significant benefit occurs when persons who drop out are included in the evaluation process. These results indicate that Crisis Intervention is a useful and effective way of responding to psychological crisis.

References

Burbach, F.R. (1991). Quality and outcome in a Community Mental Health Team. *International Journal of Health Care Quality Assurance*, **4**, 18-26.

Caccia, J. et al (1987). A counselling centre and a psychiatric out-patient clinic - A comparison. *Bulletin of the Royal College of Psychiatrists*, **II**, 182-184.

Caplan, G. (1964). *An approach to community mental health*. London: Tavistock.

Crisp, A.H., Ralph, P.C., McGuiness, B., & Harris, G. (1978). Psychoneurotic profiles in the adult population. *British Journal of Medical Psychology*. **51**, 293-301.

Crown, S. (1974). The Middlesex Hospital Questionnaire (MHQ in clinical research. A review. In P. Pichot (Ed.), *Psychological Measurements in*

Psychopharmacology. 111-24. Basel: S. Karger.

Crown, S., & Crisp, A.H. (1979). *Manual of the Crown-Crisp Experiential Index*. London: Hodder and Stoughton.

Farewell, T. (1976, September 2). Crisis intervention. *Nursing Mirror*. 60-61.

Goldberg, D.P., & Williams, P. (1988). *A user's guide to the General Health Questionnaire*. Windsor: NFER-Nelson Publishing Co Ltd.

Jacobson, G.F. (1979). Crisis-oriented therapy. *Psychiatric Classes of North America*, 2(1), 39-54.

Lindemann, E. (1944). Symptomatology and management of acute grief. *American Journal of Psychiatry*. **101**, 141-148.

O'Dwyer, T.M. (1991). *Referrals to a crisis centre and psychiatric out-patients - A comparison*. Unpublished MMSc Thesis, University of Leeds Department of Psychiatry.

Ratna, L. (1978). *The practice of psychiatric crisis intervention*. Napsbury Hospital League of Friends.

Tyrhurst, J.S. (1957). The role of transitional states - including disaster. In *Mental Illness Symposium on Preventive and Social Psychiatry*. Washington DC: Walter Reed Army Institute of Research, US Government Printing Office.

A Model of Crisis

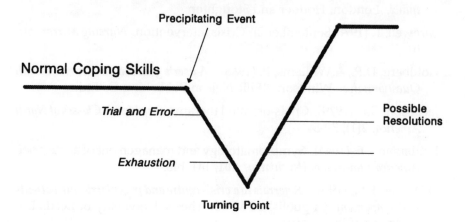

Precipitating Event

Normal Coping Skills

Trial and Error

Possible
Resolutions

Exhaustion

Turning Point

Figure 1

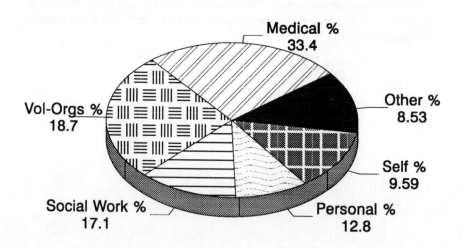

Medical %
33.4

Other %
8.53

Vol-Orgs %
18.7

Self %
9.59

Social Work %
17.1

Personal %
12.8

Figure 2   Sources of referrals   25 /6/89-24/6/92

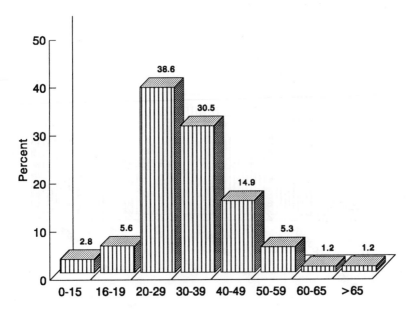

Figure 3 Ages of clients

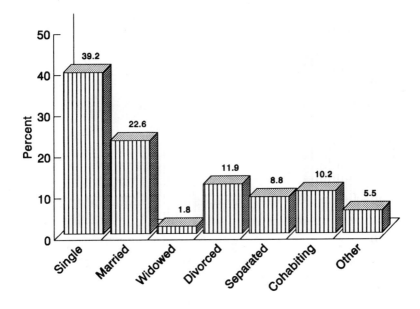

Figure 4 Marital status of clients

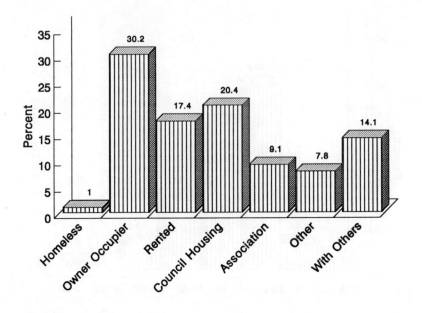

Figure 5 Accommodation status of clients

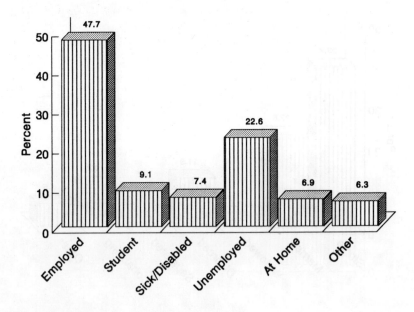

Figure 6 Employment status of clients

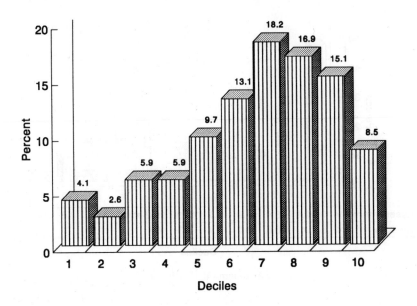

Figure 7   GHQ-60 scores at assessment by deciles

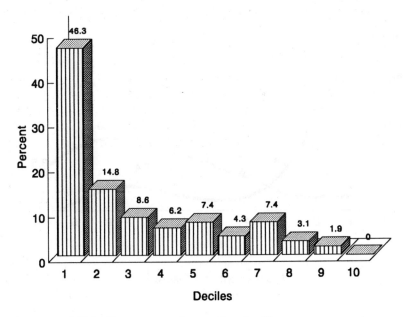

Figure 8   GHQ-60 scores at closure by deciles

445

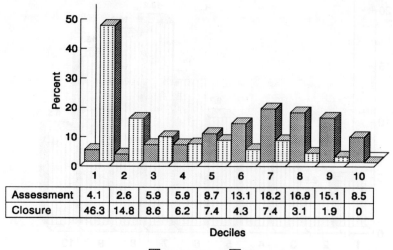

	1	2	3	4	5	6	7	8	9	10
Assessment	4.1	2.6	5.9	5.9	9.7	13.1	18.2	16.9	15.1	8.5
Closure	46.3	14.8	8.6	6.2	7.4	4.3	7.4	3.1	1.9	0

Deciles

■ Assessment ⊞ Closure

Figure 9 GHQ-60 scores at assessment and at closure

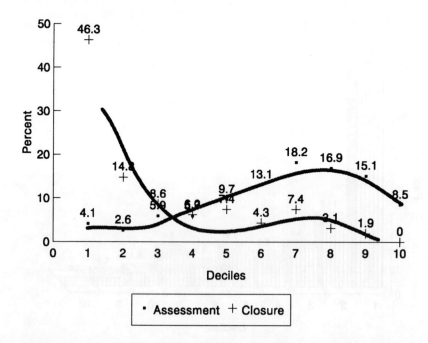

• Assessment + Closure

Figure 10 GHQ-60 scores assessment and at closure(cubic fit)

446

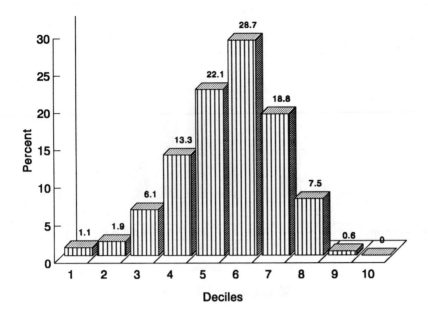

Figure 11 CCEI scores at asssessment by deciles

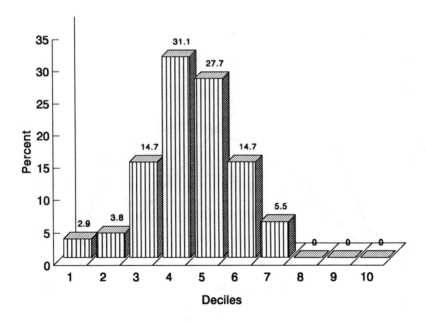

Figure 12 CCEI scores at closure by deciles

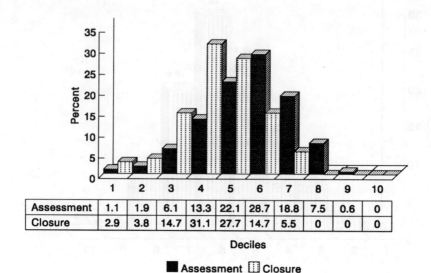

	1	2	3	4	5	6	7	8	9	10
Assessment	1.1	1.9	6.1	13.3	22.1	28.7	18.8	7.5	0.6	0
Closure	2.9	3.8	14.7	31.1	27.7	14.7	5.5	0	0	0

Deciles

■ Assessment ⊞ Closure

Figure 13 CCEI scores at assessment and at closure by deciles

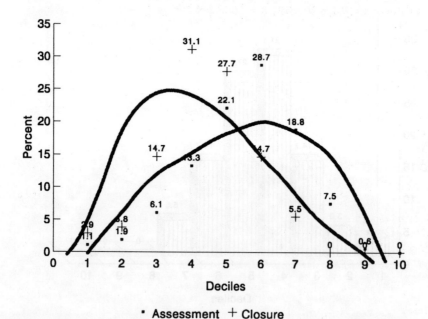

Deciles

■ Assessment + Closure

Figure 14 CCEI scores at assessment and at closure(cubic fit)

448

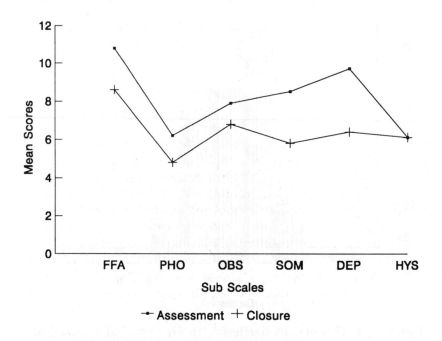

Figure 15 CCEI subscales at assessment and closure

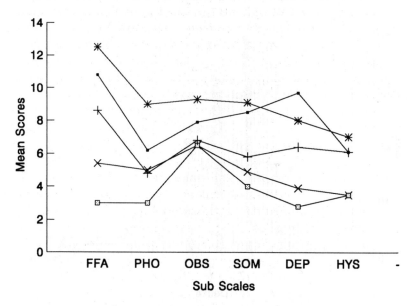

Figure 16 CCEI subscales at assessment and closure compared with normal subjects and psychiatric in-patients

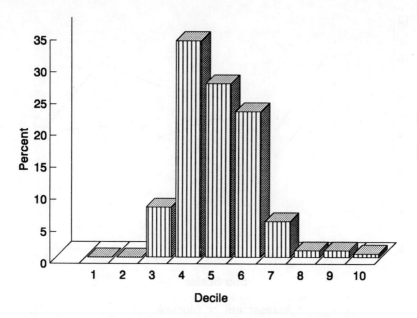

Figure 17 GAF scores by deciles(deciles reversed) at assessment

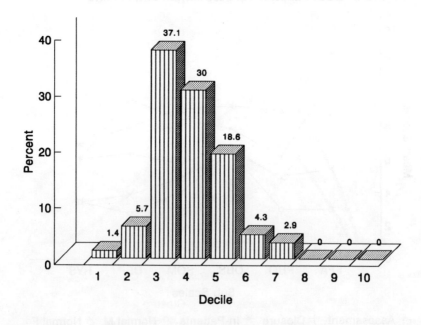

Figure 18 GAF scores at closures (deciles reversed)

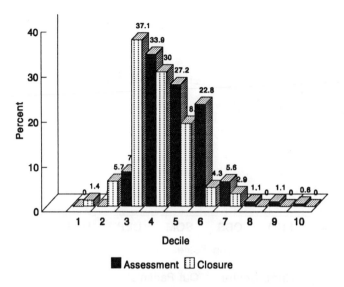

Figure 19 GAF scores at assessment and at closure(deciles reversed)

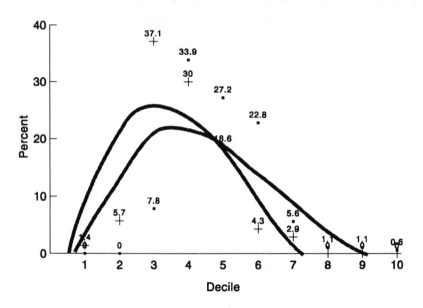

Figure 20 GAF scores at assessment and at closure
(deciles reversed) cubic fit

451

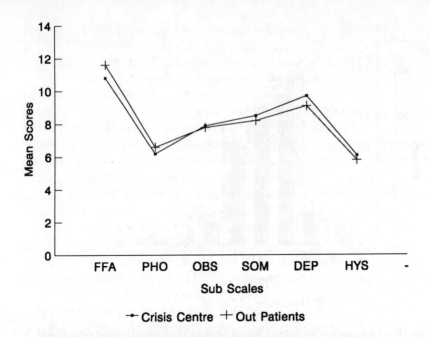

Figure 21 CCEI subscales at assessment: Crisis centre compared with psychiatric out-patients

35 The shamanic path to mental health promotion

M. Money

Abstract

The paper argues that mental health is not only fundamental to health and to health promotion, but also crierial. The concept of health must entail mental health, for all definitions of health entail notions of identity, purpose and intention which are only coherent in the context of an intact and identifiable person. All attempts to define health as substantially more than the absence of disease are therefore particularly relevant to the promotion of mental health. Current work in mental illness suggests that there is an acute problem with mental health, evidenced by the high rate of consultation for anxiety, depression, and stress-related problems. The incidence of neurosis, violence, attempted suicide, vandalism and substance abuse is also striking. It is contended that these manifestations of mental ill health may have their origin largely in a single problem. That problem is loss of meaning, the absence of a teleology - the perception of purpose and meaning in the universe. Such meaning can be recovered through what is termed the wholistic or shamanic vision. The shamanic vision is a consequence of following the shamanic path. Definitions of shamanism and the shamanic vision are discussed, and consideration is given to Achterberg's summary of its characteristics and their health promotion implications. The very opposite of pathological, it is argued that such a vision is radically and profoundly healthy. Personal unity and actualisation are enhanced by the perception of the unity of the world. The paper considers ways in which the fostering and development of the shamanic path would constitute a substantial contribution to the development of mental health promotion.

Mental health is crierial to all forms of health

Not only is mental health fundamental to health and to health promotion, it is also criterial. The concept of health must entail mental health whatever the definition of health we adopt. It does not matter whether we speak of completeness, the attainment of maximum potential, optimal adaptation, peak effectiveness, full achievement - all entail notions of integration, purpose or intention which are only coherent in the context of an intact and identifiable person who consistently expresses intention, who strives to attain, who functions optimally, who makes the healthy choice, who experiences self-actualisation. Mental health is not a post-script to health, not a gloss on its surface, it is its definandum. To be coherent, all current notions of human health must be logically predicated on the notion of a person.

This assertion is well illustrated by the findings of researchers into the psychological concomitants of complete callosal commissurotomy - the 'split-brain' operation. Following this surgical intervention several re-searchers (e.g. Bogen 1973); Sperry 1976, 1978; Gazzaniga 1967, 1970, 1975)) noted instances of conflict behaviour between the two separated cerebral hemispheres. This apparent disunity of behaviour raised ques-tions for them about the personal unity of what had survived the opera-tion. Similar discussions have taken place in attempts to make conceptual sense of certain instances of multiple personality (e.g. Prince 1906; Thigpen and Cleckley 1957). In many instances of what has been called multiple identity (Puccetti 1973) it has become clear that it is only coherent to speak of a person if we can speak of a coherent person; and that personal unity evaluated through some sort of consciousness criterion is a prerequisite for speaking of a person. Mental health must therefore be criterial for personal health, for there to be a meaningful notion of person on whom propositions about health and illness are predicated.

It follows from this that all that has been said about defining health as far more than merely the absence of disease is therefore particularly relevant to the promotion of mental health. This aspect of health espe-cially must be understood not merely as the promotion of conditions where there is an absence of clinical features or of manifest distress but as the attainment of the maximum individual human potential. And there is an obvious reciprocal relationship between the mental health of the individual and that of the community, as the notion of a community also entails the presence of individuals who have purposeful interaction.

The mental health problem

Here and now, there is a problem with mental health. In the last century Thoreau (1854; 1960) said that most men lead lives of quiet desperation. But today the desperation is no longer silent; its expression has become deafening. The high rate of GP consultation for depression and depressive episodes, the incidence of neurosis and anomie, the incidence of violence, vandalism, and substance abuse, the number of people described as TATT - tired all the time - points to an epidemic of mental ill-health. This incidence reflects a national problem. As Newton (1988) has pointed out, not only is mental illness 'more prevalent than most people realise' (p15) but determining its extent by counting in-patients (26 per cent of all hospital bed occupancy in 1980) 'gives a gross underestimation of the prevalence of disorder' (ibid).

Brenner (1976) has shown that such problems may be a reflection of economic policy, and in January 1992 the Royal College of Psychiatrists estimated the incidence of clinical depression as five per cent, affecting one person in 20. We have 4,000 suicides in Britain every year, and Hawton and Fagg (1992) have estimated that suicide attempts are made by approximately 120,000 people in Britain annually. Between 1989 and 1990 80 million working days were lost through mental illness.

Further evidence is provided by the frenetic search for utopian or millennial solutions, and while these may sometimes be bizarre the nature of the answer in no way invalidates the sincerity and even desperation of the question.

What are the most common features of mental ill-health? They include loneliness, unhappiness, isolation, depression, feelings of powerlessness and estrangement. I want to argue that these have their origin largely in one problem; that depression, for example, is a symptom rather than an illness in itself. It is a symptom of disenchantment.

The loss of meaning

The problem, the origin of disenchantment, is the loss of meaning and of purpose. We have disciplines such as theology, psychology, gerontology, and so on. But the missing -ology is teleology - the perception of purpose and meaning in the universe, and thence in the life of the individual.

Cowan (1991) has expressed this radical loss of meaning eloquently. He observes that:

Under the banner of progress we have over-exploited to the point of destruction the very things of which we're made, those four alchemical elements - earth, air, fire and water. These now are languishing in furnaces, chemical mixtures, reactors, disposable products, carcinogenic compounds and those ozonal predators that eat away at the atmosphere's protective layer. They live on as embittered exiles, condemned to support our exaggerated sense of what is required to survive. The hunter-gatherer in us has been killed off by the stock-market expert. The sage has succumbed to the economist.

I argue that if we cannot perceive purpose and meaning in the universe, and we cannot perceive it in the planet or in the natural order, then it is futile to invoke it in ourselves by some irrational act of special pleading. Meaning is not something which we can say exists only for humans but is absent from all those systems which create and maintain and accompany human existence. The discovery or rediscovery of a teleology can only be accomplished if that teleology explains not only our own purpose but - to use Buber's (1970) term - the ground of our being.

Re-enchanting the world

I believe that the key to the rediscovery of meaning is in what Berman (1981) has termed the re-enchantment of the world. It is to call an end to the 'single vision and Newton's sleep' of which Blake warned, to cease to see the universe - in a manner which itself recalls mental illness - as a giant machine mindlessly and purposelessly turning on cosmic cogs until its clockwork runs down. It may well be that the philsophical position which engendered the scientific revolution was itself a form of mental illness, for as Berman (1981) p121) observes:

Despite his eventual nervous breakdown, Newton was no psychotic; but that he bordered on a type of madness, and allayed it with a totally death-oriented view of nature, is beyond doubt. What is significant, however, is not his view of nature itself, but the broad agreement that it found, the excitement that it generated... With the acceptance of the Newtonian world view, it might be argued, Europe went collectively out of its mind.

The way in which the world is re-enchanted is by recapturing the wholistic world-view. That perspective is contained within the shamanic vision.

The shamanic vision

What is shamanism, and what are the features of the shamanic mode of perception - the shamanic vision? Shamanism is a universal human experience (Winkelman 1990) which has been termed the first spiritual discipline; 'the root from which other spiritual disciplines have issued' (Peters 1989 p 115). But in recent times, concurrent with the resurgence of interest in shamanism and its processes (Walsh 1989), the term has been used loosely, even inappropriately. McNiff (1988) reports working 'with a Native American healer who laughed at the idea of being called a shaman' (p287), and I share Johnson's (1988) concern that

Shamanism had in fact become a code word for anything that stirs passions or relates to the spiritual world - a use so broad that everything from psychotherapy to rock and roll is seen as shamanic (p270).

The shaman has been defined differently by different authorities, but Harner's definition is representative. He saw the shaman as

> a man or woman who enters an altered state of consciousness - at will - to contact and utilise an ordinarily hidden reality in order to acquire knowledge and power and to help other persons. (in Moreno 1988 p274).

However, an excellent review article by Wright (1989) suggests that Hultkrantz's somewhat more extended (1968) definition of a shaman could reasonably be adopted. That definition (p26) comprises four key features, namely

*   contact with a sacred world which interconnects with the human world. 'It is a world of spirits in animal, plant, rock, water and human form...'
*   service as intermediary between the human and sacred world
*   inspiration from guardian or helping spirits
*   experience of ecstasy

As Eliade (1964) originally indicated, shamanic techniques are all techniques of ecstasy. Ecstasy is something that is signally lacking from contemporary lives. Indeed, our lives too often are characterised by its semantic and physiological opposite, which is inertia. But the shaman who experiences it describes it in terms of a visual narrative - as the shamanic vision. Achterberg (1985) has summarised the principal features of the shamanic vision very ably. They include:

*   seeing the universe and everything inside it as being part of the same whole, of being constructed from the same fabric
*   keeping in communion with the animals and plants and stars
*   knowing about life, knowing about death, and seeing no difference
*   seeking out all the experiences of creation and turning them over and over, seeking their texture and their multiple meanings
*   expanding beyond one's singular state of consciousness to experience the waves and ripples of the universe

There are at least four respects in which I believe the Shamanic vision is relevant to issues of health and health promotion. These are:

*   The articulation of an ecological perspective
*   The use of imagery as a healing method
*   A particular familiarity with botanical agents as healing materials
*   The perception of the unity of the world and the reenchantment that this facilitates.

I shall focus only on this last aspect here, but that is not to minimise the importance of the other three. At this point I should like to anticipate and correct a possible misunderstanding. This world-view is not recovered by the ingestion of obscure botanic substances or encountering strange old Indians with piercing eyes. The shamanic vision and the path it reveals is not attained by loosening one's grasp upon reality, but by tightening it; by achieving clarity, not by dissipating it. By becoming more real - not less. Indeed, as Wolf (1991) argues, the rigorous intellectual disciplines of the new physics have led it to a world-view very similar to that of the shaman.

It should be noted that the shaman is not, as some have argued, the weak and weedy member of his society, perhaps more characterised by his own lack of mental good health than by his ability to propagate it in others. Eliade (ibid) has argued strongly to the contrary; that while traditional shamen may encounter severe illness at an early stage in their lives, their recovery marks the onset of their shamanic career.

They are thenceforward characterised by a remarkable vigour, vitality, stamina, and coherence of thought and outlook. The validity of the shamanic vision cannot be denied by belittling those who have articulated it.

Recovering the shamanic vision

The shamanic vision is recovered by the realisation, generated by many possible methods, that the individual, the world and the universe are intimately interconnected - by perceiving oneself, other humans and all other living beings as members of the same family. By identifying the oak tree as of the same lineage as oneself. Understanding Cowan's (ibid) informant, Bill Neidjie, when he explains:

'Tree, he watching you. You look at tree, he listen to you. He got no finger, he can't speak. But that leaf...he pumping, growing, growing in the night. While you sleeping you dream something. Tree and grass same thing. They grow with your body, with your feeling.'

And cherishing all human experience as informative and as potentially ecstatic. Those who experience the shamanic vision are transformed by it; a point well illustrated in the experiences of the psychotherapist Graywolf, described by Krippner (1987), who was impelled into his psychotherapeutic career by such vision.

Let us explore some of the possible implications for mental health promotion within the recovery of the shamanic vision. It is these implications I have termed the shamanic path to mental health.

458

The shamanic path to mental health

Anomie, isolation, and depression arise out of a perception of oneself as separate, valueless, and friendless. Lynch (1977) has drawn attention to the importance of human contact and social support for health. More recently, Lynch (in Ornstein & Swencionis 1990) and Argyle (1991) have demonstrated the many links between companionship, happiness, and health. An understanding of oneself as an integral part of the universal system, as a relative of all other living things, as not an aspirant but an actual member of the living community is a powerful antidote to a circumscribed view of the self. Such a perspective also adds a far broader meaning to the notion of Community Development, for the concept of community is then extended beyond the human to the animal, vegetable, the mineral members of the community.

A renewal of the relationship that exists between ourselves and other living things is already widely regarded as health-enhancing. Companion animals, for example, are well established (e.g. Friedman, 1980) as beneficial in a range of contexts that runs from Coronary Care Units via prison cells to retirement homes. And gardening, it has been argued (e.g Carse 1986), is an entirely healthy and life-enhancing activity whose benefits are at least as much mental as physical.

The fear of death is a profound cause of anxiety for some individuals. The shamanic view of death does not consist of its denial but of its acceptance and celebration as an interesting and instructive stage of human growth - a view that can be used to motivate and to reassure. Death is seen as a transition rather than an extinction; only terminal when seen from a truncated perspective. It is a transition as worthy of celebratory rites of passage as any other.

Some people are bored and disaffected with the world, and the truth is that the bored are very frequently boring, and therefore avoided, and therefore depressed. The shamanic world-view validates all experiences as intrinsically informative and potentially ecstatic, often in a number of different ways or at several levels of meaning. A person engaged in the search for a renewed meaning in the world, and who celebrates those meanings he or she discovers, can never be bored. And people who are busy and happy don't get sick. Roszak (1979) has pointed out the parallels between person and planet, and someone who sees the planet as a source of delight is more likely to be an interesting and delightful person. 'As a man is, so he sees' (Blake; in Bronowski 1958 p221).

What I am arguing for here is a vision of mental health promotion which addresses itself to fundamental issues of the meaning and purpose of life, rather than tinkering with the ingredients. Human life is enhanced and its meaning is magnified when seen as part of the life of the universe. Human existence is made more rather than less valuable when placed alongside the worth of all other living things which constitute an ecological whole. And the battle that is being fought to preserve the integrity of our ecosystem, and with it the continuance of all life on our planet, is one that can give meaning to any life. This is to follow the shamanic path to mental health promotion.

I wish to thank Janet Money for her comments on an earlier draft of this paper.

References

Achterberg, J. (1985). *Imagery in healing - Shamanism in modern medicine.* London: Shambhala

Argyle, M. (1987). *The psychology of happiness.* London & New York: Routledge

Berman, M. (1981). *The reenchantment of the world.* Ithaca: Cornell

Bogen, J.E. (1973). The other side of the brain - an appositional mind. In R. Ornstein (Ed.) *The nature of human consciousness.* San Francisco: Freeman & Co.

Brenner, (1976). *Achieving the Goals of the Employment Act of 1946 - Thirtieth Annual Review. Vol. 1 Employment.* Washington: Joint Economic Committee of the Congress of the United States.

Bronowski, J. (1958). (Ed.) *William Blake - A selection of Poems and Letters.* Harmondworth: Penguin

Buber, M. (1970). *I and Thou.* New York: Scribner's

Carse, J.P. (1987). *Finite and infinite games.* Harmondsworth:Penguin

Cowan, J. (1991). *Letters from a wild state - An Aboriginal perspective.* Shaftesbury: Element Books.

Eliade, M. (1964). *Shamanism : Archaic techniques of ecstasy.* New York: Pantheon

Friedman, E. et al. (1980). Animal companions and one year survival after discharge from a coronary care unit. *Public Health Reports* 95, 301-12

Gazzaniga, M.S. (1967). The split brain in Man, *Sc. Am.* 217:(2)

Gazzaniga, M.S. (1970). *The bisected brain.* Cambridge: Appleton Century Crofts.

Gazzaniga, M.S. (1975). Review of the split brain. *J. Neurol.* 209:(2), 75-9

Hawton, K. & Fagg, J. (1992). Trends in deliberate self poisoning and self injury in Oxford, 1976-90 *BMJ* **304**, 1409-11

Johnson, D.R. (1988). Introduction to the special issue - Creative arts therapists as contemporary shamans: Reality or romance. *Arts in Psychotherapy*, **15**, 269-270

Krippner, S. (1987). Shamanism, personal mythology, and behaviour change. *Int. J. Psychosomatics*, **34**:(4), 22-27

Lynch, J.J. (1977). *The broken heart - The medical consequences of loneliness*. New York: Basic Books Inc.

Lynch, J.J. (1990). The broken heart: The psychobiology of human contact. In R. Ornstein & C. Swencionis (Eds.) *The healing brain - A scientific reader*. New York: Guilford Press

McNiff, S. (1988). The shaman within. *Arts in Psychotherapy*, **15**, 285-291

Moreno, J.J. (1988). The music therapist: Creative arts therapist and contemporary shaman. *Arts in psychotherapy*, **15**, 271-280

Newton, J. (1988). *Preventing Mental Illness*. London: Routledge and Kegan Paul

Peters, L.G. (1989). Shamanism: Phenomenology of a spiritual discipline. *J. Transpersonal Psychol*, **21**, 1151-1137

Prince, M. (1906). *The Dissociation of a personality*. New York: Longmans, Green

Puccetti, R. (1973). Multiple Identity. *The Personalist*, **54**, 203-215

Roszak, T. (1979). *Person / Planet - The Creative Disintegration of Industrial Society*. London: Gollancz.

Royal College of Psychiatrists. (1992). *Defeat Depression*. London: RCP

Sperry, R.W. (1966). Brain bisection and mechanisms of consciousness. In J.C. Eccles (Ed) *Brain and conscious experience*. New York: Springer-Verlag

Sperry, R.W. (1968). Hemisphere deconnection and unity in conscious awareness. *Am. Psychol*, **23**, 723-733

Thigpen, C.H. & Cleckley. H.M. (1957). *The three faces of Eve*. New York: McGraw-Hill

Thoreau, H.D. (1854). In New American Library (Ed.) (1960). *Walden*. New York and Scarborough: New American Library.

Walsh, R. (1989). What is a shaman? Definition, origin and distribution. *J. Transpersonal Psychol*, **21**, 1-11

Winkelman, M.J. (1990). Shamans and other 'Magico-Religious' healers: A cross-cultural study of their origins, nature, and social transformations. *Ethos*, **18**, 308-352

Wolf, F.A. (1991). *The Eagle's Quest - A physicist's search for truth in the heart of the shamanic world*. London: Mandala

Wright, P.A. (1989). The nature of the shamanic state of consciousness: A review. *J. Psychoactive Drugs*, **21**:(1) 25-33

36 A preliminary report on an elderly and youth exchange programme

L. Moore and D. Trent

Introduction

Attitudes toward the elderly have long been the focus of investigation. Intergenerational programmes aimed at enriching the interactions between the older and younger generations and improving the view taken of the elderly by the young have abounded over the past few decades (Nash, 1968; Bagett, 1981; Tice, 1980; McGuire, 1986; Seefeldt, 1987; Corbin et al., 1989; Pratt, 1984; Cherry et al., 1985). While most of the research to date has been based on the assumption that both the young and the elderly hold negative opinions of each other, lack of contact between the two groups due, in part, to mobility within the society, has been seen as a contributing factor (Sussman and Pfeifer, 1988). Higgan and Faunce (1977) directly relate intergenerational attitudes to contact between the generations. Since few children report contact with older persons, either within or without the family (Jantz et al., 1976; Seefeldt et al., 1977), it can be concluded that the tendency for young persons to hold preconceived and unfavourable attitudes toward the elderly (Bengston, 1971) may be due to stereotyping rather than factual evidence. The assumption that increased contact will lead to more positive attitudes has support from Heider's (1958) balance theory as well as Homan's (1979) exchange theory. Research has suggested that the attitudes toward the elderly held by the young are the result of those attitudes communicated and modelled by other adults (Khan, 1973) rather than by class or one's position in society (Bennett and Eckman, 1973). Jacobs (1975) clearly argues that the appropriate time for inaugurating programmes aimed at changing attitudes is during childhood and early youth. It is also argued that while attitudes are situation specific (Lutsky, 1979; McTavish, 1971), a young person's view of the older person is better representd by a multi-dimentional array of attitudes rather than any single attitude. Therefore, any programme oriented toward the attitudes held by the young toward the elderly should be multi-faceted in design.

An Elderly and Youth Exchange (EYE) programme was set up to encourage intergenerational links between primary school children and senior citizens within the Stafford area. The purpose of the project was to determine the change in attitudes toward each other as the result of increased positive contact between the two groups. This paper will look at the preliminary results of the attitudes of youth towards the elderly.

Method

The EYE project consisted of 42 primary school children ranging in age from 10 to 11 years old. The children were taken from three classes within the same school in the county town of Stafford. The programme consisted of a taught component focusing on attitude toward the elderly, followed by a direct contact experience. The taught portion of the programme involved one session a week (9:00am to 12 Noon) for five weeks. Direct discussion teaching covered subjects such as identifying who the elderly are and aspects of aging. A brain storming exercise was aimed at helping the children explore varying aspects of age and aging. Role playing and experiential aging excercises were included.

The follow-up contacts were made with an elderly population between the ages of 64 and 92 who were resident at three sheltered housing complexes within a one mile radius of the school. The visits took place in the community centre and lasted approximately two hours, one day each week over an additional five week period. These sessions included personal and local oral histories, skills training in areas such as cooking, knitting and crocheting and modellingand observation.

The second author was present for all programme segments. An adapted Kogan (1961) Old People Scale (AKOPS) was given to the students prior to the start of the programme and then was re-administered following the completion of the programme.

Results

The three groups were combined and the results reported cover the total subject population. A comparison of the pre- and post-test results shows a mean score shift of 8.22 (pre-test mean = 129.54; Sd = 14.78; post-test mean = 137.76; Sd = 18.81). While the two are not vastly different, a two-tailed T-test was run on the means and showed a significant difference between the two (t=-2.575; p=.014; n=42). A significant difference was also found between the male and female subjects on the pre-test (t=-3.785; p=.001; n=21 males / 21 females). This would support the idea that males and females held differing attitudes toward the elderly at the beginning of the project. No significant difference was noted on the post-test (t=-1.290; p=.205; n=21 males / 21 females) suggesting that the difference in attitudes had narrowed, accounting for the significant shift in pre- and post-test scores. A comparison of means between tests within genders shows that males showed a significant shift in attitudes (t=2.6; p=.014; n=21) while the females showed no significant shift (t=.99; p=.34; n=21). Again, this would suggest that the shift in male attitudes accounts for the significant shift in overall scores.

Conclusions

Attitudes in young people toward the elderly have come under question over the years. Education has been one of the areas which is seen as having an impact on such attitudes. Likewise, the promotion of mental health has long been seen as an educative process. The current study supports the long accepted idea that early education can alter the attitudes held by children toward target populations. By establishing positive attitudes at an early age, cross support systems can be established which will give comfort and purpose to both groups as well as transferring desired skills and knowledge from the experienced to the less experienced. Projects such as EYE can go a long way toward meeting that goal.

References

Baggett, S. (1981). Attitudinal consequences of elder adult volunteers in the public school setting. *Educational Gerontology*, 7, 21-33.

Bengtzon, V. L. & Kuypers, J. A. (1971). Generational difference and the developmental stake. *Aging and Human Development*, 2, 249-260.

Bennet, R. & Eckman, J. (1973). Attitudes towards aging: A critical examination of recent literature and implications for future research. In C. Eisodorfer and M. P. Lowton (Eds.), *The psychology of adult development and aging*. Washington, D.C.: American Psychological Association.

Cherry, D. A., Benest, F. R., Gates, B. & White, J. (1985). Intergenerational service programmes: Meeting shared needs of young and old. *The*

Gerontologist, 25, 126-129.

Corbin, D. E., Metal-Corbin, J. & Borg, C. (1989). Teaching about aging in the elementary school: A one year follow-up. *Educational Gerontology,* **15,** 103-110.

Heider, F. (1958). *The psychology of interpersonal relations.* New York: Wiley.

Higgans, P. S. & Faunce, R. (1977, March). *Attitudes of Minneapolis elementary school students and senior citizens toward each other.* ERIC Document 139834, March.

Homans, G. (1974). *Social behaviour: Its elementary forms.* New York: Harcourt, Brace, Janovich

Jacobs, H., L. (1975). Education for aging in the elementary and secondary school systems. In S. Grabowski & W. D. Mason (Eds.), *Learning for aging.* Washington, D. C., Adult Education Association and ERIC.

Jantz, R. K., Seefeldt, C., Galper, A. & Serock, K. (1976). Children's attitudes toward the elderly. Final report, University of Maryland.

Khan, S. B. & Weiss, J. (1973). The teaching of affective responses. In R. M. W. Travers (Ed.), Second Handbook of Research on Teaching. Chicago: Rand McNally.

Kogan, N. (1961). Attitudes towards old people: The development of a scale and examination of correlates. *Journal of Abnormal and Social Psychology,* **62,** 1, 44-64.

Lutsky, N. S. (1979, November). *The citation and interpretation of attitude research in gerontology: A pilot study.* Presented at the meeting of the Gerontology Society, Washington, D.C.

McGuire, S. l. (1986). Promoting positive attitudes toward aging among children. *Journal of Social Health,* **56,** 322-324.

McTavish, D. G. (1971). Perceptionss of old age: A review of research methodologies and findings. *Gerontologist,* **11,** 90-101.

Nash, B. E. (1968, October). Foster grandparents in child care settings. *Public Walfare,* 272-280.

Pratt, F. (1984). Teaching today's kids - tomorrow's elders. *Aging,* **346,** 19-28.

Seefeldt, C. (1987). The effect of preschoolers' visits to a nursing home. *The Gerontologist,* **27,** 228-232.

Seefeldt, C., Jantz, C. K., Galper, A. & Serock, K. (1977). Using pictures to explore children's attitudes towards the elderly. *Gerontologist*, **17**, 506-512.

Sussman, M. B. & Pfeifer, S. K. (1988). Kin and non-kin intergenerational connecting. *Gerontology Review*, **1**, 75-84.

Tice, C. H. (1980). Creating caring communities: Linking the generations. *Aging*, **307**-308, 20-23.

37 Quality Assurance within an innovative service providing community support to people with mental health problems

C. Murray, S. Wills and J. Hughes

Introduction

This Paper sets out to describe the work of the Mental Health Community Support Team in Macclesfield Social Services District, Cheshire County Council. It is intended that the Paper be a practical guide to the service provided by the Team within a framework of innovation, community support and quality assurance. The intention in describing those components is to provide an over-view of the service which has built into its infrastructure the key elements of quality assurance.

In order to provide that over-view it has been necessary to firstly paint a general picture of the Community Support Team's work. This first section provides information about the legislative foundation of the Team through the Specific Grant for Mental Illness, (Department of Health, 1991) as well as performance outcomes and key areas. The second section describes innovatory practice, and brings together a range of methods including network development, assessment and care management processes, monitoring, evaluation and befriending. It is contended in this section that a combination of these methods is innovatory. The final section gives a theoretical summary of quality assurance and the key areas relevant to social care agencies. This is followed by a description of the practical applications of quality assurance theory within the Community Support Team practice.

It has taken energy, commitment, skill and team work to bring community support, innovatory practice and quality assurance together in one Team, and it is hoped that this Paper will stimulate and interest other social workers.

The specific Grant for mental Illness LAC (91) 19 (Department of Health, 1991) requires that the effectiveness of the work of the Community Support Team is reflected in Performance Outcomes. For the Team they have been identified thus:

> Changes in the pattern of psychiatric services received by individual clients
>
> Reduction in the frequency and length of hospital admissions
>
> Involvement of clients in the preparation of their individual Care Plan
>
> Feedback from clients during and following the intervention of the Team

From these general Performance Outcomes, it has been necessary to develop ways of measuring the extent to which these objectives are achieved. Some Performance Outcomes are easy to identify, for example, a reduction in the length and frequency of hospital admissions can be clearly demonstrated by the number of admissions to psychiatric hospital before and after referral, and a similar measure can be applied to a client's length of stay in hospital. On the other hand, it is more difficult to establish substantive feedback from clients both during and after help has been offered from the Community Support Team. In order to measure this systematically, it was decided that each client at the point of referral would be asked to complete a Quality of Life measure (Oliver, J., 1991) with the assistance of their worker. This is then repeated every six months, thus enabling a pattern to be developed of the client's perception of the effectiveness of the Team's intervention on significant aspects of their life. The Quality of Life measure was developed by Huxley et al from Manchester University (Oliver, J., 1991) and has already been used by the Community Support Teams operating within Lancashire, Rhyl, central Manchester and Boulder, Colorado, with considerable success. The incorporation of this measure (Oliver, J., 1991) into the work of Macclesfield Community Support Team will enable parallels to be drawn with the work of other Community Support Teams. A further means of obtaining objective feedback from clients is the use of the General Satisfaction Questionnaire. This also was developed by Huxley et al and in broad terms it enables the client to put on paper their thoughts and feelings about the service that they are currently receiving. (Murray, C.T., 1992) The involvement of a colleague from another Team has assisted in the objectivity of the information thus received.

The work of the Community Support Team thus builds on the Care Programming approach outlined in the Practitioner Guide to Assessment

& Care Management (Department of Health and Social Services Inspectorate, 1991) in order to meet the monitoring requirements of Central Government in respect of the monies allocated for the Specific Grant for Mental Illness. (Department of Health, 1991). This unique opportunity to recruit a new team of workers to provide a social work service to a defined group of clients with particular mental health problems, has presented many challenges and opportunities. These are highlighted in this Paper under the general headings of Innovatory Practice and Quality Assurance.

Innovatory practice

Necessity is often cited as being the mother of invention and this is truly the case within the Community Support Team. Within an environment where the notion of purchase and provider is becoming increasingly important, the situation where Teams must **provide** without the capacity to purchase is difficult. In spite of this it is profoundly possible and a quality service can be offered given the adoption, acceptance and application of certain principles.

A decision was made to respond to the monies made available under the Mental Health Specific Grant in an innovative manner. Both research and the hard evidence of our day to day work points to the social isolation of the client group with whom we work and this obviously needs to be addressed, within a substantive concept of community. Within the Community Support Team this is addressed through a combination of working practices and theoretical perspectives. Broadly, we can consider the following theoretical concepts as being those that form the basis for the Team's work; Assessment and Care Management, the application of a Quality of Life measure, the concept of Networks and Network Development, the use of befriending as a normalising concept and community support. These areas are not in themselves new, however, we would contend that the application of all as a collective whole, to assist a particular person is innovative.

As stated above, the Team has adopted an Assessment and Care Management approach. Practically this means that a Care Manager is responsible for a case from the point of acceptance and this individual will assume a co-ordinating role. In addition to this, a Key Worker is also established at this point. It is the remit of the Care Manager to gather information, for example psychiatric and social history, as well as information on existing and potential networks. Having gathered this a Network Meeting is set up. This is an opportunity for all involved to state what they are able to contribute to the care plans . This is also, very

471

importantly, an opportunity for the user to state their requirements and needs. Within this process there should be no assumptions applied about what a person should want; instead the opportunity is given to the user, within the forum of the Network Meetings (or outside of it given consideration and discussion of the user's capacities) and in subsequent Review Meetings to define the particular areas of the Care Plan. Inherent in the Team philosophy is the acceptance of the genuineness of the user's assertions in relation to their own needs and requirements. We aim to help the user to make choices and not determine what the choices should be. Having established at this stage the individual level of need and metered this against capacity to respond, a negotiated and agreed Care Plan is formulated. It is possible in the Network Meeting to establish such a Plan as all interested parties are present, thus minimising potential difficulties with availability of resources. Negotiations are overt and take place with the user present.

Care Management requires clear monitoring, and this is the role of the Care Manager and Team. It is important that the Care Manager remain abreast of the current situation in relation to a particular client between Reviews, and one means of doing this is through open channels of communication within the Team. Obviously, the main point of contact between the Community Support Team and client is the worker, and the worker's observations in relation to the Care Plan are formally canvassed weekly. Further to this, informal discussion is actively encouraged. Good communication and access to information is also enhanced through the use of standardised files. Team work is highly prized and a good deal of time and effort is contributed by all in promoting this. Communication between user and professionals is also promoted through an open access to information policy. All Care Plans, Reviews and worker summaries are given to the user to guarantee openness. This, it is felt, promotes trust, and this we contend is inherently good practice. This view has been borne out by clients in the recent Review of the Team's work. (Murray, C.T., 1992).

The work is regularly reviewed (on a 4-6 weekly basis) and at this stage all involved in the Network Meeting are again invited to take part in this process. Needs are re-considered and the service establishes those things which the client requires and are able to be addressed, hence the service continues in a clear and planned way. Social Services Inspectorate states that, '....Care Management and Assessment constitute the core business of arranging care which underpins all other elements of Community Care'. Department of Health Social Services Inspectorate, 1991).

This is an inherent part of the Team's philosophy and is thus the basis of our work.

472

As stated above, Networks provide a substantial part of the Community Support Team's method of working and these, in essence, have three main functions:

(i) The networks provide links with services, i.e. the co-ordination of the work of social workers, health professionals and all others involved.

(ii) The formalised network provides contacts with the individual's primary network. This includes family and friends who might be perceived as being close.

(iii) Networks finally provide links with activities. That is, being able to discern an interest with a client and be able to go on to pursue this, for example through the inclusion of a member of a local church group if this is an area identified as being of interest by the user.

The aim of this as well as enabling people to be more proactive in the formulation of Care Plans and giving choices in respect of any changes made, is to empower the user and to give the opportunity to contribute freely. Further aims are that the use of networks can allow people to experience and become increasingly involved in the community, and offering them the chance to become more and more involved in meaningful activities, as defined by themselves. This might include the broad area of occupation. The network by virtue of its diversity is able to provide a range of supports and specialist knowledge with a view to increasing personal effectiveness. The network is also designed to promote a positive image and encourage respect as a valued individual. A wealth of research has suggested that the client group with which we work is often living within social networks smaller than that of the majority, and kin dominated. The establishment and maintenance of new networks (or simply more extensive networks) at the onset of the Community Support Team's work, perhaps through the information gathered from other professionals or the use of network maps, can increase the size and function of an individual's social networks. This will sponsor increasing capacities, limit isolation and create the necessary changes.

Obviously the degree of change must be monitored, and as I have stated above the workers involved have a constant role in this process. The other fundamental measure applied by the Community Support Team is that of Quality of Life. (Oliver, J., 1991) It is cited in 'Caring for People' that social care,

'....will improve the Quality of Life enjoyed by a person with social care needs.' (DHSS, 1989)

This must, therefore, constitute a principal outcome measure. It is further concluded by the Government that where the new service is effectively implemented,

'....the new style of service will offer a much higher Quality of Life for people with mental illness and a service more appreciated by their families, than is possible in a traditional and often remote mental hospital.' (DHSS, 1989)

This basic instrument, the Quality of Life measure, in the case of the Community Support Team was developed by the Manchester University Mental Health Research Unit, and is used in the case of all clients close to the beginning of our work and thereafter, at six monthly intervals. The schedule covers: general well-being, work/education, leisure/participation, religion, finance, living situation, legal/safety, family relationships, social relations, health, self concept and interviewers views. It also allows the user's subjective view through the use of Cantrill's Ladder. (Oliver, J., 1991) This provides the Team with both a comparative measuring tool and a care planning instrument. Success or failure of intervention can be measured in a quantifiable way and outcomes become objective.

The facets of the Community Support Team's philosophy are not home grown and clearly a number of ideas have been collected in order to create a coherent whole. It is this coherent whole which allows a quantifiable valued service to be given, and the constant monitoring process and existence of systems which allow for continued success. It is the contention of the Community Support Team that the collection of knowledge applied to our work is, by virtue of the way methodology relates to philosophy, innovative. Moreover, the acceptance of the Team of new knowledge and practices allows for innovation to be an on-going process. The Team is presently involved in establishing a volunteer/befriending service which, it is felt, can further enhance all aspects of our work.

Quality Assurance

As already mentioned the Community Support Team is a new and innovative service and it has, by virtue of this, been possible to incorporate some of the more recent philosophies and practices which are being introduced as a consequence of the Care in the Community legislation. One of the major components of this approach is the integration of the system of managing the quality of the service provided to the client group. Quality Assurance is an integral part of the work and the Team has made application for BS 5750 accreditation. (BSI., 1987) This measure of quality assurance is being increasingly adopted within social care agencies. Within the personal social services at least one establishment has successfully applied for this standard. (Strong. S., 1991)

Quality Assurance is an effective way of managing many of the requirements of the Care in the Community legislation, including definition of standards, monitoring, reviewing, evaluation, increased service user involvement, involvement of inspection unit, team work enhancement, increasing good communication, managing recording, participation of all parties, consistency and clarity of purpose. The aim is to develop a framework of management within which quality is likely to remain consistent.

According to the British Standards Institute, Quality Assurance is setting a specification for the service, planning for its achievement, monitoring and reviewing of performance, remedial action and improvement, and the focus is on preventing problems and not correcting errors afterwards. All of those planned and systematic actions are necessary to provide adequate confidence that a product or service has satisfied given requirements. This involves service user consultation, planning, training, communication, management direction and service delivery. The British Standard also states that it is the responsibility of each organisation to understand principles of BS 5750 and adapt its operation to provide assurance that all factors affecting quality have been properly considered and dealt with. Unless a Quality System is rigorously defined and documented, it cannot be consistently effective, nor can it benefit from the analysis of results.

It is clear that a Quality Assurance system in operation should guarantee that every client has a service appropriate to their needs, at a standard that any other client could expect from the same service. In order to translate this into a helping organisation, it is important to establish the following procedures:-

Being clear about the real value of the organisation (for example the principles specified in a Community Care Plan)

> Firming up on statements about mission statement, philosophy and purpose
> Developing trained management, able to inspire and motivate workforce
> Restructuring workforce into teams

> Delegating responsibility as far down the line as possible
> Organising Performance Indicators that measure the achievements of individuals, teams and sections
> Reviewing the Quality System
> Assessing the result of internal quality audit
> Reviewing and taking corrective action

A system for monitoring records and for monitoring success or failure (Choppin, J., 1991)

These processes, if followed, should assure a quality of service to clients. Some other commentators have included the following procedures, again to ensure Quality Assurance:-

Good communication

Maintaining credibility as Service Providers by allowing full participation of all parties in developing clear policies with clear and concise procedures, so that consistent quality can be maintained.

Present and promote the service

Maintain staff morale through team work, regular meetings, recognising and sharing achievements, turning weaknesses into strengths through training, involvement, supervision and coaching

Maintain a consistent clarity of purpose

Ways of measuring quality of the service

Free up resources for in-house training

Appropriate training for all to pick up attitudes, values and standards and core performance criteria (Emery, D. J., 1992)

These are some of the more formal procedures required for the implementation of a Quality Assurance system. In terms of a very practical application it is important that any Quality Assurance system has a mission statement for the organisation and that service requirements are described along with success criteria. A process for achieving the requirements should be stated clearly, and there needs to be a system for monitoring and recording success or failure. It is essential to have an internal and external auditing process and there needs to be a means for corrective action. There also needs to be a method of reviewing the system.

It is evident from some of the considerations above that there are very many ways to both describe the components of Quality Assurance, as well as ways of implementing the same systems. So it is the responsibility of each organisation to understand the principles of Quality Assurance and adapt its operation. It is important that all factors affecting quality have been properly considered and dealt with, and unless a quality system is rigorously defined and documented, it cannot be consistently effective, nor can it benefit from the analysis of results. It is the belief within the Community Support Team that a Quality Assurance process has been established and has been maintained, and that all clients receive a service which maintains a consistent quality. However, there are occasions when other service providers make it difficult to maintain a Quality Assurance and this is a problem which has to be addressed continually in the most appropriate manner. The remainder of this Paper describes the way the Community Support Team operates a Quality Assurance system within the frameworks mentioned above.

The Team has a very clear mission statement based on the Specific Grant for Mental Illness,

'....to contribute to the health and social care needs of people whose mental illness is so severe that they have been accepted for treatment by the specialist psychiatric services (i.e. those covered by the care programme approach.)' (Department of Health, 1991)

Service requirements with success criteria are defined within the performance outcomes and key tasks listed at the beginning of the Paper were agreed within the District Advisory Committee for Social Services. The process for achieving requirements is contained mainly within the Assessment and Care Management process, as identified within the Care in the Community legislation. This process begins with an informal enquiry to the Team followed by a screening process for every client. The aim of this is to identify the client as someone who is suitable to receive community support. A pro-forma is used which encapsulates the key tasks and performance outcomes identified at the start of the project. This prevents arbitrary decisions being made about eligibility for service. Assessment continues and information including a Social History and Psychiatric History, is sought in order to monitor and evaluate performance criteria. At this stage a check is made to ensure that client need is within the two highest priority bands identified within the Cheshire Social Services group. These include:-

1. Rapid and sudden deterioration of mental health
2. Significant/gradual deterioration

Following the Screening Meeting either further information is requested or a Network Meeting is requested of the referrer, who would normally become the Key Worker. The client is asked about their preference for both numbers and place of the Network Meeting. At this Meeting, the Care Plan is discussed, and one of the two Community Support Team Care Managers will take responsibility to both manage that Meeting and administer the Care Plan, a copy of which is sent to all involved, including the client. The Care Plan will include specific short term intervention goals, as well as ways of measuring outcome.

Following the implementation of the Care Plan, four to six-weekly review meetings take place, again including the client. The aim is to review the previous four to six weeks' care and to make new aims, or to continue existing aims until the next review meeting. Copies of documentation are provided to the client and other workers and Service Providers. In clerical terms, the Team uses a software system developed within Cheshire for Care Management, which allows fairly easy administration of the Care Plan, both in narrative form and in terms of a weekly Service Provider chart. It is also possible to manage budgetary control within this system.

The Assessment and Care Management system also includes systems for monitoring and recording success or failure. As soon as is practicable the support workers will go through the Quality of Life measure with clients. (Oliver, J., 1991) This has shown to be a reasonable measure of the clients' own perception of their quality of life, and is used on a 'one-off' basis to enhance the Care Plan process. It is also used on a six-monthly basis to allow some comparison of change, or no change, in the clients' Quality of Life. This information is also shared with the client. The fact that the Care Plan and the workers' report sheets are given to the clients, allows them and the Team Supervisor to monitor that the actual work undertaken fits into the Care Plan. The information required for the Performance Outcomes is put into a software package so that changes in pattern of care including hospital admission, crisis referrals, before and after referral to the Team, can be monitored. This allows us to take correcting action if necessary. The regular contact which the Team have with clients can be two or three times a day, seven days a week on occasions, and allows changes in the clients' well-being, symptoms and quality of life to be noted, so that if any action needs to be taken to either prevent an admission or plan an admission, this can be done effectively and quickly. A further system for monitoring is a fortnightly Case Discussion where the Team as a whole will go through the work with clients, and talk about what goes well and what needs to change. Supervision also provides another system for monitoring the work with the clients.

Success or failure is recorded in a variety of ways. Regular Reports to the District Advisory Committee detail progress in relation to the previously determined performance outcomes. Repetition of the Quality of Life measures (Oliver, J., 1991) at regular intervals gives a visual and statistical indication of change. Workers' recordings giving summaries of interventions and Care Plans are also methods of recording success or failure. The Team has been recently involved in auditing and evaluating their work. This has taken the form of a Review process which will become an annual event in the Team, although this does not exclude the day-to-day monitoring as mentioned above. The intention is that auditing, monitoring and evaluation become part of the infrastructure of the Team. The Review includes the use of a General Satisfaction Questionnaire completed with clients, by a colleague from another team. A General Satisfaction Questionnaire was sent to professionals who have made referrals to the Team. A Review Day was set aside for the workers in the Team to sit down and formally discuss what it does well and what needs to change, making use of the information from the client and professionals' General Satisfaction Questionnaire. That process has recently been completed and a report will follow giving background to the Team and providing review information, as well as action plans for change. The information will again be provided to clients, (with guidance if necessary) and to other professionals, and any major changes that need to be made will be communicated to all the relevant people.

At the present time our system for monitoring records within the Team is the responsibility of the Team Leader. The Team Leader monitors client Report Sheets and other information in the file and the monitoring of Care Plans is shared between the two Care Managers. The Team Secretary monitors the records which are kept on the computer, but these are also checked by clients and other professionals who receive copies, and again monitored by the Care Managers. It is also hoped that the process of application for BS 5750 will enhance the monitoring of records. A recent request has been made to an Independent Consultant to review our methodology and systems.

As an on-going process staff development and training provides a basis for harnessing skills and unlocking talents. We are able to meet some of those needs within the Team and by bringing other people in to provide training. Providing extra responsibility, increasing co-operation, communication and participation within the Team and, as the Team develops, to bring clients more and more into that participatory process, has an impact on aspects of Quality Assurance. The support workers are enrolled within the National Vocational Qualification scheme which enables them to demonstrate competencies in relation to key tasks and this is significant in the concept of Quality Assurance.

One of the overall philosophies of the Team that ensures the whole process of Quality Assurance, is open communication and information exchange. There is no information kept within the office that is not available to anyone else, and information kept in the file, with the exception of third party information, is made available and provided to the client with explanation if necessary.

As already mentioned, the Review system is something which is incorporated into the monitoring and evaluation process. It is clear at the moment that having set a Team up from new has made it easier to incorporate a monitoring, evaluating and review culture. It is evident from the feedback from Team members, that they have taken this on with relish. Team members are clear about what they are doing, how they are meant to do it, what success and failure means and how to measure this. Quality Assurance is now an integral part of the work of the Community Support Team. The feedback from clients and Team members and professionals from the first Review has been positive. There are few areas that need to be corrected, and these are being addressed at the present time. The system allows for open communication, exchange of information and clarity of purpose.

Acknowledgements

Thank you to all of the Community Support Team workers without whom the excellence of practice shown in this paper would not have been possible. The commitment of the team workers to implementing Quality Assurance and Innovative practice has been very high.

Debby McGuinness, Support Worker

Anne Neve, Support Worker

Ann Harrison, Support Worker

Christina Swindells, Support Worker

Sharon Beesley, Team Secretary. (especially for typing this paper)

Reference

BSI., (1987). BS 5750/150 900:1987 A positive contribution to better business.

Choppin, J. (1991, June). Forward with a fighting retreat. *Industrial Management*.

Department of Health, (1991, November). Specific Grant for the Development of social care services for people with a Mental Illness. *Local Authority Circular LAC (91) 19*.

Department of Health and Social Services Inspectorate (1991). Practitioners Guide 5.

DHSS (1989). Caring for People, 10-55

Emery, D. J. (1992, January 31). Quality Management report on workshop. *Cheshire County Council, Macclesfield District*.

Murray, C.T. (1992). Community support team review. *Cheshire County Council, Macclesfield District*. (unpublished)

Oliver, J. (1991). The Social Care Directive: Development of a quality of life profile for use in community services for the mentally ill. *Social Work and Social Science Review*. 3 (1)

Strong, S. (1991, November 1). Home with an official seal of approval. *Care Weekly*, 10.

38 The Caring Together Scheme

M. Murray

'Ageing is associated with health unless there is a sickness or disability. Some ill health and disability can be prevented. When this is not possible, the majority of problems are dealt with through self-care, with support from relatives or friends. When these support systems fail, proper diagnosis and treatment may be required.

The main focus of health promotion in old age rests, therefore, with individuals within their own environment, with health professionals playing a vital role in transferring knowledge and adopting skills so as to enhance the possibility of meaningful, autonomous and satisfying lives for elderly people within the communities.'

Taken from the Preface of:
'Promoting Health Among Elderly People'
King Edward's Hospital Fund for London 1988

Introduction

Mental health problems of the elderly are enormously diverse. Not only are problems extremely varied, but so are the settings in which they occur, the range of professionals who may help the elderly cope and finally the kinds of services that can be provided to respond to these diverse needs. Prevention of mental illness and promotion of mental health in the elderly requires innovative approaches. In contrast to younger people for whom prevention efforts are initiated before the expression of the disease, prevention and promotional activities for the elderly tend to be directed at persons who have one or more chronic disease conditions and may be at risk of acute illness.[1] Consequently, health promotion initiatives for the elderly need to be aimed at delaying further decline and/or motivating the person rather than attempting to cure, totally reverse, or completely prevent disease conditions.

Although inextricably linked with physical health problems, mental health problems are a particular concern because of the high risk situation of the elderly.[2] Older persons find themselves having to make major decisions in later life as a result of changes in role status, financial difficulties, new leisure life-styles, changes in relationships, loss of loved ones, experiences of loneliness and isolation and alterations in health and physical appearance.[3] However, specific problems of later life can be alleviated or reduced through particular interventions and service delivery systems.[4] For example, the development and implementation of programmes that address specific problems can reduce the elderly person's risk of poor health. Reducing stress can reduce the risk of poor health of the individual. Programmes of this type are designed to try to improve the health and well-being of both the individual and group by enhancing the skill, knowledge and support required to increase positive changes in lifestyles. Such an approach, holistic in nature, embraces both the whole person and the environmental systems that influence the life of the individual and group.[5]

For such schemes to be successful there is the need for the elderly person to have both knowledge of and access to the programmes. Although many facilities now exist for the care of the elderly it is without question that in numerous cases the older person has little knowledge of and/or makes little use of these facilities. Many schemes are in operation, including those provided by statutory and voluntary agencies but are perhaps not fully co-ordinated or well publicised. The result is that a number of elderly people remain 'at risk'. Eventually the elderly person may require premature institutional care when earlier intervention and support would allow many to live at home for even longer periods of their life.[6]

It is well established by statistics and clinical experience that the elderly do in fact under-utilise mental health services. T. E. Bryant noted that older adults remain under-represented in both public and private practice[7] while Eisdorfer has estimated that as many as eighty per cent of the elderly who have mental health problems receive no service at all from mental health professionals.[8]

However, the needs of the elderly are generally acknowledged to be at least as great as those of other adult age groups and the fact that therapeutic interventions are useful with the elderly is well established clinically, if not accepted popularly.[9]

Even if we accept

'The older among us certainly have a right to enjoy the best possible health and hence the highest quality of life for all the years they live. Further, older people in optimum health, living and working, participating in all aspects of community life constitute a national resource we can ill afford to waste. Programmes and policies which operate to enhance the health and well-being of older persons enhance the health of the nation'[10]

elderly people will ultimately benefit only if they have:

    i) a knowledge of existing services

    ii) adequate services to meet their needs, and

    iii) access to service(s) appropriate to their needs.

Within Mid Staffordshire, prior to the introduction of the Caring Together Scheme, a number of developments had taken place to try and enhance the level of service provided for the elderly mentally ill. Following the agreement of the Joint Strategy[11] a specialist team of Community Psychiatric Nurses was appointed to care specifically for the elderly mentally ill, more day places and hospital beds were provided and transport facilities were improved to enable both in-patient and day patients to have improved access to health services and recreational facilities.

However, in discussions between representatives from the Mental Health Unit and other agencies (both statutory and voluntary) a number of deficiencies in service provision were identified. These included:

* lack of public education regarding dementia and mental illness in general;
* lack of assistance in emergency situations;
* lack of knowledge about available facilities, such as the incontinence laundry service and respite care beds;
* problems in identifying elderly people at risk and in bringing them into the area of care provision;
* the need for assessment by a specialist team in the early stages of dementia and the need for an holistic approach rather than the assessment of a person as to his or her suitability for a specific facility;
* the need to develop community networks to replace the reducing levels of social support from family and friends;

* lack of co-ordination between service providers;
* lack of evaluation of the professionals and care staff working in this area of care.

In recognising the above needs, consideration had also to be given to the then prevailing financial situation and the need to ensure effective use of resources. Furthermore, analysis of the above deficiencies also highlighted that it may have been possible to overcome a number of problem areas by better use of existing resources, i.e. improvements in co-ordination and accessibility of service.

Following discussions it was agreed that a pilot project would be established to

"identify whether there were substantial numbers of elderly people who required assistance and were not in receipt of these required service(s) and if so were there sufficient existing services to meet these needs'.[12]

The area chosen for the piloting of this was in an urban area with limited mental health service resources. The pilot scheme was subsequently implemented on a permanent basis and now operates as:

The Caring Together Scheme

The main focus of the Caring Together Scheme is to help the elderly at risk to make better use of existing resources. Although many resources do exist to provide help to the elderly, more effective use of these resources will lead to benefits for the elderly people. Consequently, the Caring Together Scheme co-ordinates the efforts of many different groups to improve services for the elderly.

Objectives

    i) Co-ordinate (a) a community based care system and (b) a long-term care system for the elderly.

    ii) Prevent premature institutional placement of the elderly.

    iii) Maintain older persons in their own homes when this meets the wishes/needs of the elderly person and the carers of the elderly person.

Strategic aims

    i) To marshall and direct long-term care resources in the community

    ii) To increase access to a wider range of services than is currently available.

    iii) To match service use to the identified needs of the elderly persons.

iv) To stimulate the development of needed in-home and community services.

v) To reduce the need for costly medical and institutional long-term care services.

vi) To promote efficiency and quality in community long-term care services.

vii) To promote reasonable division of labour among informal support systems (including families, neighbours and friends) privately financed services and publicly financed care.

ix) To maintain or enhance outcomes for the elderly person including physical and mental functioning and quality of life.

x) To co-ordinate services and promote quality standards in institutions responsible for the provision of long-term care.

Programmes

Interventions used in this project to arrange and co-ordinate services include the following:

i) Outreach to identify and attract the target population.

ii) Screening to determine whether the older person is part of the targeted population.

iii) Comprehensive assessment to determine individual problems, resources available and service needs.

iv) Care planning to specify the types of care to meet the need of the individual elderly person.

v) Service arrangements to implement the care plan through both formal and informal providers. vi) Monitoring to ensure that services are provided as planned and modified as necessary.

vii) Reassessment of care plans in response to changing needs.

There are four main elements of the scheme:-

A) the Gatekeepers approach

B) Assessment Evaluation Unit

C) the Community Network, and

D) Mental Health Promotion

A) The Gatekeepers approach:

is based upon the simple consideration that the best people to identify the elderly at risk are those who go into elderly people's homes, e.g. gas meter readers, insurance collectors, police, etc. However, although those at risk may be identified, notification to appropriate agencies is often not forthcoming because the identifier may not be aware of who is best to help and/or they may fear that action taken by themselves could lead to a deeper commitment.

The Gatekeepers approach seeks to avoid the above problems by adopting the following approaches:

1) The appointment of two experienced and trained personnel, i.e. liaison officers. Of the two liaison officers appointed, one had experience from a medical background and in particular dealing with elderly people with dementia. The second liaison officer was from a professional background in social services.

In additional to the above professional staff, there is secretarial support. The tasks to be carried out by the liaison officers includes:

   i) The management of a centre from which they themselves work and operate a telephone help-line. Furthermore the centre provides advice and resource material for use by carers, voluntary groups, etc.

   ii) Identifying gatekeepers by liaising with such groups as the Gas Board, Police, etc.

   iii) Arranging the training of gatekeepers

   iv) Publicising the service.

   v) Developing and maintaining a directory of available services. (This involves contacting all services who work with the elderly)

2) The programme operates by allowing any gatekeeper who feels that an elderly person is at risk to contact a liaison officer. The involvement of the gatekeeper then ceases although they may wish to be kept informed of the outcome and in certain cases become involved in the care of the elderly person.

3) Liaison officers visit the elderly person and after assessing the situation contact the appropriate agencies.

It is essential that the liaison officers have the experience and training which enables them to communicate with elderly persons who may be resentful or frightened of other people entering their homes.

(In all cases the general medical practitioner of the elderly person at risk is informed. This ensures that appropriate medical assessment and treatment becomes available)

4) After onward referral to the most appropriate agencies the liaison

officer reviews the care programme of the individual elderly person concerned and the liaison officer maintains an 'at risk' register.

In addition to the above the liaison officer is intimately concerned with a Community Network.

B) The assessment evaluation unit:

consists of the following; Psychogeriatrician, Community Psychiatric Nurse and a Social Worker.

Referrals are made on an open basis but it is the responsibility of the Assessment Team to contact the appropriate general practitioner to ensure the general practitioner institutes the required referral and medical history, etc.

Whenever possible the assessment is carried out in the home of the elderly person concerned but it is necessary on occasions for the elderly person to attend hospital where there are in-patient and out-patient facilities so that further medical examination/tests can be performed.

It is the responsibility of the assessment team to arrange further treatment programmes, obtain support, etc. and to ensure that the necessary monitoring and follow-up of the treatment/care programme is carried out.

C) The community network:

is designed to encourage the use of existing services for the elderly. These services may not be well known or co-ordinated and in certain localities elderly persons may not be aware of the services that can be used. Therefore on a neighbourhood or village basis the liaison officers contact a particular 'group leader'. This may be a local minister or doctor or leader of a voluntary service. Working through the neighbourhood leader, the liaison officer identifies all existing services for the elderly in that neighbourhood and arranges for 'group leaders' of these agencies to meet on a regular basis. In this way a community network of services can be promoted, organised, publicised and co-ordinated with support provided by the liaison officers.

An example of a promotional programme is to organise a neighbourhood care scheme whereby a neighbour would agree to keep a watchful eye on an elderly person living nearby and act as befriender.

In addition the liaison officers maintain a point of contact with the particular neighbourhood so that if any problems occur then those within the neighbourhood can have immediate access to the liaison officers.

The value of the scheme is that the liaison officer(s) can act as a facilitator in bringing together local groups who use existing local facilities for the benefit of the elderly population in that area. Often all that is needed within a community is an initial catalyst to help undoubtedly willing volunteers to pool their resources towards a common goal.

A further important feature of the neighbourhood Community Network is to compile an 'at risk' register outlined above for the elderly and this list will be maintained on a central data storage system held on a confidential basis by the liaison officers. In winter, for example, the elderly at risk will already be identified.

D) Mental health promotion:

In relation to promoting the well-being of the elderly, the liaison officers work in conjunction with other agencies (e.g.Mental Health Promotion Unit at the base hospital) to arrange education and training courses for the elderly, their carers and other professionals, arrange exhibitions, publicise local and national initiatives and assist local voluntary groups.

Summary

Although the schemes outlined are described on an individual basis, it must be appreciated that each is but a part of the whole in providing facilities to help the elderly have a fuller and more rewarding lifestyle. The Caring Together Scheme itself is but an initiative which contributes to the total service provided for elderly people.

Since the Caring Together Scheme was introduced further facilities and resources have been commissioned in the area covered by the Scheme. However, referrals by the Gatekeepers have continued to increase and further developments of the Scheme been implemented while it is also planned to commission the Scheme in other areas.

References

1. Filner, B. & Williams, T. (1981). Health Promotion for the elderly. In A. Somers, & D. Fabian, (Eds.), *The Geriatric Imperatives* (pp187-204). New York: Appleton Century-Crofts.

2. Brusse, E. E. & Blazer, D. G. (1980). *Handbook of geriatric psychiatry*. New York: Jan Nostrand Reinhold.

3. Davis, J. (1983 Spring). Mental well being of elders. Seeking positive solutions. *Generation 7*.

4. Birren, J. & Sloane, R. B. Prevention aspects of mental illness in later life. In J. Birren, & R. B. Sloane, (Eds.), *Handbook of mental health and ageing*. Prentice Hall: Englewood Cliffe N.J.

5. Wellness, & Dychtwald, K. (Ed.) (1983 Spring). Health promotion for elders. *Generation 7*.

6. M. Murray, (1988). Mental Health Promotion for Elderly People. King's Fund College Travelling Fellowship to USA.

7. Bryant, T. E. Report to the President from the President's Commission on Mental Health Washington D. C. Government Printing Office. Edited by Michael A. Amyer, & Margaret Gatz.

8. Eisdorfer, C. (1989). Evaluation of the quality of psychiatric care for the aged. *American Journal of Psychiatry*, **135**, 315-317.

9. Assessing a Mobile Outreach Team. Bob Knight. Mental Health & Ageing Programs and Evaluations Sage Publications Inc. 1993.

10. Fallcreek, S. & Mettler, M. (1982). *A healthy old age: A sourcebook for health promotion with older adults*. Seattle Centre for Social Work Research: University of Washington.

11. A Joint Strategy for the Development of Mental Health Services. Mental Health Unit of Mid Staffordshire Health Authority and Social Services Department of Staffordshire County Council. May 1989.

12. An Evaluation Study of the Caring Together Scheme: A unique initiative in preventative mental health for the Elderly. Funded by West Midlands Regional Health Services Research Committee 1990.

39 The promotion of mental health for black women users

Z. Nadirshaw

The paper is presented in two parts:
1. a) Highlighting issues within current mainstream psychiatric psychology services
   b) Presentation of psychological problems/distress
   c) Implicity Euro and ethnocentric assumptions underlying cur rent psychiatric and related mental health services (Classification, Diagnosis etc.) without taking into account other world views of psychology and psychiatry.
   d) Racist Assessment Base
   e) Challenging ideology and philosophy of Normalization (Wolfensberger) with service planning, service delivery.

2. Looking at and identifying essential features of good practice for mental health services for black women.
   a) Need to redefine mental health concept in keeping with African and Asian psychiatry and psychology.
   b) Alternatives to current traditional medical (drug) treatments to be provided within mainstream services.
   c) Development of empowerment and consciousness-raising strat egies for black women.
   d) Preparing guidelines on sexual and physical abuse for black women in hospitals as well as on black women's rights.

Issues to be addressed

1. Clarification of term black minority ethnic women

We are addressing problems relating to women of African and Asian (including SE Asia descent).

2. Presentation of psychological and other mental health problems ascribed to:

   (a) **The raging hormone theory** which emphasizes connection between the womb and the brain and women's constitutional vulnerability to it. Exacerbated for black women, who are also told that their 'genes' are at fault.

   (b) **Black women as mothers**. Combination of reality of motherhood (combined effects of racism, poverty, tiredness, isolation, loss of personal and racial identity) with myth of superwoman/madonna resulting in later depression and stress. Statutory organizations with their controlling nature see black women as unfit to be looking after children and therefore place children in care.

   (c) **Conditioned response of black women blaming themselves** for the oppression. Directing guilt and blame towards themselves. Seeing themselves as 'sick'. Internalized oppression/repression.

   (d) **Position of black women** as an oppressed group in society, being denied proper resources and facilities, and access to money and employment. Personalized and institutionalized oppression leading to powerlessness and lack of control over one's life.

   (e) **Triple discrimination** of race (colour), ageism and sexism. Being defined as redundant and useless. Being Black seen as a 'deviancy'. Caught in a circle of viciousness-> powerlessness -> hopelessness -> lack of worth.

   (f) Black women being traditionally **defined through their relationships** rather than through their own worth and playing their own role. Difficulties in relationships ascribed to them, causing them to question their role.

   (g) **Archetype of good/bad women**. The madonna/whore dichotomy. Continues to have a negative effect on black women's identity.

3. Medicalization of black women's distressed experiences.

Based on several factors:

   (a) 'Pathology' ascribed in black women rather than the system which create/produces it. Assumptions made about this pathology are then perpetuated within the black woman and her family.

(NB White women and their families are not a homogenous group. Why should such presumptions be made about black people?)

(b) **Ethno and Eurocentric assumption** that Western modes of thought and ways of analysing people, minds and cultures are superior to modes and ways that are not derived from the West. These assumptions underlie the mental health services guiding mental health practices which are then undertaken in a similar manner. Distress and other symptoms being 'culture bound', with illness/health being defined and classified within the main Western psychiatric classification system, no acknowledgement of other world views, e.g., religious and spiritual aspects, are integrated with medicine and psychiatry.

Contemporary psychiatry and psychology based on these assumptions and an implied and implicit suggestion that they are superior models to the so-called underdeveloped cultures of Africa and Asia.

(c) **Racist Assessment Base**: wherein the methods used and the actual process of assessment disadvantages black women. Need to question its objectivity and ask 'Who benefits from current assessment? Whose needs are really being met? Who assesses the assessor?'

Conflict exists between black women's **real** needs for mental health services versus needs as assessed and prescribed by the professionals and the system.

(d) **Imbalance of power and control.** Solely in hands of the controlling aspects of white (majority) organizations and services. (Psychiatrists, GPs, Psychologists and Social Workers.) Powerful professionals exerting further control leading to self-doubt, learned helplessness and dependence on statutory organizations and services.

(e) **Challenging normality base** of 'Normalization' philosophy and ideology (Wolfensberger). What is not considered near to mainstream norm and values is seen as 'different' with a negative value attached to the 'differentness'. Seen as 'deviant', 'odd', 'undesirable' (e.g. skin colour), resulting in negative images, prejudiced beliefs and stereotyped views (e.g. Asians are psychologically more robust, they care for their own, don't suffer mental health problems as they somatize it, etc, etc.)

Black women need to say they are different and that positive value is attached to that 'differentness'.

(f) **'Guinea-pigging' experimentation** done on black women's mental health (more on Afro-Caribbean than Asian women). Images of black women to be experimented on Mental Health Service is not about healing, but social and medical control. Black women continue to see themselves as ill as a consequence, rather than as women first.

(g) **Over-subscription to Medical Treatment** Drugs rather than the use of other 'softer' treatment, e.g. psychotherapy, counselling, etc. Black women not seen or thought sufficiently intelligent or articulate to respond to such approaches!

(h) **Effects of medication** Besides the more obvious and overt ones, lack of knowledge about effect on hair and skin care and weight gain with black women leading to lowered self-esteem.

4. *Black professional women*

Conflicts of role and loyalties on part of **black women service providers**. They practice within mainstream psychiatric and mental health services. This conflicts with loyalty to black women service users. Problem further reinforced by professional black women staff being undermined and not valued. How to get white professionals to accept black women as equal colleagues representing customers/clients is a particular problem. Burn out problems leading to demoralization and working in a crisis-oriented manner all the time becomes the issue.

5. *Physical violence and abuse*

Continued abuse and violation of black women in hospital settings leading to further stress and distress.

Recommendations for good practices

1) Style of service
2) Style of working
3) Training
4) Support for Black women as mental health workers

1) Style of service

the key issues are:

a) **Alternatives to medical treatment**. This to be offered within mainstream services e.g. herbalists, acupuncture, healers, etc. To be offered in a responsible and flexible manner.

b) **Open referral system**: with self referral in particular.

c) **Location of service**: in comfortable, non-stigmatizing, localized settings, e.g. health centres/community centres.

d) **Flexibility of service** so that women can be seen out of hours or at home as necessary. Provision of child care facilities should also be made.

e) **Access to written information:** copies of reports or letters sent to others should be accessed by the woman user.

f) **A 'Sensitive' service** which provides services that are specific to a woman's ethnic background, age or sexual orientation wherever possible; if this is not possible then it should be identified as a deficiency within the services. Services should establish policies which adhere to strict guidelines and code of conduct (e.g. guidelines on sexual and physical abuse of black women in special and ordinary psychiatric hospitals/institutions).

g) **Accountability to service user:** through systems or membership of management groups who plan and dictate policies.

2) *Style of working*

the key issues are:

a) **Professional detachment** and to avoid its negative effects. Breaking away from the more 'distancing' professional role as also from the relatively unfamiliar and foreboding context of 'patient' and 'therapist' roles or expert and recipient.

b) **Demedicalizing 'the problem'** and locating it within the social context and sources of oppression in black women's lives. Need to make these links explicit at both individual and social level.

c) **Empowerment** of black women. To understand and learn about power and control, to challenge the notion of the professional being the expert, and to promote styles of working which minimize powerlessness and dependency. Development of consciousness.

d) **Skills development** in developing assertive power, learning to say 'No', child management work, work related skills, confidence building in the strength and knowledge about resourcefulness of black women, rights, stress and stress management, etc.

e) **Clear acknowledgement of different style of working and thinking.** Taking an ecological perspective to the 'problem', relating to women as women - both personal and in terms of approach to working with women. Sensitive practices which validate reality of black women's lives in multi-racial Britain should be developed, (e.g. women's groups, users groups, self-help or therapy

497

groups), or by facilitating access to groups and activities provided by and for women by voluntary organizations in the community.

3) Training

a) **Redefining mental health concepts**. Training should be reviewed from a frame of reference which is not derived from Western cultures alone. Definitions of mental health, mental illness, disease are different and different cultures (e.g. mind-body split, effects of religious and spiritual influences within medicine, etc). Black women should not be 'compartmentalized' within an organic/biological model. Need to be seen as a 'whole'. Person first, mental health second.

b) **Developing knowledge and awareness of 'black' issues within mainstream psychiatry, psychology, etc.** avoiding assumptions about ethnocentricism, i.e. things developed within Western culture for Westerners being applied to non-western cultures without much by way of adaptation to new and other cultures.

c) **Effect of personal and institutional racism**. To understand the negative effect of such practices resulting in very negative attitudes and belief systems and images about black women. To develop strategies which get rid of devaluing words like 'deviance', 'victim', 'sick', etc. Substitute words like growth, development, and empowerment. The importance of working in this way and raising the key issues for women regarding mental health services, i.e. stereotyping, oppression, psychiatric ideology, etc.

d) **Health Promotion campaigns** to be established targeting GPs as one of the main sources (GPs in the new world of purchaser-provider and fund holders, are the first port of call within mental health services). Police, legal and other statutory services also need to be targeted.

4) Support for black women as mental health workers

a) **Black women workers valued** Black women workers experience harassment and sexism in, as well as, out of the workplace, have conflicts between their roles in and out of the work. Problem is further reinforced by white professionals, including women not accepting them as equal colleagues. Burn-out problems, demoralization and segregation/marginalization are serious issues.

b) **Access to further training and career development**. Black women mental health workers do not receive recognition for their work at all levels within the organisation. The knowledge that they do not have equal access to opportunities for further training or career/ personal development is well documented. Management recognition and support, systems for reviewing personal development, effective policies on sexual harassment at work need to be available to black women staff.

40 Effects of father-loss upon psychological well-being and academic performance of Iranian secondary school students

B. Najarian

Abstract

This study was aimed at investigating the effects of father-loss upon academic performance and psychological well-being of Iranian students who had lost their fathers during the 8-year Iraq-Iran war. Subjects were 239 (133 male and 106 female) third-year students studying at four different secondary schools in Ahwaz, Iran. The sample consisted of 110 students belonging to the martyr families (the experimental group) and 129 students from the non-martyr families (the control group). The Children Depression Scale (CDS - Tisher and Lang, 1978), recently revised and standardized for the Iranian population (Golzari, 1991), was used to assess subjects' depression and self-esteem, while grade point averages (GPAs) for the first and second years at secondary school were used as indices of academic performance. Results showed that while GPA scores were unrelated to any of the CDS subscales, the experimental group's GPAs were significantly lower than those for the control group. The duration of father-absence (DUR) was also unrelated to GPA scores. But DUR did show significant negative associations with the Affective Response, Sickness/Death, Social Problems, Miscellaneous Depression, Depression, and Lack of Self-Esteem subscales of the CDS. Finally, no significant differences were found between the experimental and control groups regarding their scores on Lack of Self-Esteem, Pleasure, Guilt, Miscellaneous Depression and Miscellaneous Pleasure subscales, but the experimental group did score significantly higher than the control group on the Affective Response, Sickness/ Death, and Social Problems subscales.

Introduction

An intact nuclear family is thought to contribute significantly to the normal development of children's psychological functioning and academic achievement (Kelly & Wallerstein, 1980; Atkinson & Ogston, 1974), and in general the literature suggest that father-loss leads to a higher incidence of psychological problems, particularly depression and scholastic disruption in children (Roy & Fuqua, 1983; Shinn, 1978). However, nearly half of all children may experience the absence of a parent, mostly absence of the father (Bane, 1976). It is claimed that one-fifth of all children under 18 live in homes where the father is absent (Goldstein, 1983), and in the USA, at least 20 million children live in single-parent families (Roy & Fuqua, 1983).

In comparison to the children from intact families, children of single parents have been reported to exhibit lower self-esteem, lower tolerance for delay of gratification, lower social coping skills, and higher incidences of neurosis and suicide (Fry & Scher, 1984; Roy & Fuqua, 1983). Lancaster and Richmond (1982) have shown that death of the father causes more disruptions in children's life than divorce. They also claim that following father-loss, the child's locus of control tends to shift to an external orientation. The literature suggests that children (in particular, boys) from father-absent homes exhibit more depression (Roy & Fuqua, 1983), and experience more difficulty in moral development than children from intact families (see Hoffman, 1971). Depressed children in turn usually report a negative self-concept, poor concentration, loss of appetite, and a diminished interest in life (Brown, Andrews, Harris, et al., 1986; Beck, 1967), and children's affective problems may take the form of behavioural disorders, particularly a disruptive behaviour disorders, like conduct or oppositional-defiant disorders (Kaplan & Sadock, 1990; Quay & Routh, 1987).

Children's cognitive development may also be profoundly influenced by the experience of father-loss (Fowler & Richards, 1978; Parish & Copeland, 1977). Parish and Taylor (1979) reported that father-absent students show a number of educational problems, and Hetherington and Parkes (1975) claim that children who experience father-loss have more difficulty with their school work. Sutherland (1973) and Deutsch and Brown (1964) showed that father-absent students score significantly lower on intellectual tests than do those who are father-present, and Crescimbein (1965) found significantly lower scores on achievement tests among father-absent elementary school students than among children from intact families (also see Blanchard & Biller, 1971). The National Association of Elementary School Principals (NASEP) (1980) found that children from single-parent families were more likely to obtain D and F grades than A, B or C grades. Some studies have pointed to the lack of positive father-child interaction being associated both with children's general academic underachievement (Grunebaum, Hurwitz, Prentice & Sperry, 1962) and with psychological problems (Carlsmith, 1964).

In view of the fact that thousands of lives were lost during the eight-year Iraq-Iran war, and the finding that Iranian children have very strong emotional ties with their parents (Golzari, 1991), a growing concern for the academic achievement and normal development of psychological functioning of those Iranian children who have lost their fathers during the war (i.e., martyr students) has repeatedly been expressed. In an earlier study, Najarian, Liami, Shahedi et al. (1991) compared the scores of martyr and non-martyr high school students on the Beck Depression Inventory (BDI - Beck, 1967) and the Coopersmith Self-Esteem Scale (1967). These authors found no differences between groups on the two scales. However, the failure to support the predicted differences may well be attributable to psychometric problems, such as the clinical nature of the Beck scale (see also Burns, 1979). The present study was conducted to investigate the effects of father-loss upon secondary school students' psychological well-being and their academic performance, using a similar procedure to that employed by Najarian et al. However, in view of their findings, the Children Depression Scale (CDS - Tisher and Lang, 1978) was used instead of the earlier scales; the CDS includes subscales for both depression and self-esteem, and has a less clinical bias than the BDI (see Golzari, 1991).

Subjects

The sample consisted of 239 (133 male and 106 female) third-year secondary students studying at four different schools of Ahwaz, Iran. There are six secondary schools for martyr families at Ahwaz (known as Martyr or Shahed Schools), four of which were randomly selected for this study. At these schools, nearly half of the students come from the martyr families and the other half are regular students. There were 47 males and 63 females belonging to the martyr families (the experimental group) and 43 males and 86 females from the non-martyr families (the control group) in the sample. The mean ages of the experimental and control groups were 14.19 (sd=1.14) and 13.49 (sd=.67) years, respectively.

Dependent variables (the CDS and GPAs)

The CDS was originally constructed by Tisher and Lang (1978) and later revised in 1983). The revised version has been translated into a number of languages including Spanish, Italian, German and Japanese. It is claimed that even 11 year old children have no difficulty in completing the questionnaire (Golzari, 1991). Since its development, the CDS has been employed in a large number of studies (e.g., Kazdin, Esveldt-Dawson, Sherick, & Colbus, 1985; Kovacs, 1981).

The scale comprises 66 items, of which 18 are related to positive characteristics (e.g., pleasure) and 48 are concerned with depression and negative psychological aspects. Subjects are instructed to select one of the five choices available to them. These options are 'Absolutely incorrect' (1), 'Incorrect' (2), 'I do not know, I'm not sure' (3), 'Correct' (4) and 'Absolutely correct' (5). Each item is included in only one subscale. The eight Subscales of the CDS have been formed on the basis of theoretical grounds; CDS produces 11 scores for each subject, one for each of its eight subscales and three combined scores.

The CDS subscales are: Affective Response (AR- 8 items), Social Problems (SP- 8 items), Lack of Self-Esteem (SE- 8 items), Sickness/Death (SD- 7 items), Guilt (GL- 8 items), Pleasure PE- 8 items), Miscellaneous Depression (MD- 10 items), Miscellaneous Pleasure (MP- 9 items), TOTDEP (sum of all subscales but the latter two), TOTPE (sum of the PE and MP subscales), and DEPRES (the difference score between TOTDEP and TOTPE). The latter score has been suggested as the best index of depression.

The Farsi version of CDS has been standardized for the general population of Iran by Golzari (1991). The test-retest reliability of the scale, as assessed over a 6-week period, is .82. By using Cronbach's Alpha Test, its internal consistency is reported to be .96. The construct and concurrent validity of CDS have also been reported to be very satisfactory (see Golzari, 1991). In order to obtain an index reflecting students' academic performance, GPAs for the first and second years at secondary school were derived from each student's academic file.

Procedure

Researchers attended every third-year class of the four randomly selected Martyr Schools at Ahwaz, Iran, and administered the CDS. Subjects were told that the research project was concerned with the quality of teaching at Martyr schools, and the researchers did not give any detailed information about the objectives of the study nor about the CDS items.

Data analysis and results

A 2(Sex) X 2(Group) analysis of variance applied to the age of subjects indicated no significant difference between male and female subjects

504

(F=2.13; df[1, 237]; p=N.S.). However, the control group were found to be significantly older than the experimental group (F=37.1; df[1, 237]; p<.001). Golzari (1991) has shown that older children normally report more depression symptoms than younger ones, and ANCOVA tests, controlling for the age of subjects, were therefore used for the analysis of scores on the CDS subscales as well as the GPAs. An ANCOVA performed on GPAs showed that the experimental group's GPAs were significantly lower than the control group both for the first year (F=119.84; df[1,237]; p<.001) and the second year (F=127.14; df[1, 237]; p<.001). Furthermore, it was found that the female students' GPAs were significantly greater than the males: first year (F=19.27; df[1, 237]; p<.001), second year (F=21.58; df[1, 237]; p<.001). There were no significant 2-way interactions in these analyses. A series of Pearson correlation tests indicated no significant association between GPAs and any of the CDS subscales. Table 1 presents the mean and standard deviation for the age and GPAs of both groups.

Table 1
Mean and standard deviation of age and GPA's

Group	Sex	N	Age	1st Year GPA	2nd Year GPA
				Mean (sd)	
	Female	63	14.05	14.95	14.61
			(.98)	(2.05)	(1.95)
Martyr	Males	47	14.38	13.69	13.25
			(1.31)	(1.48)	1.47)
	Both	110	14.19	14.41	14.12
			(1.14)	(1.93)	(1.87)
	Female	43	13.47	17.80	17.57
			(.55)	(1.49)	(1.59)
Non- Martyr	Males	86	13.5	16.89	16.67
			(.73)	(1.70)	(1.94)
	Both	129	13.49	17.19	16.95
			(.67)	(1.68)	(1.87)

A series of ANCOVAs carried out on the CDS data indicated that the experimental group have scored significantly higher than the control group on AR (F=4.28; df[1, 217], p=.04), SD (F=12.59; df[1, 218]; p=.001), DEPRES (F=3.81; df[1, 145]; p=.05), SP (F=6.56; df[1, 219]; p=.01), and TOTDEP (F=4.7; df[1, 166]; p=.03). However, the two groups did not differ significantly from one another with regard to their scores on SE (F=2.3; df[1, 217]; p=.13), MP (F=1.74; df[1, 206]; p=.19), GL (F=.85; df[1, 219]; p=.36), PE (F=.12; df[1, 220]; p=.73), MD)F=3.12; df[1, 221]; p=.08), and TOTPE (F=.26; df[1, 193]; p=.61). The difference between the two

Table 2
Summary results of ANCOVA's performed on CDS

Dep Var.	Indep. Var.	Level	Mean	sd	df	F (p)
AR	Sex	Female	24.83	(7.95)	1, 217	14.82
		Male	20.49	(6.77)		(.001)
	Group	Martyr	24.44	(7.92)	1, 217	4.28
		Non-Martyr	20.64	(6.89)		(.04)
SD	Sex	Female	20.44	(6.11)	1, 218	2.71
		Male	18.56	(5.49)		(.1)
	Group	Martyr	21.36	(5.52)	1, 218	12.59
		Non-Martyr	17.67	(5.57)		(.001)
SE	Sex	Female	24.86	(7.13)	1, 217	.31
		Male	23.98	(6.55)		(.58)
	Group	Martyr	25.59	(6.88)	1, 217	2.3
		Non-Martyr	23.39	(6.62)		(.13)
MP	Sex	Female	36.42	(5.16)	1, 206	.01
		Male	36.14	(5.06)		(.91)
	Group	Martyr	36.51	(4.76)	1, 206	1.74
		Non-Martyr	36.08	(5.37)		(.19)
GL	Sex	Female	23.30	(5.89)	1, 219	1.88
		Male	24.19	(5.97)		(.17)
	Group	Martyr	24.40	(6.10)	1, 219	.85
		Non-Martyr	23.28	(5.78)		(.36)

Table 2
Continued

Dep Var.	Indep. Var.	Level	Mean	sd	df	F (p)
SP	Sex	Female	25.91	(8.06)	1, 219	5.45
		Male	22.86	(7.23)		(.02)
	Group	Martyr	26.58	(7.52)	1, 219	6.56
		Non-Martyr	22,16	(7.34)		(.01)
PE	Sex	Female	29.73	(4.47)	1, 220	4.40
		Male	28.38	(5.04)		(.04)
	Group	Martyr	28.71	(4.88)	1, 220	.12
		Non-Martyr	29.20	(4.80)		(.73)
MD	Sex	Female	33.03	(4.46)	1, 221	7.07
		Male	30.55	(5.49)		(.01)
	Group	Martyr	32.83	(5.73	1, 221	3.12
		Non-Martyr	30.56	(6.12)		(.08)
TOTDEP	Sex	Female	153.50	(38.18)	1, 166	1.99
		Male	143.56	(32.62)		(.16)
	Group	Martyr	158.46	(35,51)	1, 166	4.70
		Non-Martyr	139.03	(32.88)		(.03)
TOTPE	Sex	Female	66.15	(8.47)	1, 193	1.08
		Male	64.72	(8.97)		(.30)
	Group	Martyr	65.44	(8.21)	1,193	.26
		Non-Martyr	65.35	(9.19)		(.61)
DEPRES	Sex	Female	89.14	(42.19	1, 145	.9
		Male	78.49	(38.63)		(.34)
	Group	Martyr	95.69	(38.76)	1,217	3.81
		Non-Martyr	74.21	(39.49)		(.05)

sexes was statistically significant for AR (F=14.82; df[1, 217]; p=.001), SP (F=5.45; df[1, 219]; p=.02), PE (F=4.4; df[1, 220]; p=.04), and MD (F=7.07; df[1, 221]; p=.01). No significant difference between males and females was found with regard to their scores on SD (F=2.71; df[1, 218]; p=.1), SE (F=0.31; df[1, 217]; p=.58), MP (F=.13; df[1, 206]; p=.91), GL (F=1.85; df[1, 219]; p=.17), DEPRES (f=.9; df[1, 145]; p=.34), TOTDEP (F=1.99; df[1, 166]; p=.14), and TOTPE (F=1.08; df[1, 193]; p=.3). These analyses yielded no significant 2-way interaction. The summary results of these ANCOVAs are reported in Table 2.

A frequency test revealed that the mean age for the duration of father-loss (DUR) is 8.72 (sd=2.6 years). The minimum and maximum values for DUR were 3 years (one case) and 13 years (three cases), respectively, with a range of 10 years. The distribution for this variable was found to be bimodal at values of 11 (36 cases) and 5 years (22 cases). No significant difference was found between boys and girls with regard to DUR. DUR showed no significant associations with GPAs; first year (r=-.05; df=102; p=n.s.), second year (r=-.01; df=101; p=n.s.). However, it correlated significantly negatively with scores on a number of CDS subscales. These findings indicate that shorter duration of father-loss is associated with lower self-esteem and more depression symptoms. Table 3 shows the

Table 3
Correlation coefficients between duration of
father-loss and CDS subscales

CDS Subscales	Duration of Father-Loss (DUR)		
	Girls	Boys	Both
	(N=36)	(n=21)	(n=57)
AR	-.29 *	-.46 *	-.38 **
SD	-.22	-.43 *	-.30 *
SP	-.20	-.52 **	-.33 **
MD	-.30 *	-.35 *	-.34 **
MP	-.08	-.21	-.13
PE	.05	.23	.11
SE	-.36 *	-.46 *	-.41 ***
TOTPE	-.02	.01	-.02
TOTDEP	-.27 *	-.59 **	-.40 **
DEPRES	-.25	-.57 **	-.37 **

*** p= .001

** p= .01

* p=.05

508

summary results of Pearson correlation tests applied to the data for DUR and CDS subscales.

In a further exploration of the contributory role of the duration of the students' father-loss to their mental health, a median-split criterion was employed to divide the experimental group into two subgroups (short vs. long DUR). subjects with DUR of nine years or less were allocated to the short DUR subgroup, and those with DUR of longer than nine years were placed into the long-DUR subgroup. A number of t-tests applied to the data (using short vs. long DUR as independent variables and scores on CDS subscales as dependent variables indicated no significant differences between the two subgroups concerning their age (t=.06; df=99; p=.952), first year GPA (t=.51; df=100; p=.614), second year GPA (t=.04; df=100; p=.971), MD (t=1.76; df=93; p=.08), PE (t=.49; df=91; p=.624), TOTPE (t=.89; df=77; p=.375), and MP(t=.27; df=84; p=.786). However, the subgroup with shorter DUR scored significantly higher than the other

Table 4
Summary of results of t-tests carried out od
duration of father-loss and CDS data

Variable	Group	N	Mean	(sd)	t-value (p)
AR	Short DUR	45	26.78	7.53	2.52
	Long DUR	48	22.73	7.92	(.01)
SD	Short DUR	43	22.77	5.05	1.99
	Long DUR	52	20.50	5.87	(.05)
SP	Short DUR	46	28.28	7.40	2.01
	Long DUR	47	25.17	7.54	(.05)
MD	Short DUR	48	34.02	5.78	1.76
	Long DUR	47	31.96	5.64	(.08)
MP	Short DUR	42	36.07	5.00	0.27
	Long DUR	44	36.34	4.17	(.79)
PE	Short DUR	46	28.28	4.25	0.49
	Long DUR	47	28.77	5.18	(.62)
SE	Short DUR	42	27.88	6.35	2.91
	Long DUR	49	23.76	7.04	(.005)
TOTPE	Short DUR	39	64.15	8.01	0.89
	Long DUR	40	65.70	7.38	(.38)
TOTDEP	Short DUR	34	170.74	33.74	2.56
	Long DUR	37	149.95	34.70	(.01)
DEPRES	Short DUR	28	112.54	33.73	2.91
	Long DUR	30	84.87	37.90	(.005)

subgroup on AR (t=2.52; df=91; p=.01), SD (t=1.99; df=93; p=.05), SP (t=2.01; df=91; p=.05), DEPRES (t=2.91; df=56; p=.005), TOTDEP (t=2.56; df=69; p=.01), and SE (t=2.91; df=89; p=.005). The summary results of these t-tests are presented in Table 4.

A number of Pearson correlation coefficients were calculated to examine the association between subjects' scores on CDS subscales and their scores on the 'lack of self-esteem' (SE) subscale (for each group separately). For the non-martyr students, all of the derived associations were statistically significant at p<.01. However, for the martyr students, the correlation between SE and MP, and TOTPE did not reach the level of significance. As expected, for both groups, the subscales related to depression showed

Table 5
Correlation coefficients between lack of self esteem and other CDS subscales

CDS Subscales	Lack of Self-Esteem	
	Martyr Subjects (n=62)	Non-Martyr Subjects (n=85)
AR	.79 ***	.60 ***
MD	.71 ***	.53 ***
MP	-.01	-.42 ***
PE	-.40 ***	-.51 ***
SD	.73 ***	.65 ***
SP	.74 ***	.65 ***
TOTPE	-.22	-.53 ***
TOTDEP	.88 ***	.83 ***
DEPRES	.87 ***	.82 ***

*** P=.001

** P=.01

* P=.05

positive, and subscales associated with pleasure (i.e., MP, PE, TOTPE) exhibited negative correlations with SE. Table 5 presents a summary result of these analyses.

510

Subsidiary study

In view of the non-representativeness of the academic performance of non-martyr students at martyr schools reported by Makaremi, Khoda-Rahimi, Pouravaz, et al. (1991), a subsidiary investigation was carried out to assess the validity of the present findings and to attempt to replicate the findings of Makaremi and his associates. Makaremi et al. (1991) compared a large sample of students studying at martyr schools with a group of students studying at public schools in Shiraz, Iran (each sample was comprised of both martyr and non-martyr students), and found that GPAs of non-martyr students studying at martyr schools were significantly higher than both martyr students at the same schools and non-martyr students at public schools. Furthermore, they found no significant difference between GPAs of martyr students studying at martyr schools and non-martyr students studying at non-martyr (i.e. public) schools. These findings thus suggested that academic performance of non-martyr students at martyr schools may not appropriately represent the scholastic status of the general population of students.

For the subsidiary study, four public schools were randomly selected

Table 6
Mean and standard deviation of age and GPA's

Group	N	Age	Mean (sd) 1st Year GPA	2nd Year GPA
Martyr Students at Martyr Schools	110	14.19	14.41	14.12
		(1.14)	(1.93)	(1.87)
Non-Martyr Students at Martyr Schools	129	13.49	17.19	16.95
		(0.67)	(1.68)	(1.87)
Non-Martyr Students at Non-Martyr Schools	120	14.33	13.96	14.33
		(1.29)	(1.87)	(1.95)

from the total number of public schools in the same regions of Ahwaz as those for the martyr schools. The GPAs for 120 randomly selected students at these schools were then collected, using exactly the same procedure as that explained earlier. The mean and standard deviation of the age, and first year and second year's GPAs for these students are presented in Table 6.

Two Group (3) X Sex (2) ANCOVAs (while controlling for the subjects' age) were carried out on the first and second year GPAs (groups were martyr students at martyr schools, non-martyr students at martyr schools, and non-martyr at non-martyr schools). These analyses revealed no significant 2-way interactions between Group and Sex factors. However, in both cases, the main effects for sex were statistically significant for the first year ($F=21.56$; $df[1, 357]$; $p<.001$) and the second year ($F=25.78$; $df[1, 357]$; $p<.001$), indicating that GPAs for female students were higher than for males. The main effects for first year GPAs ($F=97.35$; $df[2, 357]$; $p<.001$) and second year GPAs ($F=79.76$; $[2, 357]$; $p<.001$) were statistically significant. A number of Tukey's HDS tests were performed to explore the simple main effects for these results. In both cases, it was revealed that the difference between GPAs of non-martyr students at martyr schools is statistically significantly higher than those for martyr students at the same schools and non-martyr students at non-martyr schools. No significant difference was found between the GPAs for the martyr students at martyr schools and non-martyr students at non-martyr schools.

The present study was aimed at investigating the effects of father-loss upon psychological characteristics and academic performance of Iranian secondary school students. Martyr students were found to be significantly more depressed than non-martyr students (as measured by several of the CDS subscales; i.e., AR, SD, MD, TOTDEP, and DEPRES), but they did not differ significantly from non-martyr students regarding their scores on scales related to self-esteem (SE), guilt (GL) and pleasure (MP, PE, and TOTPE). These findings are less contradictory than they seem when viewed in the light of the general cultural, social and religious backgrounds of martyr students: Despite being depressed over the loss of their fathers, the special respectful treatment the martyr children receive for their status in the community (i.e., loss of father in the war) may even strengthen their self-esteem. Relatedly, it is claimed that self-esteem usually remains relatively undamaged in people suffering from grief reaction or bereavement (see Kaplan & Sadock, 1990).

Duration of father-loss (DUR) showed negative significant associations with all of the psychological measures assessing depression symptoms

512

(except Guilt subscale) in father-absent children, while DUR showed no significant correlations with those variables related to pleasure. These findings may imply that:1) Depression symptoms following the father-loss are self-limiting, and that the longer this period, the less depressed children will be (perhaps as a result of employing coping mechanisms that eventually succeed), or 2) Younger children recover more effectively than older ones from negative impacts of father-loss. Age of the child during the father's absence has repeatedly been pointed to as an important variable in determining these effects (e.g., Goldstein, 1983). Koocher (1974), for example, has claimed that children do not grasp the concept of death until they reach seven years of age, and Santrock (1972) found that father-absence is most detrimental when it occurs in the 6-9 year period of life.

The distinctly superior academic performance of non-martyr students at martyr schools may be due to a number of factors, the most important of which are:

1) Since Iran's martyr schools generally offer better educational opportunities to their students than the public schools, many non-martyr families prefer to send their children to these schools, even though they may have to make a considerable effort to register their child at these schools. Therefore, it may well be that non-martyr students at martyr schools are not representative of the general student population at Ahwaz.

2) Teachers may unintentionally have impeded martyr children's academic performance by having a negative bias towards them. Relatedly, Barclay, Stilwell, and Barclay (1972) have shown that, in comparison with father-present elementary school children, father-absent children were rated by their teachers as lower on a number of personality dimensions and on personal and social adjustment. In addition, teachers almost universally expect less personal effort and work from these children.

3) Martyr students may indeed have weaker intellectual potentials or poorer school performance than non-martyr students studying at martyr schools, an implication which receives some support from the finding that GPAs were significantly associated with neither duration of father-loss nor with scores on CDS subscales.

A number of factors have been proposed to explain the negative associations between father-absence and children's cognitive performance (Roy and Fuqua, 1983; Shinn, 1978). It seems that these effects may be mediated by socioeconomic status, age at parental loss and sex of the child (Roy & Fuqua, 1983). Lessing, Zagorin, and Nelson (1970), for example, found a generalised deficit on WISC subtest scores among father-absent working-class children, whereas middle class father-absent

513

children showed only limited and partial deficits. The present finding that girls scored significantly higher than boys on almost all of the CDS subscales, provides additional support for the contributory role of child's gender in coping with the adverse effects of father-loss (see Golzari, 1991).

Roy and Fuqua (1983) showed that an adequate social support system may mediate the negative effects of single-parent family status on children's academic performance. The social support available to the single-parent families at the time of loss and thereafter, appear to help them to deal more effectively with the loss of spouse and difficulties associated with raising the children (Roy & Fuqua, 1983; Shinn, 1978). Children whose fathers have been martyred may therefore show fewer disruptions in their lives than those who have lost their fathers for other reasons (e.g., divorce). Ethnic membership is another factor that seem to be associated with differential effects of parental absence (Montare and Boone, 1980). It should be noted that Iranian father-martyred families may not be representative of all father-absent families, for they normally receive significant financial, moral, and social support from the government and their relatives. It is worth mentioning that in the Islamic Republic of Iran, martyrdom is socially and ideologically considered as a privilege (i.e., a type of spiritual promotion) which transcends the family's honour and dignity. As a result, people usually have a sense of social and religious duty for the martyr families and are very sympathetic and supportive towards them, particularly towards the martyr's children.

The subsidiary investigation clearly replicates the earlier findings reported by Makaremi et al., (1991) by suggesting that non-martyr students studying at martyr schools show scholastic qualities and academic performance significantly superior to both martyr students at martyr schools and non-martyr students at public schools. An important implication from this study is that the educational settings at martyr schools are likely to cause unfair academic comparisons between martyr students and non-martyr students, and the depression symptoms reported by non-martyr students may thus partially be attributable to this unfair and biased educational circumstance. In comparison with non-martyr students, martyr students may perceive themselves as failures and underachievers, while such comparisons are unjustified owing to the non-representativeness of non-martyr students at martyr schools. Furthermore, the psychological characteristics of non-martyr students at martyr schools may not represent the psychological profile of the general population of students. Although lack of any association between duration of father-loss and GPAs provides additional support for this interpretation, this hypothesis remains to be examined at further studies.

Limitations and suggestions

The authors believe that future studies should compare four groups: martyr students at martyr schools, martyr students at public schools, non-martyr students at martyr schools, and non-martyr students studying at public schools. The authors suggest that a 2(school) X 2(student) design should be employed, if possible, in order to examine the representativeness of martyr and non-martyr samples studying at martyr schools. In addition, the samples used in future studies should be drawn from populations with varied socioeconomic backgrounds so that the confounding effects of cognitive potentials can be precluded; as a further check, measures of intelligence and other indices of cognitive functioning should be used where possible. This was not possible in the present study because there are too few martyr students studying at Ahwaz public secondary schools.

Acknowledgements

The authors would like to thank F. Liami, B. Dabbagh, and M. Pouravaz for their collaborations in data collection, and Ahwaz Martyr Foundation for its support.

References

Atkinson, B. R., & Ogston, D. G. (1974). The effects of father-absence on male children in the home and school. *Journal of School Psychology*, **12** (3), 213-221.

Bane, M. J. (1976). Marital disrupion and lives of children. *Journal of Social Issues*, **32**, 103-117.

Barclay, J R., Stilwell, W. E., & Barclay, L. K. (1972). The influence of parental occupation on social interaction measures on elementary school children. *Journal of Vocational Behaviour*, **2**, 433-446.

Beck, A. T. (1967). *Depression: Clinical, experimental, and theoretical aspects*. New York: Harper and Row.

Blanchard, R. W., & Biller, H. B. (1971). Father availability and academic performance among third-grade boys. *Developmental Psychology*, **4**, 301-305.

Brown, W., Andrews, B., Harris, S. et al. (1986). Social support, self-esteem and depression. *Psychological Medicine* **16**(4), 813-831.

Burns, R. B. (1979). *The self-concept*. London: Longman.

Carlsmith, L. (1964). Effect of early father absence on scholastic aptitude. *Journal of Educational Review*, **34**, 3-21.

Coopersmith, S. (1967). *Antecedents of self-esteem*. San Francisco: Freeman.

Crescimbein, J. (1965). Broken homes do affect academic achievement. *Child and Family*, **4**(2), 24-28.

Deutch, M. & Brown, B. (1964). Social influences in Negro-White intelligence differences. *The Journal of Social Issues*, **30**(2), 2-35.

Fowler, P. C., & Richards, H. C. (1978). Father absence, educational preparedness, and academic achievement: A test of confluence model. *Journal of Educational Psychology*, **10**(4), 595-601.

Fry, P. S., & Scher, A. (1984). The effects of father-absence on children's achievement motivation, ego-strength and locus of control orientation: A five-year longitudinal assessment. *British Journal of Developmental Psychology*, **2**(2), 167-178.

Goldstein, H. S. (1983). Fathers's absence and cognitive development of children over a 3 to 5 year period. *Psychological Report*, **52**, 971-976.

Golzari, M. (1991). Standardization of a scale for the measurement of childhood depression. *Unpublished M.A. Dissertation, Medical Science University of Iran*, Tehran, Iran.

Grunebaum, M. G., Hurwitz, I., Prentice, N. M., & Sperry, B. M. (1962). Fathers of sons with primary neurotic learning inhibition. *American Journal of Orthopsychiatry*, **32**, 462-473.

Hetherington, E. M. & Parkes, R. D. (1975). *Child psychology*. New York: McGraw-Hill.

Hoffman, M. L. (1971). Father-absence and conscience development. *Developmental Psychology*, **4**(3), 400-406.

Kaplan, H. I., & Sadock, B. J. (1990). *Clinical Psychiatry*. London: Williams and Wilkins.

Kazdin, A. E., Esveldt-Dawson, K., Sherick, R. B., & Colbus, D. (1985). The hopelessness scale for children: Psychometrics and concurrent validity. *Journal of Consulting and Clinical Psychology*, **54**(2), 241-245.

Kelly, J. B., & Wallerston, J.S. (1980). *Surviving the breakup: How parents and children cope with divorce*. New York: Basic Books.

Koocher, G. (1974). Talking with children about death. *American Journal of Orthopsychiatry*, **44**, 404-411.

Kovacs, M. (1981). Affective disorders in children and adolescents. *American Psychologist*, **46**(2), 19-29.

Lancaster, W. W., & Richmond, R. O., (1983). Perceived locus of control as a function of father-absence, age, and geographic location. *Journal of Genetic Psychology*, **143**, 51-56.

Lessing, E. G., Zagorin, S. W., & Nelson, D. (1970). WISC subsetand IQ score correlates of father absence. The *Journal of Genetic Psychology*, **117**, 187-195.

Makaremi, A., Khoda-Rahimi, S., Pouravaz, E., Zahli-Nezhad, Z., & Jahedi, A. (1991). Comparison of academic achievement of students studying at Shiraz Martyr Schools with those studying at non-martyr schools. *Journal of Shahed Centre for Research and Psychological Services*, Shiraz, Iran.

Montare, A., & Boone, S. L. (1980). Aggression and parental absence, racial-ethnic differences among inner-city boys. *The Journal of Genetic Psychology*, **137**(2), 223-232.

Najarian, B., Liami, F., Shahedi, I. S., Mahmoudi, A., & Pour Faraji, S. F. (1991). The relationship between self-esteem and depression in a sample of high school students from Martyr families in Ahwaz, Iran. *Journal of Education*, No. 1, 53-68, Tehran, Iran.

National Association of Elementary School Principals (1980). One-parent families and their children: The school's most significant minority. *Principal*, 31-36.

Parish, R. S., & Copeland, T. F. (1980). Locus of control and father-loss. *The Journal of Genetic Psychology*, **136**, 147-148.

Parish, T. S., & Taylor, J. C., (1979). The impact of divorce and subsequent father-absence on children and adolescent's self-concept. *Journal of Youth and Adolescence*, **8**, 491-531.

Quay, H. C., Routh, D. K., & Shapiro, S. K. (1987). Psychopathology of childhood. *Annual Review of Psychology*, **38**, 491-531.

Roy, C. M., & Fuqua, D. A. (1983). Social support may mediate effects of single parent performance. *The School Chancellor*, January, 183-190.

Santrock, J. W. (1972). The relations of type and onset of father-absence to cognitive development. *Child Development*, **44**, 455-469.

Sarason, I. G., & Sarason, B. R. (1987). *Abnormal psychology* (Fifth Edn.).

New Jersey: Prentice-Hall.

Shinn, M. (1978). Father-absence and children's cognitive development. *Psychological Bulletin*, 85(2), 295-324.

Sutherland, H. E. G. (1930). The relationship between IQ and size of family in the ease of fatherless children. *Journal of Genetic Psychology*, 161-170.

Tisher, M. & Lang, M. (1978). The Children's Depression Scale: Review and further developments. In D. P. Cantwell & G. A. Carlson (Eds.), *Affective disorders in childhood and adolescence: An update*. New York: Spectrum Publications, In.

41 The primary healthcare team

C.W.D. Phillips

There are 3,300 patients in our practice, and 3 Doctors who all work less than full-time. Our team includes the Practice staff who are employed by the Doctors, i.e. District Nurses, Health Visitors, Community Psychiatric Nurse and in our case we have a Clinical Psychologist working in our Health Centre. We also have an attached Social Worker, and our meetings are sometimes attended by the Home Care Organiser.

Whose mental health do we promote? 90% of the population consult their Doctors at least once per year. People may also see other members of the Team directly, such as the Practice Nurse, and Community Psychiatric Nurse. We now have to offer health checks to the whole population. There are financial incentives to run Health Promotion Clinics, and although we are sceptical about the stated purpose of these clinics, they may provide opportunities for broaching issues related to mental health. The practice Team is thus likely to have contact with over 90% of their practice population in any one year.

When patients come to see us, we try to understand why. We do not necessarily fit them into medical diagnoses, although this is the popular conception of the Doctor's work, and presenting problems often do fit neatly into diagnostic categories. Accidents resulting in broken bones probably require referral to the Hospital, but we might also reflect on what caused the accidents and whether they could have been avoided. Certainly our antennae perk up, when a child is injured in an accident. We make diagnosis in physical, psychological and social terms.

One third of patients who see us, and one sixth of the general population, have problems which Psychiatrists recognise as Psychiatric problems.

Obviously it would be inappropriate for GPs to refer one sixth of the people on their lists, or every third person they see, to a Psychiatrist. The vast majority of these cases are within the capability of the Primary Health Care Team, as are the majority of patients with physical problems.

Psychiatric illness, through no fault of Psychiatrists, continues to have associated stigma. Patients generally prefer to be seen at the health Centre rather than the Psychiatric Department. The Health Centre and the Primary Health Care Team who work there have the advantage of familiarity, background knowledge, accessibility and continuity. The GP is often in a position to deal with a mental health problem before it is perceived as such by the patient.

The GP is a facilitator rather than a load-carrier. GPs and other Health Care workers have mental health needs like everybody else, so it's important that we avoid carrying other people's burdens. However, we are often in a position to help people shed their loads. They sometimes seem to need our permission, and we may be able to liberate them from fears of misconceptions. We listen, and pick up cues which we reflect back to the patient. We notice change in patients whom we may have known for a long time, and ask ourselves (and possibly the patient also) why. We show them options, and facilitate their decisions. Sometimes we do nothing more than await events.

Balint talked about the Doctor as a drug, which may be sufficient for the patient's needs. Sometimes people laugh on their way out of the consulting room. This is not because doctors are humorous people, but our role enables people to express their concerns and thus feel relieved.

To do this kind of work, motivation rather than brilliance is needed. Of course we have to be properly trained. I need hardly say that clinical competence is paramount. Clinical competence depends on attentiveness and accurate observation, the same characteristics which we need for promoting mental health. Put another way, sound medical practice incorporates a degree of mental health promotion.

Charisma may be O.K. for those who have it, but we avoid pretending to be charismatic if we're not. Patients may see through that. They are more likely to appreciate our interest and concern, although not necessarily so. They may disagree with or object to the direction of our interest. A parent who brings a child with abdominal pain may not be too happy at probing into family dynamics. If not handled skilfully and sensitively these situations can end up with distressed or angry parents.

We try to promote a friendly atmosphere in the Health Centre. There are no spaces reserved in the car park. The receptionists realise how important their job is, and that the treatment starts with them. The patient is often feeling better, by the time he or she sees the Doctors (and that's **not** because they have to wait long for an appointment).

Adult relationships require mutual respect and responsibility. They can't be one-sided. This applies within the Team where members support each other and have high professional expectations of each other. It also applies between patients and health-care workers. If the patient appears to be using our services inappropriately, he or she may need some explanation of just what we have to offer, and what is expected of the patient. Patients have responsibilities, not only in the use of the National Health Service, but more importantly in looking after their own health.

Autonomy carries responsibility. Child-like dependence is incompatible with control of one's own destiny.

Primary Health Care Team meetings offer a convenient venue for eating our lunchtime sandwiches on Monday and Wednesdays. Our aim is our patients health. Our method is to present cases. After team discussion, responsibility may be shared with another member such as the C.P.N. or it may revert to the presenting member. The Clinical Psychologist is especially skilful at helping us to see how to proceed.

The team is involved with:-

1. Tertiary prevention of Psychosis and severe personality disorder.
2. On-going support of vulnerable people e.g. C.P.N's group.
3. Encapsulated neuroses in people otherwise well. e.g. phobias.
4. Reactions to life events.
5. Somatization. Helping people to see the connection between their symptoms and life-events, including their own expectations and beliefs.
6. Drug-related problems including alcohol.
7. Helping the team to help each other.

'Leadership' of the Primary Health Care Team is shared, and moves around the team. There are two rules - only one conversation at a time is encouraged, and we direct our conversation to patient care.

I said earlier that Mental Health promotion depended on motivation rather than brilliance. We need to be patient-centred. We have to start from where the patient is. Judgemental attitudes have to be avoided. We have to avoid regarding some patients as 'genuine', and others as somehow less worthy of our attention. Mental Health problems should be accorded their real priority in differential diagnosis, rather than having 'Functional' added on at the end. 'Functional' problems are genuine.

Mental Health Promotion is not something we dole out. It is an integral part of Primary Health Care, and takes into account the patient's views and his or her readiness to look at what is on offer.

This talk should not have been given by me. It would have been more convincing if it had been given by an outside observer. I acknowledge the lack of research on my part. I must confess I have been more interested in attempting to describe the whole, rather than submit fragments of our practice to scientific scrutiny. Suggestions for a way forward would be most welcome.

42 Changing patterns of mental healthcare: The role of support staff in developing local services

J. Powell

Introduction

Although providing care in the community for people with mental health problems is not new, there has been a growing emphasis over the last decade or more on providing the best possible service within a necessarily limited budget. Thus the development of good quality community mental health services constitutes a major challenge for policy makers, planners and direct service providers alike, particularly with more widespread understanding that this is not necessarily a cheap option, and when restricting public expenditure is a priority in the policies of national governments.

The current debate concerning the role of non-professionally qualified staff or paid support workers in the development of mental health services may be seen in this context (Chowcat, 1992; Qureshi et al., 1989). Drawing on the findings of a recently completed study of a developing community mental health service, this paper identifies various ways in which non-professionally qualified staff have contributed to the overall development of a locally based service, and highlights some of the implications for professional practice and service development.

Our two-year evaluative study of the process of moving an overall service away from a parent hospital focused primarily on the development of community based mental health services, rather than on hospital closure (Powell and Lovelock, 1991; 1992). As a case study giving attention both to the organisational/managerial context and to front-line delivery issues, this project exemplifies an approach to evaluation which recognises pluralism of interests and criteria of success, research as a process, and the value of partnership between researchers and service providers (Powell and Lovelock, 1989). The study explicitly combined several research methods and thereby brought different perspectives to bear. A prominent place was given to the views and experiences of direct service users, carers, GPs, and the multidisciplinary staff team. This approach is mirrored in the way that the present paper draws on a range of different sorts and sources of data to explore the contribution that support workers made to the developing service.

In outlining a blueprint for 'a good community mental health service', Jones (1988) identifies its main characteristics as diversity, informality, outreach and feedback. In our detailed study of a decentralising mental health service, there was much evidence of these key characteristics (Powell and Lovelock, 1992). Although subject to the constraints imposed by limited resources, there was a growing diversity within the overall service. Some aspects of the service showed a highly developed level of informality; others had made less progress on this front. Outreach activities, embodying collaboration with other agencies and networks, had been a growing area of activity for the service throughout the period of our study.

The major and positive developments charted in the overall study took place over a relatively short timescale and were largely achieved through the coming together of the 'community' and 'residential' teams, and the development of collaborative activity and joint working with other local agencies. The involvement of support workers in these two areas of activity forms the main focus of this paper.

The overall service

To understand more about the changing nature of the service and the impact on those providing the service on a day-to-day basis, we encouraged all team members to participate in a logging exercise. All staff kept a record of their work activities during three separate weeks, roughly one month apart, in the period prior to the move away from the main hospital site. At this time the residential unit was located in separate accommodation within the hospital grounds. This exercise was repeated again some fourteen months later, after the whole service had come together in its new community base.

These data were analysed first from the perspective of where staff spent their time, and then in terms of their day-by-day activities. The second approach served to complement and extend the understanding of the operation of the service provided by the first.

The first logging exercise clearly revealed the multi-faceted nature of the service; this was further underlined by the second phase of recording. Together, the data present a diverse picture of activities within the overall developing service. The complex interplay between the different aspects of the service in the context of providing residential care, developing services for continuing care clients, assessing new referrals, and sustaining a range of client interventions, was revealed in a number of ways.

The new building itself brought together what have frequently been perceived as traditionally separate and distinct alternatives to providing care. It also facilitated interaction between the many members of the multidisciplinary team.

The 'non-traditional' community role of those staff based in the residential unit was evident in both the logging studies, highlighting an important area of overlapping activity between the 'residential' and 'community' arms of the service. Once united on a shared site, these activities remained focused around work with individual clients. This primarily involved the assessment of newly referred clients, who were seen either at home or in the newly integrated unit, once established.

The more detailed data on where staff members spent their time are described and discussed elsewhere (Powell and Lovelock, 1991;1992). However, an example based on information recorded by two staff members, both nurses based in the residential unit, illustrates how their work

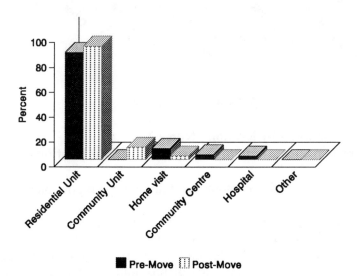

■ Pre-Move ▦ Post-Move

Figure 1 Analysis by location - Nurse 1
Average percentage of total time spent at various locations

involved contact with both resident and non-resident users of the service (see figs.1 and 2).

Both figures illustrate how residentially based staff spent a small but significant amount of their time away from the residential unit. This pattern remained relatively stable over time. Following the move into the shared community base, use was made of its interviewing facilities. In the case of nurse 1, it appeared that this venue largely replaced clients' homes as a community location.

However, actual percentages shown in the figures must be treated with caution. With the introduction of the support workers some changes in staff activities, not necessarily associated with a change of location, could

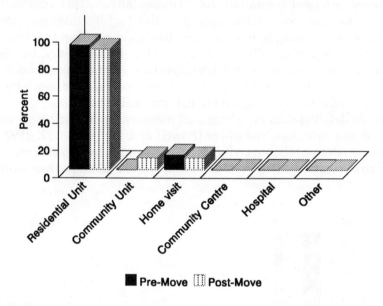

Pre-Move **Post-Move**

Figure 2 Analysis by location - Nurse 2
Average percentage of total time spent at various locations

be anticipated. Further exploration of this issue was possible using more detailed descriptive data.

In the residential unit, the introduction of the support workers, sharing the day-to-day running of the residential unit with the duty nurse, had only a minimal effect on the life and routine of the unit and its residents. There appeared to be a high degree of informality in the contacts between all staff and residents, as they shared in the daily life of the unit. There was considerable overlap between many of the tasks undertaken by the nurses and the support staff. However, alongside this overlapping of tasks, there were some clear divisions of responsibility. The duty nurse was in charge of the unit and had administrative and professional responsibilities to carry out. Supervision of medication, handling specific enquiries about a resident's well-being, and contact with other professional colleagues, took up substantial proportions of the duty therapist's time, along with supervising the support workers. These tasks were inevitably interwoven with other activities; more informal contacts with residents and staff, supervision of a student nurse, and some administrative work.

The more ordinary, routine and regular interactions of domestic life essentially took place between the support workers and residents. For example, the housekeeper was usually involved in the preparation of meals and this frequently provided a time for talking informally with some of the residents, who might join him in this task. Time was also spent sitting with residents, sharing in their conversations, or joining in a game of cards. Whereas previously this in-house support had been provided wherever possible by the nurses, it was now an activity which was being carried out and developed by the support workers. There were several recorded accounts of a support worker accompanying residents to local shops, to a nearby drop-in centre, or in one case on an appearance at the local court.

These more qualitative data also suggested an increased involvement of residentially based staff in one-to-one client contact during the second logging period, reflecting in turn the contribution made by the introduction of support workers into the residential unit. The gradual withdrawal from routine involvement in the residential unit allowed residentially based staff to become involved in working with clients living in their own homes. This shift in focus represented a substantial contribution to the overall work of the team in the local community, particularly in responding to new referrals to the service. In addition, through the introduction of support workers, the residential unit was able to develop and sustain a more informal homely setting, where residents were encouraged to participate more in the daily domestic life of the unit.

Continuing care services

Developing greater informality, in terms of wider accessibility and acceptability, was also a feature of other aspects of the overall service, particularly in the area of daycare (Echlin, 1989). The setting up of a joint day care initiative, which involved several agencies, statutory and voluntary, represented an important step forward in this respect. It also played a part in stimulating wider interest in working with people with longer term mental health problems and to some extent encouraged the setting up of an identified 'continuing care team' within the overall service.

Our logging study highlighted an increasing use of local community facilities, particularly in the development of services for continuing care clients. Furthermore, many of the developments indicated by the first set of logging data continued to operate on a regular basis, although relying to a considerable extent on the increasing involvement of the OT helper and other non-professionally qualified staff. The team members who had previously been actively supporting these ventures on a day-to-day basis, now spent increasingly large proportions of their time involved in the planning and development of other service innovations. This was evident from the analysis of staff activities by location, and in particular, the recorded activities of the senior OT helper (see figs. 3 and 4).

Prior to the move the OT made a substantial contribution to

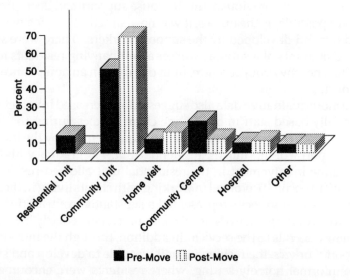

Figure 3 Analysis by location - Occupational therapists
Average percentage of time spent at various locations

activitieslocated at both the residential unit and at various community centre settings. This pattern changed following the move, suggesting less direct contact with clients and more time spent in the community office.

For the OT helper the pattern of change over time was reversed. Following the move of the overall service to its community base, the OT helper spent less time in the office and substantially more time at community centre locations. This increase in time spent in the local community reflected the expansion of the day-care development, set up prior to the move with a substantial involvement from the OT as well as the OT helper.

To gain a fuller understanding of these changing patterns of service use and professional practice, we sought the views and experiences both staff

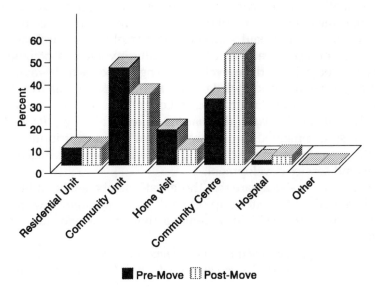

Pre-Move **Post-Move**

Figure 4 Analysis by location - O T helper
Average percentage of total time spent at various locations

and users. Once again, these findings are presented in detail elsewhere (Powell and Lovelock, 1992; Powell, 1991). However, reference to some of these comments provides other perspectives on the changing role of professional workers and the contribution of both paid support workers and volunteers.

In general, staff members were keen to develop services for people with longer term mental health problems, but they were also concerned about the impact of these developments on their own professional practice. For example, this team member was not alone in voicing her concern:

'*I do find it tremendously stimulating being involved in developments ... but as a service is it right that a clinician - a nurse, an OT or whatever - should abandon their clinical work to take on this work? There are different views about this. Is it a personal choice or is it what the service needs, and who makes the choice?'*

The shift from direct work with clients to service planning and management at a local level was mirrored in the day-to-day running of the newly established daycare initiative referred to previously. Whilst several members of the team continued to maintain some regular contact with club members, volunteers and the co-ordinator, day-to-day professional back-up passed to the duty officer system. Furthermore, the six volunteers, working closely with both the co-ordinator and the OT helper, (subsequently renamed community officer to reflect her 'out-reach' activities), came to provide regular and consistent help in the club.

The volunteers and paid support staff, namely the co-ordinator and community officer, were aware of the lessening involvement of these team members, but welcomed the level of ongoing support which was offered. They appreciated the knowledge that some back-up was available if needed from the duty officer at Acorn Lodge. This back-up was seen as:

'The important link ... but at the same time a feeling of being quite separate.'

They also commented on the professional staff's contribution to the overall management of the club, and their associated activities in fund-raising and service development.

The users were also aware that those staff members who initially had been involved in the setting up of the daycare initiative, now had less involvement in the club's day-to-day activities. As one club member commented:

'They used to spend a lot of time here, but now it allows them time to go off and perhaps visit other clients who are housebound. The volunteers have relieved them a bit.'

Club members saw both the co-ordinator and the community officer as important people, to whom they could turn if they had any difficulties. Many valued having the choice of either a man or a woman and the different styles they brought to their work. For example:

'If we have any problem, we can go to (co-ordinator or community officer) even Acorn Lodge (the formal services) to get help if we need it. That's what this is for; you can get help. Although we don't talk about our problems, they can refer to someone else.'

As the previous quotation illustrates, members tended to see both the co-ordinator and the community officer as access points to the more formal mental health services, should they need them. One member explained how she had been able to get professional help when she had needed it:

'... had a few problems recently and managed to get help through the club. I mentioned it to [community officer], who got me an appointment at Acorn Lodge (the formal services). They are there to help if you need it, but coming here they

don't discuss problems, only if you want to.'

The views of both service users and providers serve to illustrate the importance of ensuring access to professional staff, both in terms of expert help for individual users, and professional support and supervision for those directly engaged in the demanding task of the day-to-day running of the service. This access to professional support, as Qureshi (1989) suggests, also has the advantage of giving the paid support worker more freedom to develop relationships with service users in the context of a limited responsibility for the total care provided.

Discussion

Achieving such changes in the overall service as those outlined above has involved a major cultural shift in the organisation as a whole. This has been evident from the changing attitude on the part of professionally qualified staff to the potential use of support workers in the provision of services. They are no longer seen exclusively as amateurs whose contribution could be improved with professional training (MIND, 1982). Many innovations in the service have, to a considerable extent, been sustained by the greater involvement of support workers, both within the residential unit and in the day-to-day running of services for continuing care clients. This greater use of non-professionally qualified staff, evident from our logging studies and elaborated through the views of both service users and providers, has significant implications for professional practice.

A shift in emphasis away from direct work with clients to the management and development of services took place over our study period. In addition to these changes in professional practice, the logging exercise also revealed that in one form or another the supervision of the growing number of support workers had become an increasingly significant activity undertaken by many team members. This task was seen as important both in terms of staff support and development and as a way of ensuring good quality care.

To some extent the successful involvement of support staff in the maintenance and development of any service rests with the quality of supervision provided by the professionally qualified team members. However, in addressing the needs of individual workers, it is also important to consider the development needs of the team as a whole. Team building and the development of a service philosophy shared by managers and service providers, both professional practitioners and direct care staff, are essential to the development of a high quality service (Lemmer and Braisby, 1991).

Our study leaves little doubt about the value of introducing support workers into various settings within a locally based community mental health service. As other schemes have shown (Leat and Gay, 1987), support workers can offer a quality of 'ordinariness' which has the benefit of making some aspects of the service more accessible to its users. they cannot, however, be seen as an alternative to the professional input. Support workers are an additional resource, without whom the service would be less diverse, flexible and creative in responding to individual needs.

Finally, on a cautionary note, it is important to emphasise that the greater involvement of support workers, in the ways outlined in this paper, does not provide a cheap option. Traditionally, in all the caring professions, support workers, whether described as aides, assistants or auxiliaries, have received little support and few opportunities for acquiring training or formal qualifications (Hancock, 1989; Hugman, 1991). Most, but not all, are women. They are also relatively poorly paid on the basis that caring is unskilled work and is undertaken primarily for love rather than money (Dalley, 1988; Becker, 1990). The contribution that support workers, in their many guises, can and do make to 'care in the community' is now beginning to be better understood and appreciated (Jones, 1989). The needs of support workers for a supportive staff network and access to training is now being acknowledged as part of the true cost of developing high quality locally based services (DoH, 1991). Without this, as Lavender and Holloway (1988, p. 299) confirm.

... there is no reason to believe that the quality of care outside the traditional institution will be any better than within it.

References

Becker, S. (1990, April 12). The sting in the tail. *Community care*, (pp.22-4).

Chowcat, J. (1992, January). Skill mix in the Health Service: The case for a code of practice. *An MSF (Manufacturing, Science & Finance Union) Discussion Paper.*

Dalley, G. (1988). *Ideologies of caring: Rethinking community and collectivism.* Basingstoke: Macmillan.

Department of Health (Social Services Inspectorate). (1991). *Training for community care: A joint approach.* London: HMSO

Echlin, R. (1989). *Daycare Information Pack.* London: Good Practices in Mental Health.

Hancock, C. (1989). The NHS: evolution or dissolution? In M. Jolley & P. Allan (Eds.), *Current issues in nursing.* London: Chapman & Hall.

Hugman, R. (1991). *Power in caring professions*. Basingstoke: Macmillan.

Jones, G. (1989). Women in social care: the invisible army. In C. Hamlet (Ed.), *Women and Social Services Departments*, Hemel Hempstead: Harvester Wheatsheaf.

Jones, K. (1988). *Experience in Mental Health: Community care and Social Policy*. London: Sage.

Lavender, A. & Holloway, F. (Eds.), (1988). *Community care in practice: Services for the continuing care client*. Chichester: John Wiley & Sons.

Leat, D. & Gay, P. (1987). *Paying for care: A study of policy and practice in Paid Care Schemes*. London: Policy Studies Institute.

Lemmer, B. & Braisby, D. (1991, January 3). Bridging the training gap. *Health Service Journal*, 22-23.

MIND. (1982). *Working together? Voluntary and statutory mental health services*. London: MIND Publications.

Qureshi, H., Challis, D. & Davies, B. (1989). *Helpers in case managed community care*. Aldershot: Gower.

Powell, J. (1991). *The Sevenoaks Club: A joint initiative in daycare*. Southampton: CEDR, Department of Social Work Studies, University of Southampton.

Powell, J. & Lovelock, R. (1989). The development of community-based adult mental health services - a research contribution. *Bulletin of the Royal College of Psychiatrists*. 13 (12), 662-6.

Powell, J. & Lovelock, R. (1991). *An evaluation of a developing community mental health service*. Southampton: CEDR, Department of Social Work Studies, University of Southampton.

Powell, J. & Lovelock, R. (1992). *Changing patterns of mental health care: a case study in the development of local services*. Aldershot: Avebury.

43 The tip of the iceberg: Promoting good mental health practice with social services staff

J. Pritlove

Non-medical primary care in mental health

Community care for people with mental health problems can be represented as a continuum of services along which those who use these services, or have need of them, move. At one end of the continuum are the traditional, medically-oriented, psychiatric services; at the other, the ordinary networks of community life. In between these two extremes lies a range of services, some better defined than others, and among them is primary care.

Primary care in mental health is usually seen as a medical service. However, its key qualification is that it is the service which the person in need of help goes to first, rather than that it is based on any definition allied to the type of help received. In this sense it is identified mainly in relation to secondary or tertiary care, to which the primary care practitioner may refer the service user for specialist care or treatment (Williams, 1985).

When understood in this sense, primary care in mental health is also clearly a function of the work of Social Services Departments. People with mental health problems, and their carers, receive assessment and care from a variety of social services staff who are not part of the secondary specialist mental health service. Such staff include neighbourhood team social workers, social welfare officers, home care/home help staff, family nursery centre staff, and staff in aged persons' homes. As in medical primary care, these staff are not specialists in mental health work, and often service users are referred directly to them; referral on to specialist care (for example, to the specialist mental health social worker) will often only take place via one of these primary care workers.

Social services staff in primary mental health care

The primary care role of social services staff in mental health is very important, for two main reasons: firstly, because social services clients are a group especially at risk of poor mental health; and secondly, because it is often the most efficient way of offering help.

There is plenty of evidence that social services clients are especially at risk of poor mental health (Cohen and Fisher, 1988). The most basic link is that between social deprivation and mental health problems (Royal College of Psychiatrists, 1986). The majority of social services clients suffer social deprivation, almost by definition.

Furthermore, significant groups of social services clients are especially vulnerable to mental ill-heath (Newton, 1988). Many social services clients are elderly: older people are at increased risk. Cohen and Fisher's study of social services clients in North Yorkshire found that 70% of elderly clients had an identifiable mental health problem (Cohen and Fisher, 1988). Another important group of clients comprises young mothers with small children, suffering isolation. Research shows that this group is very vulnerable to depression (Brown and Harris, 1978). A further group which figures highly in social services caseloads is the parents of children in care. Again, research indicates that these frequently suffer mental health problems (Isaacs et al., 1986). Finally, primary carers are often involved with social services care, and again are greatly at risk of mental health problems: in one study, 56% were found to be so affected (Cohen and Fisher, 1988).

These findings mean that the majority of social services staff are inevitably involved, in a primary care sense, with mental health problems in many of their clients, whether they choose this or not.

However, although this state of affairs is inevitable, it is also potentially extremely beneficial for the clients concerned and their families. This is firstly because the help which these clients receive from social services staff may be the only help available to them for their mental health problem. The numbers of people suffering mental ill-health in the community are very large, but the resources of the specialist mental health services are very small (Goldberg and Huxley, 1980). Consequently, the only kind of help available for many will be that provided by primary care. Medical primary care, moreover, often cannot provide the kind of time input which many social services staff can supply, and which is the essential ingredient in the care of many people with severe mental health problems.

The work of social services staff in mental health primary care is also important because it can have a key preventive role.

Social services staff often see people with mental health problems, and their carers, before the specialist services do, and in less stigmatised settings. They are also often closer to the network of ordinary help in the local neighbourhood. They are therefore able to intervene in a vital way to detect mental ill-health and help those affected, and this may prevent deterioration or allow early referral on to other kinds of help. The North Yorkshire study showed that social services staff detected identifiable mental health problems which were not detected by the general practitioner involved, in 20% of the most severe cases of functional mental illness, and in 22% of cases where there was severe dementia (Cohen and Fisher, 1988).

The Leeds project: basic approach

Social services staff can therefore, be seen as a key part of primary care in mental health. It is doubtful, however, whether this is widely known or understood either within social services or within other parts of the mental health service. All too often social services departments have been seen as the 'handmaidens of psychiatry', with no specific expertise of their own, dependent upon medical services, with 'mental health work' meaning solely that carried out by specialist staff.

This ignores the clear messages of the facts described above. Failure to recognise the vital role and the great potential represented by social services staff in mental health community care means that people with mental health problems, and their carers, will miss out on help which should be available to them.

Consideration of these issues has led Leeds Social Services Department to set up a major action-research project, the aim of which is to assess, support and improve the mental health work done by non-specialist staff. The project is known as 'The Tip of the Iceberg', the iceberg being the mental health work done by non-specialist staff, of which often only the tip is visible officially (Pritlove, 1990).

The project began in 1985, when three of the Department's area-based Specialist Mental Health Social Workers met to consider the common issues which they were facing in dealing with cases brought to them for advice and support by non-specialist staff such as generic social workers and social welfare officers. They decided to carry out a survey of mental health work done by non-specialist staff. The survey was done over a period of 6 months, and the result indicated a high level of mental health work being undertaken, but with little recognition, support or training.

As a result of the survey report, the Director decided to widen the scope of the project to include the whole Department, and it has been operating, in different forms, up to the present.

The project has two objectives: to identify the mental health work done by non-specialist staff; and to improve this work by training and supporting staff who do it and by encouraging its expansion and development to meet the needs of people with mental health problems and their carers.

The design and operation of the project has been based on the principle of relating it as closely as possible to the day-to-day work of the staff concerned. For this reason, the research method has used a simple 'low technology' approach rather than a more 'scientific' one. The work has been carried out, wherever possible, by specialist staff who work in the same office as the non-specialist staff concerned. The use of extra resources has been minimal, with no outside agency involved, and the normal resources of area offices and the Department's training section alone being used. Wherever possible, the training has been based upon the actual work being done by staff.

The Leeds project: people with mental health problems who receive help from non-specialist staff

To meet the first of the project's objectives, the identification of the mental health work carried out by non-specialist staff, two large-scale surveys have been carried out by Specialist Mental Health Social Workers. The first was in 1985-6, and covered three of the city's nine social services areas. The second was in 1988-1989, and formed a six-month study of referrals and cases in another area office. In total, these surveys looked at 1,518 cases and 1,088 referrals, a very large sample.

Overall, 22% of cases and 18% of referrals were assessed as having a mental health problem. The definition of 'mental health problem' was partly based upon that used by Fisher and colleagues in their study of mental health work in a Social Services Department (Fisher, Newton and Sainsbury, 1984). This is a social work, rather than a medical, definition of a mental health problem. It was chosen because it was relevant to the issues faced by the staff and was easy to use.

A sub-sample of cases was examined in terms of the characteristics of the clients concerned. This showed that three-quarters of clients with mental health problems were women, and half were aged under 40. However, a further third were aged over 70.

The severity of the mental health problems was demonstrated by the fact that half were assessed as 'marked' or 'severe'; 30% of these clients had been, or were, psychiatric in-patients, 29% were currently receiving help

538

from the psychiatric services, and 20% had been subject to compulsory admission under the Mental Health Act.

A very important aspect of the mental health problems was their impact upon the family as a whole. In over half the cases, this was judged to have a severe or marked effect. 43% of those with mental health problems were living with a child or children aged under 18, and 59% of the cases were officially designated 'child care' or 'family problem' cases. 29% involved statutory child care, and in 85% of these the social worker's assessment was that the mental health problem had contributed materially to the statutory action.

The Leeds project: the work of non-specialist staff

Two main issues emerged in the project for the mental health work done by non-specialist staff. These are the recognition of mental health problems; and the issues in work carried out with clients, such as knowledge, attitudes, and resources.

The problem of recognition of mental health problems is not confined to social services staff: it exists also in medical primary care (Goldberg and Huxley, 1980). In Leeds, as in other Social Services Departments, the problem begins with the Departmental statistics, which refer to 0.8% of referrals and 1.8% of cases as 'mental illness'. The reason for this, of course, is that 'child care', 'family problem', and 'elderly' are prime classifications: if any of these apply to a case, it receives that classification whether or not there is a mental health problem present. In fact, as shown above, staff working with clients identify 18% of referrals and 22% of cases as having a mental health problem.

These misleading Departmental statistics matter for two reasons: they can be used as an excuse for not giving mental health work the resources which are required, and they may influence staff by blocking potential recognition of mental health problems in their cases.

Recognition by staff is clearly vital. Research with general practitioners has shown that recognition of mental health problems aids in their treatment (Cohen and Fisher, 1988). It is clear from the research in Leeds, and from other studies, that sometimes mental health problems are not recognised by non-specialist staff. This is often a matter of 'mental set': a social worker who maintains that 'there are not mental health problems in my caseload' may simply be thinking along the traditional lines where a 'child care' case is not seen as anything else, and 'mental health' means a case where there is only one problem, and that is a mental health one.

Studies of social services clients using medical research instruments such as the General Health Questionnaire have shown that at least half of clients have an identifiable mental health problem (Cohen and Fisher, 1988). On this basis, the Leeds surveys, in which social services staff assessed 22% of their clients as having such a problem, indicate some probable failure in recognition. Moreover, the Leeds surveys showed that the proportions of referrals assessed as having a mental health problem were much lower than for ongoing cases, especially when the assessment was carried out by the team leader rather than the Specialist Mental Health Social Worker. This reinforces another finding by Cohen and Fisher, that mental health problems fare worse at referral than in ongoing cases.

Nevertheless, despite these obvious problems with recognition, it was clear that in many cases the worker had accurately identified a mental health problem, sometimes in the face of some disbelief by, for example, medical colleagues. There was certainly evidence of social services staff recognising a mental health problem where the medical services had not, as Cohen and Fisher found. The importance of this process of recognition, in an environment which often gives little formal encouragement to it, should not be underestimated.

Thus the overall conclusion of the project is that the main issue here is not recognition but how social services staff can help with the problem once it is recognised.

This consists mainly of two problems: knowledge and attitudes; and resources. Much of the situation with regard to knowledge and attitudes can be summed up by the comment of the social worker in the project who described a very difficult case involving a mother suffering from schizo-phrenia and her two children. The social worker had very effectively acted as counsellor, advocate and mobiliser of community resources for the mother, while officially only being involved because of the children. Having described all his work with the mother, he added: 'I haven't got a lot to provide'.

As Cohen and Fisher found, social services staff frequently provide very effective and imaginative help to clients with mental health problems, but because of a set of attitudes within the Department, and, perhaps, within themselves, they feel very little confidence in dealing with people with mental health problems, and continue to believe that only medical staff have the necessary knowledge to intervene.

An important aspect of this problem is the fact that the surveys showed that social welfare officers, who may have received very little training about mental health, frequently carry some of the most difficult mental health cases. In one area office, 36% of social welfare officers' caseloads had mental health problems, compared to 23% of social workers' caseloads. Social welfare officers are often acutely aware of their 'unqualified' status when dealing with, for example, doctors, and have inappropriately low levels of confidence about their role in mental health. In fact, the surveys showed them dealing very effectively with extremely difficult mental health problems.

Just as important as knowledge and attitudes is resources. Social services staff in the project felt that they lacked adequate resources to provide help to clients with mental health problems. Their resources consist of training and support; time; and non-stigmatised, locally based facilities for people with mental health problems.

In view of what has been said above about knowledge and attitudes, the need for training and support is self-evident. Time is a particular issue when Departmental priorities put statutory child care work ahead of most other duties. Often a social worker may be involved with a family where there is a mental health problem only because of the child care needs of the case; he or she may feel that they wish to help with the mental health problem, but are constrained by time from doing so adequately.

A third aspect of resources is that what many clients with mental health problems are looking for is not access to traditional mental health services but help which ties in more naturally with the less stigmatising networks of community help with which area-based staff often work. A good example of such a resource is a group for mothers under stress attached to a family nursery centre. However, such resources are often not available.

In terms of the needs of social services staff in recognition of mental health problems, and help for clients who suffer from them, the project has carried out a series of training and support initiatives across the city. These have included the six-month action-research scheme at one area office, already referred to, as well as a variety of training and support schemes with different groups of staff. There has been a particular emphasis on providing training for team leaders, who play a crucial role in supervising the mental health work done by non-specialist staff. The training and education process has also included senior management.

Although the project has been primarily aimed at social workers and social welfare officers, a direct link has been with the large mental health training programme run by Specialist Social Workers and the Training Section with home care (home help) staff.

Non-medical primary care in mental health: implications for the future

The importance of primary care in community care for people with mental health problems and their families cannot be overemphasised. Specialist (secondary or tertiary mental health services) provide for only 7% of all those with mental health problems (Goldberg and Huxley, 1980); the only source of help for the remaining 93% of sufferers and their carers is primary care. This statistic will be come even more pronounced as fewer and fewer live in long-stay hospital care.

Primary care has several key advantages: it can be more accessible, can be less stigmatising, and it can provide a much higher input of staff time for each client than does secondary or specialist care.

However, it will only work at all if it is seen as complementary to specialist services. The Leeds project was based upon the idea that primary care workers could only carry out their work effectively in mental health if they had the right relationship with specialist staff such as mental health social workers, and community psychiatric nurses.

There are in fact three models for the relationship between primary and secondary care services in mental health (Williams, 1985). The first is the 'replacements' model, where primary care is simply replaced by secondary care. For the obvious reasons given above, this is not acceptable. In the second model, 'increased throughput', primary care practitioners refer more patients/clients to the secondary services. Again, for reasons stated throughout this paper, this would make no sense. It is the third model, 'liaison/attachment' which is relevant here. In this model, secondary services work closely with primary care services through training, provision of advice, assessment, support and supervision, with easy access to referral to specialist help where it is appropriate.

In Leeds, a good example of this approach has been the development of the Home Care service for people with mental health problems. Five schemes have been set up across the city in which Home Care staff work intensively with people with severe mental health problems. Assessment, training, support and regular supervision are provided by the local Specialist Mental Health Social Worker. These schemes have been found to be very successful: the quality of life of a number of severely disabled people has been significantly improved, and the cycle of continuous readmissions to psychiatric hospital, which had previously obtained for the clients, has been broken.

Overall, in fact, the 'Tip of the Iceberg' project has demonstrated the crucial role of area-based Specialist Mental Health Social Workers in developing and supporting the primary care role of departmental staff. There are ten of these specialists, based in neighbourhood offices across the city. They embody 'liaison/attachment' model described above, by providing a comprehensive and appropriate range of help for primary care staff abut mental health work: training, advice about cases, joint assessment of need, and regular support and supervision.

The Leeds project has demonstrated the vital role of non-medical primary care, working in conjunction with the appropriate secondary services. However, this will only be fully effective if it receives the resources necessary to do the job. Primary care is grossly underfunded compared to secondary care: mental health in-patient care costs £26,250 per person per year, and all community services cost £107 per person per year (Mental Health Foundation, 1990). In view of the clear importance of primary care, this imbalance needs to be rectified.

The results of the Leeds project have shown that the resources required are: more time for primary care staff to work on the mental health aspects of their clients' situations; more time for specialist staff to provide training, support and supervision; and funding for small-scale, locally based resources to meet the needs of key at-risk groups such as isolated young mothers, carers, and unemployed people.

In this context, a comment by Chris Heginbotham, former Director of MIND, is appropriate. He noticed that the proportion of expenditure in social services departments on specialist mental health services matched their 'official' referral rate for mental health cases: about 2%. The Leeds project, and other research, has shown that the real proportion of mental health in referrals is more like 18%.

While it is unrealistic to expect that the proportion of spending on mental health will change in line with the reality of the situation, this analysis reaffirms the basic point: that social services departments carry out a vital primary care role in mental health with completely inadequate resources.

This conclusion is especially relevant in terms of the changes which are due to take place in community care funding in 1993. Case assessment and case management for people with mental health problems and their carers will depend to a great extent on the contributions of primary care staff in social service. If, then, the changes are to work effectively, the input of these staff will have to be properly resourced and supported.

If 1993 sees this message understood and acted upon, the needs of many people with mental health problems, and their carers, will be better met.

Acknowledgements

The 'Tip of the Iceberg' project has been designed and carried out by:
Norman Barker, Specialist Social Worker (Mental Health)
Chris Copeland, Principal Social Worker
Sue Naidu, Specialist Social Worker (Mental Health)
Ron Pratt, Specialist Social Worker (Mental Health)
The development of the Mental Health Home Care Schemes has been

carried out by:

Linda Atkins, Specialist Social Worker (Mental Health)

Peter Dwyer, Neighbourhood Team Manager

Barbara Fenwick, Home Care Manager

Sue Naidu, Specialist Social Worker (Mental Health)

References

Brown, G. W., & Harris, T. (1978). *The social origins of depression.* London: Tavistock.

Cohen, J., & Fisher, M. (1988). *The tip of the iceberg.* Bradford: University of Bradford.

Fisher, M., Newton, C., & Sainsbury, E. (1984). *Mental health social work observed.* London: Allen and Unwin.

Goldberg, D., & Huxley, P. (1980). *Mental illness in the community.* London: Tavistock

Isaacs, B.C., Minty, E.B., & Morrison, R.M. (1986). Children in care - the association with mental disorder in the parents. *British Journal of Social Work*, **16**, 325 - 339.

Mental Health Foundation (1990). *Mental illness: the fundamental facts.* London: Mental Health Foundation.

Newton, J. (1988). *Preventing mental illness.* London: Routledge.

Pritlove, J., (1990, May 10). A general practice? *Community Care.*

Royal College of Psychiatrists (1986). *Report of working party on bed norms and resources.* London: Royal College of Psychiatrists.

Williams, P. (1985). Psychiatric disorder in the community and in primary care. In G. Horobin (Ed.), *Responding to mental illness* (pp.12 -26). London: Kogan Page.

44 The promotion of mental health as seen from the user perspective

D. Richards and W. Poppleton

The London Borough of Richmond upon Thames is an Outer London Borough which straddles the River Thames in South West London. It was formed in 1965 bringing together Barnes, Richmond, Twickenham and Hampton. The borough, in its thinking, retains the previous parish land boundaries and often village identity. The river creates a natural boundary and the three major parks, Bushy, Richmond, and Old Deer, give open space to what is seen as an affluent middle-class area.

The borough has a population of 154,600. The unemployment rate is low, around 5.4%, there being close access to Heathrow Airport and developments on the main route to the West and good commuter links into London.

The health needs of the borough are covered by the Richmond, Twickenham and Roehampton Health Authority; its boundaries are not co-terminous with that of the borough. Roehampton is part of the London Borough of Wandsworth, which includes a vast high-rise council estate, and the only hospital for the district, Queen Mary's. Most in-patient mental health services for Richmond are in a hospital at Epsom eleven miles away which, in line with community care policies, is being closed in 1996, but with higher costs this may well be earlier.

The Director of Public Health Medicine suggests that 43% of the Adult population in the Health Authority being seen by their GP, more than half of these will have a disorder with a conspicuous psychiatric component. We have a joint mental health strategy; the vision statement reads, 'All residents of the Borough with mental health needs should be valued and respected as individuals and have access to a range of comprehensive, high quality, locally based services. There should be a choice of flexible, integrated services which are co-ordinated and responsible to people's need for prevention, care, support and treatment.'

The strategy was drawn up between the Health Authority, Local Authority and voluntary organisations in 1989/90.

When I came into this post of Principal Officer, Mental Health Services three years ago, at each of the residential and day care service appraisal days I attended, service users would tell me what I had to obtain for them. Believing that together we can achieve, I began asking for their help and support, and offering suggestions as to how they became involved in making their needs heard.

In the early summer of 1990 a White Paper Grant Scheme from the Kings Fund 'Local and Vocal' gave us our first formal opportunity to assist service users in developing their own voice. The secretary from the Community Health Council, a psychologist and myself, with support from the local MIND group, put together a bid entitled ' Initiating User Involvement in the Community'. The aim was to employ a worker to assist service users to form their own group and voice their own opinions.

We did not succeed, instead the Community Health Council provided money from its own budgets to employ a worker and the aim of a service users group began to take shape.

The 'Being Vocal' project, started in July 1990 was a local project funded by Richmond, Twickenham & Roehampton Community Health Council and the Joint Care Planning Team. The aims set for the Project Worker were to produce a report and to organise a conference. I applied for the post, but was not successful, however the Community Health Council approached me and asked if I would consider helping out with the group discussions and interviewing of users, I agreed.

A Project Group was formed by Community Health Council, Local Authority, Health Authority and Voluntary Organisations to oversee its work.

The aims of 'Being Vocal' were to provide a compendium of users' views of their first ever contact with services, through admission, in-patient life to aftercare and beyond, to using community based services.

A questionnaire was used to interview service users, along with taped group discussions. The questionnaire enabled the sharing of negative as well as positive experiences and I would just like to read out to you a few of the comments from 'Being Vocal'. First a few comments about users' worst experiences of using services:-

'Lying on the floor of the ward with my whole body in spasms because of the drugs, while being ignored or criticised by the psychiatric nurse'.

'My opinions were not significant in my treatment - there is no negotiation, it's not equal' and

'Sometimes you're not in a fit state to ask, you're in an emotional state. They just issue out the tablets and you have no idea what they are for, or of the side effects'.

And now some of the positive experiences of being in contact with psychiatric services:-

'This meant having experienced good supporting staff and getting their attention, help and appropriate treatment and care when I needed it, from doctors, nurses, CPNs, social workers and occupational therapists'.

'Staff are for the most part OK people. A doctor let me stop medication, he gave me a chance and he was quite lenient. He had a liberal attitude'.

- A few copies of 'Being Vocal' are available here today.

Once the report was finalised in January 1991, it was distributed and I was asked to present it with one of the local psychologists, to Richmond, Twickenham & Roehampton Health Authority. I believe the professionals in our locality found this a very novel experience. People were asked to consider the report as an open and honest compendium of users' views on which to act as a springboard for future decisions.

From 'Being Vocal' our locality progressed to a conference - 'Creating a Local Voice', held in November 1990. This again was the initiative of the Community Health Council. A steering group of users and professionals organised the event. The conference was specifically for users and carers only, because it was felt that some users may find it intimidating to have members of staff present. Users would be able to express their views freely.

Approximately 50 people attended. The 'Being Vocal' project survey results were presented and two users, one from Survivors Speak Out and one from Nottingham Patients Council, spoke on the subject of users' involvement.

Once there was the momentum and interest, users and carers decided to set up their own local groups. Because users and carers had different aims and objectives, it was agreed that the groups should be formed separately. The carers group decided to be a support group for each other. The users group called 'Ease Your Mind' decided they would be about user involvement and personal support. I am the co-chair of the group.

In the initial stages of setting up the users group we got together on producing a leaflet to hand out to other users to promote out aims and objectives. It was a brief introduction to the group - we also decided to have membership cards. This made people feel they belonged.

Ease Your Mind meetings take place twice a month and we meet at the local CHC offices. Our numbers at meetings range from 5-12 people and we mail out to approximately 28 people. Any tasks undertaken by group members are shared so that mutual support is given. We did experience difficulties in the initial setting up of the group regarding budgeting, we therefore decided to become a project of Richmond & Barnes MIND, although we wanted it clearly stated that we wished to retain our own identity. They have asked us, if we are going to the press on a particular subject, to brief them in advance. This so far has not been a problem.

One other problem that we came up against in the group was continuity - as we users acknowledge that we are not the most reliable of people, and it has been difficult to maintain momentum. Funding has also been difficult. We found that most organisations we approached were prepared to fund specific events, but they were not prepared to fund running costs. To ease this problem we were able to do some fund raising for ourselves. Also recently the group made an application to the joint care planning team to fund our next conference and we asked at the same time if they would be willing to put £200 towards our running costs, otherwise the group could not continue. I am pleased to say it was forthcoming.

The users group has now been running since December 1990 - we have user representatives attending community mental health team meetings and Council for Voluntary Service forums. We have also been involved in the setting up of the community care plans and a pilot workshop involving the education of society in mental health. We have yet to pierce the barrier around our local Joint Care Planning Team, Joint Steering Group, and our Social Services Committee.

The group has experienced frustrations in so far as the implementation of change takes forever. Users have been met in some areas with resentment and fear. Professionals often use language that can confuse, whether as shorthand or deliberately. Richmond, Twickenham & Roehampton Health Authority have yet to truly believe in user-led services. I have been challenged by planners and psychiatrists as to how representative I am of users, I tell them that I am as representative of users as they are of psychiatrists and planners.

Our most recent venture was a conference 'Partners in Innovation' which took place in March 1992. This event was funded by the joint finance Research & Development monies. This conference gave users, carers and professionals alike the opportunity of getting together under one roof to share ideas and experiences and also break down some of the barriers that exist. It was attended by 30 users/carers and 30 professionals and was by invitation only. For this conference it was agreed that the split in numbers of professionals and users/carers should be equal, therefore everyone attending was meeting rather more on equal terms.

It was decided to hold this conference at a comfortable venue and to have a good buffet as we felt that users are always on the cheap receiving end of services and we wanted this to be different. A Video called 'Partners in Innovation' compiled by the London School of Economics was shown and then people split into five groups to discuss national issues arising from the video; they included advocacy, work, involving users in planning, medication and talking help. The afternoon session began with a panel consisting of a user, a psychiatrist, a carer, a CPN and a social worker talking on the topic of what community care meant to them. People were then asked to go into their groups and discuss how they could personally influence working together. The day finished with the panel being asked their views on how they would like the situation to be in a years time. The day was enjoyed by all and everyone was keen to make this an annual event.

In our locality users have been accustomed to being parented by services, therefore user involvement is a whole new venture for them. They have found it quite difficult to adjust to the idea of user-led services and having their voices heard.

Some professionals appear to have been in a comfortable rut and are not used to being challenged - especially by a user!

Perhaps by attending meetings and by being a representative I myself can go some way to challenging the stigma attached to mental illness/and yes, I do feel it is an illness.

On a more personal note I feel that it is the responsibility of users and professionals alike to overcome their differences and work together to provide a healthier environment and attitude regarding mental illness.

Ease Your Mind as a user group has grown and developed its own style, in the absence of any paid worker; but supported by staff from a variety of disciplines and established voluntary organisations. A model perhaps we might emulate when addressing the needs-led, customer choice aspect of community care implementation.

We believe that a group such as Ease Your Mind assists in the transfer to service users, of the power to determine their own care and treatment and to be an integral part of the management of services, which after all, should be responsive to their identified needs.

Ease Your Mind by its very activities, gives to its members self-esteem and self-confidence, the ability to engage and challenge from a clear support base. By keeping those of us who are paid to manage and provide services in touch with the reality of the service users' needs and perspectives, it promotes the mental health of its own members.

45 A staff support service following major incidents at work

K. Sullivan

Introduction

There has been increasing acknowledgement over recent years of the existence and significance of stress in the health service and caring professions (Parks 1982). The effect of stress on such general psychological characteristics as work motivation and satisfaction are well documented (e.g. Hackman and Oldman 1980).

One of the earliest studies to attract attention was Menzies work on defence against anxiety, which looked at defence mechanisms among nurses as a response to stressful situations (1960). Revons (1962) examined the relationship between staff morale and patient turnover and found staff morale to be an important factor in patient recovery.

The Briggs report (HMSO 1972) made a strong plea for personnel counselling services for nurses.

George (1986) argued for NHS managers to pay attention to the need for caring for the carers and recognised a place for organised support networks.

Over the years these calls for staff care within the health service have been taken up and there is now a variety of services available (Owen 1991). These services can be seen as falling into four main but overlapping categories of staff care provision.

1. A counselling service

Usually where at least one full time counsellor is in post, offering one to one interviewing and group facilities. They tend to offer a wide range of preventative programmes for the teaching of coping strategies e.g. relaxation and self awareness.

2. Support groups

> often facilitated by external experts
> arranged for vulnerable groups
> also peer support groups.

3. Crisis intervention

> provide services following major disasters.
> distress at work
> bereavement counselling.

4. Teaching of coping strategies

> 'on going' in service provision for interested staff
> built in education programmes.

Background to the present service

The present service began with a recognition, on the part of the clinical director, of the need for some form of staff support service within the organisation.

The clinical director convened a work party to consider:
- the types of problems for which staff required support
- whether support was being provided at present
- to consider what models of service provision would be desirable and practicable.

Three main areas of staff problems emerged from the group.
> (1)Traumatic incidents at work e.g. physical assault, suicide of a patient.
> (2) Work related problems e.g. difficulties with colleagues.
> (3) Personal, family and social problems.

It also emerged that some staff counselling was already taking place. Some staff members when faced with difficulties were approaching individual chaplians, nurses or psychiatrists for assistance. However, these services were informal, very much reliant on the individuals initiative and occurred on an ad hoc basis.

When considering possible models of staff support service provisions, the group agreed a fully comprehensive counselling service would be the best and most appropriate. However, the group was also aware that, at least initially, the financial situation precluded such an option.

The group then considered what would be the most appropriate form of service provision that could be provided within present resources, taking into account the staff needs and the organisations moral obligations.

It was in this context that the idea of providing a staff support service following major incidents at work emerged.

The term 'major incidents at work' was to include incidents such as physical assaults by patients, the suicide of a patient, a fire within the working environment, etc. Any incident which was identifiable, likely to cause stress, and encountered as a result of work and the working environment.

Whilst there was strong anecdotal evidence for the need for staff support services in these areas, there were some initial scepticisms.

A search of the literature covering the area was enough to allay these.

Consider the incidence and effects of physical assault alone:

Llewelyn and Fielding (1987) interviewing British nurses found that 'violence or threatened violence from patients or relatives' was one of the most stressful areas of their work.

A survey by the Health Service Advisory Committee (HSAC 1987) of 3000 hospital and community staff revealed that 11% had received minor injuries from assault at work in the previous 12 months: Rogers and Salvage (1988) cite a recent National Association of Health Authorities report of a 47% increase in violent attacks on health service staff in some specialities in recent years.

Over a quarter of assaults in the HSAC survey took place in a psychiatric setting, the largest single category. Studies of violence specifically in this sector repeatedly show that the majority of reported assaults on staff by in-patients are against nurses (Fottrell 1980, Armond 1982, Aiken 1984, Hodgkinson et al.1985, Pearson et al. 1986). Moreover, this is not just due to the greater numerical superiority of nurses over other staff groups. Roscoe (1987) found that, while only 48% of staff in his survey were nurses, 83% of assaults reported to him were on nurses.

It has been estimated that actual levels of violence may be five times greater than official levels due to underreporting (Lion et al. 1981). Risk rates were highest for nursing assistants, charge nurses and clinical nurse managers. Managers who had reported being assaulted once could expect to be assaulted again every 19 days.

It is often pointed out (e.g. Haller & Deluty 1988) that, although this sort of violence is obviously widespread, the vast majority of incidents are classified as 'minor'. For instance, in Pearson et al.'s (1986) survey, nearly

70% of assaults resulted in no visible injury. However, any complacency is at odds with the concerns of nurses expressed to Llewelyn & Fielding (1987) above and the growing literature on the psychological consequences of trauma (e.g. Mezey & Taylor 1988).

In one of the two studies to have addressed the psychological consequences on psychiatric staff of being assaulted at work, Conn & Lion (1983) found that 'almost unanimously the victims of assault agreed that the emotional impact of having been attacked far exceeded the impact of physical injury'. This emotional impact sometimes resulted in symptoms resembling those of post-traumatic stress disorder (PTSD)-insomnia, eating disturbances, anxiety, an exaggerated startle response, etc. Other work-related responses included fear of working with dangerous patients, anger at the aggressor leading to conflict with the 'caring' role, guilt and self-doubt about the incident and their competency.

Lanza (1983) surveyed nurses who had been assaulted at work. Most often they reported 'minimal' reactions to the incident (which Lanza felt reflected an element of denial). However, many remained preoccupied with the incident itself and their feelings of self-blame and somatic reactions over the long term. These effects were not overcome quickly for the majority; 65% took more than a week to recover from the incident, and 28% had not fully recovered within 24 weeks. Nearly half lost time as a result of the assault and some thought of a different career.

Whittingham, R. & Wykes, T. (1992) interviewed 24 psychiatric workers who had been assaulted and twice more within two weeks of the assault.

Some of these subjects reported high levels of strain which persisted well beyond the incident, while four subjects reported symptoms that would have been consistent with a diagnosis of post traumatic stress disorder.

It is important to note in their admittedly small study, that nearly all the assaults resulted in no apparent physical injury to the victim. They were the sort of 'petty' violence which many psychiatric nurses are subjected to on a very frequent basis and which they themselves often dismiss as insignificant.

An outline of the service

Aims

The aim of the service is to offer an accessible, available, confidential, high quality and immediate staff support service to staff who experience major incidents at work.

The service is pro-active and offers short term support. If further help is agreed to be appropriate, assistance will be given to identify and arrange it.

Personnel

The service consists of 12 voluntary counsellors who were recruited from across the organisation. They were chosen for their experience in counselling, although they are not all professionally qualified in this area. The selection procedure endeavoured to ensure a professional, geographical and gender balance to the service.

The staff are supported with regular supervision from the service co-ordinator and three monthly feedback, support and training sessions.

The service provision has been endorsed by the Board. The organisation management have agreed to allow the counsellors time to undertake the work and to provide the rooms where the counselling may take place.

The information process

A series of meetings were undertaken by members of the working party to ensure that all members of staff were aware of the new service. Folded A4 information leaflets were distributed to all work settings within the organisation with instructions that they be prominently displayed and easily available. Details of the service are included in the induction programme and a leaflet included in induction information packs so that all new staff will be aware of the service.

Service procedure

The service procedure is as outlined on Fig.1.

(A) Once a senior manager, e.g. an assistant director of nursing services, has been informed of an incident in their area, e.g. a physical assault on a staff member by a patient

(B) They take three courses of action within 24 hours

(1)They ensure that the staff member is aware of the Staff Support Service. They ensure that they have a copy of the leaflet and attached to the leaflet is a copy of the counsellors' names, work place and work phone numbers.

(2)A member of the Staff Support Service is informed of the incident and the names of those involved.

(3)Where appropriate, the line managers of other areas are told of the incident, e.g. if a domestic worker was involved in an incident the domestic services manager would be informed so that they could ensure their staff were aware of the service.

(C)The staff member is then able to choose a counsellor from the list if they wish.

(D)A member of the Staff Support team will contact the staff member within 48 hours to ensure that they are aware of the service and to remind them that they can use it now or at a later date if they wish.

In the event of support being needed on an emergency basis out of hours, the home numbers of the counsellors are available in the Hospital Co-ordinator's bag.

Service monitoring

As this is a confidential service, the names of those seeking contact with the counsellors are not kept. A minimum amount of information to monitor the use of the service is however collected.

Each counsellor fills in monthly returns on -
- the number of initial contacts
- the number of subsequent contacts
- the nature of the incident
- the profession of the persons involved and who made the referral

These figures are compiled and reviewed quarterly in the Training Session.

Use of service

Statistics for the first six months of the service are available and are as follows:

No of initial contacts	44
No of subsequent contacts	50
Nature of incidents	
Work based problems	41%
Work and home based problems	18%
Family/home problems	9%
Major incidents	32%
Professional referred	
Nursing	95%
Administration	5%
Who referred?	
Nurse management	41%
Self referral	59%

There has been no consumer satisfaction survey undertaken to date. However, the anecdotal feedback has been very positive.

STAFF SUPPORT for MAJOR INCIDENTS at WORK

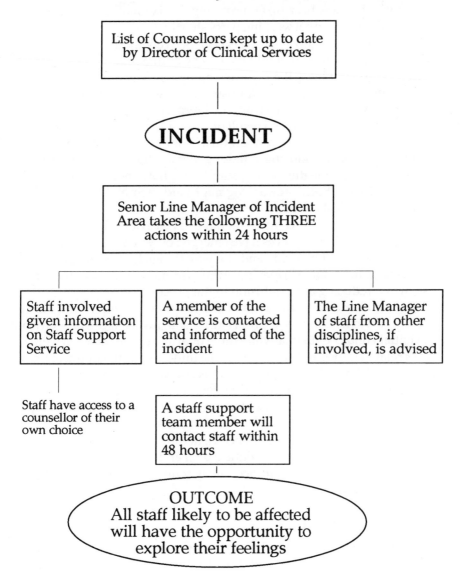

Figure 1 The service procedure

Future service development

The service has now been up and running for six months and is due to be reviewed by the original working party shortly. Overall the service seems to have been well received and has been actively used. However, there are a number of issues that will have to be addressed.

On a peripheral level the service's name will have to be considered. Some staff members have been unsure as to what constitutes a 'Major Incident'. Also the evidence from the literature suggests that traumatic responses may also occur as a result of 'minor incidents' and perhaps we should ensure the service reflects this. Along these lines perhaps we should consider introducing a more general educational aspect to the service, possibly a leaflet letting staff know how they may feel after a violent incident. Such prewarning might aid their ability to cope with such psychological effects.

The service access procedure will have to be reviewed. As the service has got underway differences have emerged between the envisaged way the contacts would be made and the way things have gone in practice. Efforts need to be made to maximise the ease and efficiency of the service use, while reducing any confusion in the process.

More fundamentally the review will have to consider whether the present service is the most appropriate for staff needs. It can be seen from the initial contact data that while three quarters of the referrals were for work related issues, only one third came under the initial target of 'major incidents'. The review will have to reflect on whether the service should be broadened or whether more than one service is necessary.

Perhaps in the light of the use staff are clearly making of a staff support service, we may even review the financing of such a service.

Whatever the outcome this has been a helpful 'first shot' at providing a focused staff support service. Future data and review should allow the service to be modified to more accurately reflect the needs of staff within the organisation.

Acknowledgement

I would like to acknowledge the hard work, enthusiasm and commitment of the members of the Staff Support Development Team and the Staff Support Service Counsellors whose efforts have enabled this paper to be compiled.

References

Aiken, G. I. M. (1984). Assaults on staff in a locked ward: Prediction and consequences. *Medicine, Science and the Law*, **24**, 199-207.

Armond, A. D. (1982). Violence in the semisecure ward of a psychiatric hospital. *Medicine, Science and the Law* **22**, 203-209.

Conn, L. M. & Lion, J. R. (1983). Assaults in a university hospital. In J.R. Lion, & W.H. Reid (Eds.), *Assaults within Psychiatric Facilities*. Orlando, Florida:Grune & Stratton

Fottrell, E. (1980). A study of violent behaviour among patients in a Psychiatric hospital. *British Journal of Psychiatry*, **136**, 216-221.

George, J. (1986). Needed - care for the carers. *Health and Social Service Journal* **96**, (1).

Hackman, J. R. & Oldham, G. R. (1980). Word redesign, Reading, MA,: Addison-Wesley

Haller, R. M. & Deluty, R. H. (1988). Assaults on staff by psychiatric in-patients: A critical review. *British Journal of Psychiatry*, **152**, 174 - 179.

Health Service Advisory Committee (1987). *Violence in staff in the Health Service*, London: HMSO

Hodgkinson, P. E., McIvor, L. & Phillips, M. (1985). Patient assaults on staff in a psychiatric hospital: 2 year retrospective study. *Medicine, Science and the Law*, **25**, 288 - 294.

Lanza, M. (1983). The reactions of nursing staff to physical assault by a patient. *Hospital and Community Psychiatry*, **34**, 44 - 47.

Lion, J. R., Snyder, W. & Merrill, G. L. (1981). Underreporting of assaults on staff in a state hospital. *Hospital and Community Psychiatry*, **32**, 497 - 498.

Llewelyn, S. P. & Fielding, R. G. (1987). Nurses: Training for new job demands. Work and *Stress*, 1, 221-237.

Menzies, I. (1960). *A case study on the functioning of social systems as a defence against anxiety in human relations*. London:Tavistock.

Mezey, G. & Taylor, P. J. (1988). Psychological reactions of women who have been raped: A descriptive and comparative study. *British Journal of Psychiatry*, **152**, 330 - 339.

Owen. G, M, (1991). *'Taking the Strain'*, *stress, coping mechanisms and support networks*. National Association for staff support, 9 Caradon Close,

Woking, Surrey.

Parkes, K. (1982). Occupational stress among student nurses: a national experiment. *Journal of Applied Psychology,* **67**, 784 - 796.

Pearson, M., Wilmot, E. & Padi, M. (1986). A study of violent behaviour among inpatients in a psychiatric hospital. *British Journal of Psychiatry,* **149**, 232 - 235.

Revans, R. (1962). Hospital attitudes and communication. *Sociological Review* Monograph 5.

Rogers, R. & Salvage, J. (1988). Nurses at risk. A guide to health and safety at work. London:Heinemann

Roscoe, J. (1987). *Survey on the incidence and nature of violence occurring in the Joint Hospital.* Unpublished report to the Working Party on Violence. Bethlem Royal and Maudsley Hospital Special Health Authority, London.

Whittingham. R, & Wykes, T. (1992). Staff strain and social support in a psychiatric hospital following assault by a patient. *Journal of Advanced Nursing,* **17**, 480-486.

46 The promotion of mental health: Fallacies of current thinking

D. Trent

The promotion of mental health is difficult at best. We are constantly enjoined to promote mental health within our given communities with little or no guidance. Frequently we are levied with the task as an additive duty to the other bits and pieces which we are required to do during the course of the day. We are told that it is important but we are expected to 'get on with the job' with little more than moral support.

Part of the difficulty that many of us experience is due to one of two problems. The first is the way in which we define mental health. The second is the manner by which we then attempt to promote the concept of mental health.

Definition in absence

The primary difficulty in promoting mental health is due in no small part to the lack of any reasonable definition of what mental health is, within the professions and the general public at large. Keith Tudor speaks frequently of the varying definitions which have been attempted to encompass the concept of mental health. These range from '...the ability to live happily...' to '...socially considerate behaviour...' The vast majority of the attempts to define mental health are positive and tend to focus on the strengths of the individual.

Unfortunately, within many of the areas dealing with mental health and mental illness, there is still the assumption that mental health is the absence of mental illness. A brief excursion into any one of our cities, towns or villages will immediately show that clearly anecdotal evidence

561

suggests that the general public continues to hold this view.

It is easy to see why. Mental health and mental illness are self-defining as medical assumptions by the use of the terms health and illness. Since the purpose of medicine is to cure illnesses, then health becomes the absence of illness. The two become inextricable linked to each other. As the old song says, 'They go together like a horse and carriage.'

If mental health is defined as the absence of mental illness, either directly or by implication, it is impossible to think of mental health without thinking of mental illness. It is rather like defining your left hand as being similar to but somewhat different from your right hand. It would be impossible to explain the idea to someone who had no hands and had never seen a hand what a left hand was like without describing in some detail what a right hand was like.

The difficulty can easily be demonstrated. Close your eyes and imagine, if you will, a rablotz. In order to do so, you need to have some idea of what a rablotz is unless you have already seen one. This may be difficult since, to the best of my knowledge no such item exists. So let me define a rablotz for you in some detail. It is approximately twice the height of a siblotz and almost half again as long. It has twice the number of curves, but they are all at the opposite end of the main spine. The legs are shorter and the colour is somewhat darker than a siblotz. In fact, in many ways a rablotz looks like a slightly altered mirror image of a siblotz.

Now you can begin to see the problem. Until you know what a siblotz looks like, you will have no idea of what a rablotz looks like. This is because one has been defined based on the other. If I define mental health as the absence of mental illness, I must have a knowledge and understanding of mental illness in order to understand mental health.

The concept

The concept of mental health as the absence of mental illness is easily understood. The idea of a straight line continuum with health at one end and illness at the other is easily conceptualised by most people. It also dichotomizes mental health and mental illness. Anyone who has studied cognitive processes is aware that if I can group information into convenient and easily defined boxes, it makes understanding the information far easier. This is one of the underlying concepts of statistical analysis. I can easily identify and understand the concepts of black and white, while it may be more difficult to either identify or understand the conceptual difference between two shades within a wide range of greys. The assumption of 'us' and 'them' has been the basis for many of our sports as well as nationalism and most of the wars throughout history.

We all use this process and can recognise it in processes such as stereotyping. By grouping people or things together based on one or two characteristics, we can allow ourselves to weed through a great deal of information in a very short time. Needless to say, when we group information in this manner we lose a great deal of the richness of the group which we are focusing on and can frequently jump to conclusions which are unsupportable.

By fitting information into stereotypes, however, we will often make comparisons whether they are valid or not. In many ways, mental illness has fallen victim to this practice and has suffered greatly from it. Mental illness is frequently seen in the same way as an unwanted pregnancy. We did not plan for it, but it must be dealt with and hopefully we can do so without the neighbours finding out about it. I may sympathise or even empathise with Aunt Martha, but I still may not wish to discuss it outside the family or with the children.

I may also use the comparison to establish my own sense of mental health or illness. I may not know where I am on the line, but I still may tell myself that I am farther toward the health end than you are.

There is another problem with the idea that mental health is the absence of illness in addition to the ease with which we can create errors in judgement and comparisons. By creating health as the absence of illness, it tends to 'professionalize' the idea of mental health. It becomes a concept that is not available to those of us walking along the street or leading 'normal' lives.

I remember seeing a cartoon in *Punch* a few years ago which showed a man walking out of a psychiatrist's office. (It's always a psychiatrist, isn't it?) The man's shoulders were slumped and his face showed a sad expression. He obviously was not happy. The Psychiatrist was leaning out of the door and was speaking to the departing man. The caption read, 'Now Mr. Jones, don't go trying to cheer yourself up. These things are best left to us professionals.'

I have found over the years, however, that while almost everyone is interested in psychology at some level, not everyone wants to be a psychologist. There are many people who do not want to study psychology as an academic pursuit. They want to know more about themselves and their friends and how and why they do what they do, but they want to do other things with their professional lives. If a person had to be a professional psychologist in order to be happy, there would not be very many happy people in the world.

563

A 'no win' situation

The second problem is that if we define mental health as the absence of illness, then the only way we can be healthy is to be missing something. We cannot, in theory, *gain* mental health since it is the *absence* of illness. We can only lose mental illness. While this may be a subtle distinction and may be seen only as a manipulation of words, it does have a large impact at the implication level.

It places us in a very subtle 'no win' situation. I have to lose to win. It also suggests at a very subtle level that since health is the absence of illness, I have to do something to be healthy. Illness, then, rather than health, is the natural state of the individual. I must not only do something to become healthy, I must do something which will cause me to lose something. I have no place to go. If I do nothing I am ill. If I do something, I am forced to get rid of something. Either way, I will lose.

It also fits our cultural assumptions. I am told not to be selfish, to give is better than to receive. I am told to think of others first, not to brag. Pride is one of the seven deadly sins. In short I am told not to consider myself and not to do for me. Yet if I am to be healthy I must do something, and that is ultimately centred on me. Now I am in violation of all of the cultural injunctions against selfishness.

While I recognise that this is a very concrete way of framing the concept of mental health, it is important to remember that the very people who need most to take a more flexible view are frequently those who are least likely or able to do so. You or I probably do not think this way on a day to day basis. We are more likely to ignore the idea altogether. We will put it out of our minds. It will, like mental illness, approach the realm of taboo. It will be far easier to use mental health as a replacement term for mental illness.

Health promotion

If the problem, then, with definition of mental health is fraught with subtle minefields, the difficulty in promoting mental health is even more difficult to traverse. Again here we get bound up in subtleties. Health promotion and mental health promotion in particular is frequently seen as determined by the degree of prevention or intervention required.

Primary prevention is aimed at those who are seen as fairly stable and well. They make up the vast majority of what we may see as the general population. They are able to cope with their worlds and seldom, if ever, come into contact with the mental health services. When they do, they frequently do so in an ancillary manner. This section of the population is unlikely to require much more than just information.

Secondary prevention is aimed at those within the general population who are deemed to be at risk. These are individuals who could be described as having sub-clinical disorders or who are exposed to stressors or environments which may overpower their ability to cope. Individuals within this group are seen as having increased likelihood of experiencing mental difficulties and have an increased likelihood of entering the mental health system.

Tertiary prevention is targeted at those who are actively experiencing difficulties beyond their ability to resolve on their own. It is what is commonly referred to as the ill sector of the population. This sector requires support and help in getting through their day.

It is readily seen that these are not discrete categories, and that movement between categories is likely to be the rule rather than the exception. Most of us will agree with those assumptions and the use of the primary, secondary and tertiary terms. The problem for mental health promotion is similar to the idea of defining mental health by the presence or absence of mental illness. We are defining what we do based upon the health or illness of those at which we are aiming our efforts. This can only lead to difficulties similar to those we have experienced in separating mental health and mental illness. We are attempting to qualify what we do based on criteria outside the limits of our efforts. It might be more helpful to focus on what we are doing rather than defining what we do by the anticipated outcome.

We can continue to use the same terminology, albeit I would tend to use it in reverse order. We can continue to argue that there are three levels of mental health promotion. Instead, however, of arguing that they are targeted at three different populations or that they are designed to accomplish three different goals, they can be seen as three different methods designed to accomplish the same goal, that is to improve mental health within the population at large.

Primary mental health promotion

Primary mental health promotion focuses on the removal of illness, regardless of how great or small that illness is. While the two concepts are unique and distinct, they remain closely linked and any change in one will generate an effect on the other. The more illness we remove, the healthier our populations become. That is not to say that they become healthy, only that they become healthier. While the two are linked, they are not the opposite ends of the same continuum.

This is currently being done. Those of us that work under the mental health umbrella are only too aware that for many years that has been all we have done. We have created great institutions over the years which have been designed to remove mental illness from our societies either by removing the illness from the individual or the individual from the society.

There is nothing wrong with removing illness. Psychiatry has been founded on the idea of removing illness. The entire profession of clinical psychology is aimed at the same goal, as well as numerous other professions. Within the UK we spend millions each year to remove illness from our patients. The removal of illness fits very easily into the medical model. It is a natural function of those within the NHS to attempt to remove or cure illness. Primary mental health promotion has been around for a while now and although we have not always gotten it right, we have, for the most part, had the very best of intentions. While the cost of primary mental health promotion is significant, it is a cost that most of us feel is well worth paying.

Secondary mental health promotion

Secondary mental health promotion has come into its own over the past few decades. Secondary mental health promotion includes the targeting of skills and knowledge deficits. It is aimed at helping individuals to improve the quality of their lives not by removing illness, but by teaching individuals skills and increasing their repertoire of usable and effective strategies for improving the quality of their lives.

Secondary mental health promotion is the most easily quantified. Regardless of the measure we choose to use, be it monetary or attendance, since much of it takes place in workshop and classroom like arenas, quantification of the results amounts only to keeping count. Records are easily maintained and information is readily accessible at most any time.

Likewise, it is the most easily monitored. By quantifying the data, it can readily be placed into numerical databases and computer or hand analyzed. Targets are set with a minimum of difficulty, and the degree to which they are met is a simple matter to determine. Because the information is so accessible, reports can be accomplished on a repetitive basis with little or no disruption to the parent organisation.

Additionally, secondary mental health promotion is the most lucrative. While primary mental health promotion is resourced from the government, or from third party sources, secondary mental health promotion is resourced from those receiving the information. That is, while few patients in mental hospitals pay for their own treatment directly, most people attending secondary mental health promotion activities pay their own way. It is money which is additional to any fiscal budget established by government. It is also lucrative in terms of attendance. For agencies which do not charge, there are great gains to be made both politically and monetarily by showing that increasing numbers of people are gaining from a given service. Budgets are increased and status and expertise are established throughout the professional circles.

Finally, because it is so easily quantified and monitored and because it is so lucrative either in monetary or attendance terms, it is currently the most popular. Courses are springing up within virtually every organisation and facility. Private organisations are establishing themselves with national coverage. There are companies which focus totally on stress management or on assertiveness training. Many of these groups have been around for a considerable period of time but are now coming into their own. Open courses are being given by established organizations such as the Workers Educational Authority (WEA) as well as by private individuals. Industry is becoming a greater and greater consumer. In many ways, secondary mental health promotion is truly the 'flavour of the month.'

Tertiary mental health promotion

The third and final form is the tertiary level of mental health promotion. Tertiary mental health promotion is aimed at trying to change the attitudes, opinions and beliefs of the general population concerning mental health and mental illness. It is concerned with trying to get the subject de-stigmatised so that it can be freely and openly discussed.

This level is by far the most difficult to quantify. While I can easily tell you how many patients I have treated or how many people have attended my anger management course, I have great difficulty in telling you how many people now think differently about mental health and mental illness than did yesterday. Likewise, I cannot tell you how great any given change was. At best, I can only look at secondary indicators over a period of time. I can begin to track how many people are using a service and how soon they avail themselves of that service. I can also look at the number of supportive public references to the subject which have taken place over a given time. In any case, the quantification of either my efforts or their results is of questionable accuracy at best.

By the same token, it is the least easily monitored form of mental health promotion. Since the results are difficult to quantify, the monitoring of any effort is extremely difficult. It is difficult to set targets and to monitor any progress toward those targets. Efforts in most cases can only be judged successful months or possibly years after a given effort has been initiated.

This makes tertiary mental health promotion the most expensive. There is little direct payback. The benefits are deeply hidden within other more recognisable parameters and are seldom seen as a benefit of the efforts undertaken. Unlike primary mental health promotion, there is little government funding specifically for tertiary mental health promotion. At best, most of it is tacked on as an additive to either health promotion or to mental illness prevention. It is expensive in both direct costs as well as in time, and yet, it is the provision of tertiary mental health promotion which will determine the future of both primary and secondary mental health promotion. Without a change in attitudes toward mental health, we will insure that we will always have an abundant requirement for both primary and secondary mental health promotion activities.

Fallacies

The fallacies of current thinking, then, are not in what we do, but in the way in which we formulate the ideas. If we leave mental health as a poorly defined concept which relies on mental illness for its validity and if we continue to focus on the illness level of the population served rather than on the service we are trying to provide, we will always have difficulty in trying to promote mental health. We will know what it is not and we will know at whom it is aimed, but we will not know what it is or how we will do it.

47 Mentally disordered offenders

I. White

Traditionally, those appearing before the Courts with mental health problems have received a less than satisfactory service, not least because of arguments over who should make the necessary provision. Criminal Justice agencies, including the Home Office, have argued that the primary responsibility lies with health providers whereas the Department of Health has taken the opposing view. The outcome has been that such a service has therefore been given low priority and has undoubtedly led to many mentally disordered offenders being inappropriately brought into the criminal justice system, and then incarcerated in prison department custody. Research from Professor Gunn in his recent survey of prison population has demonstrated a not insignificant proportion of prison inmates with mental health problems.

However, the publication of Home Office Circular 66/90 on the 3rd September 1990 provided a welcome sense of direction in terms of resolving the impasse. Its purpose was to 'draw the attention of the courts and those services responsible for dealing with mentally disordered persons who commit or are suspected of committing criminal offences to (a) legal powers which exist (b) the desirability of ensuring effective co-operation between agencies to ensure that the best use is made of resources and that mentally disordered persons are not prosecuted where this is not required by the public interest'.

It was made explicit that Government policy is that, wherever possible, mentally disordered offenders should receive care and treatment from the Health and Social Services. It spelt out the implications of such a policy for the Police, the Crown Prosecution Service, Courts, the Probation

Service and the Prison Medical Service and laid specific responsibilities on Chief Officers of Police, Courts, Chief Probation Officers and Prison Medical Officers. It also, in the annexes to the circular, drew attention to examples of good practice from around the country. Unusually, in my experience, agencies were written to about a year after the publication of the document asking what action had resulted from the publication of the circular.

Within the Northumbria Probation area, an extremely large geographical area stretching from the Scottish borders some 70 miles south and over to the west bordering Cumbria, we responded by establishing a working party to clarify our response and to determine what initiatives we should be taking. On national level, the Department of Health and the Home Office established a review of health and social services for mentally disordered offenders and others requiring similar services on the 30th November 1990 under the chairmanship of Dr. John Reed, Senior Principal Medical Officer, Department of Health. This produced separate reports from its Community Advisory Group, Hospital Advisory Group and Prison Advisory Group as well as an overview document. The Reed Committee have reported and we are currently awaiting indications as to whether or not funding is to be made available to translate the good intentions into reality and I briefly refer to the current state of discussions towards the end of this paper.

Within Northumbria the Probation Service decided, as one of the smaller services with maybe relatively few axes to grind, that we would take it upon ourselves to act as a catalyst and we therefore took a number of initiatives:

a) Drawing on one of the examples of good practice detailed in H.O.C. 66/90 an invitation was extended to representatives of the assessment panel scheme in North West Hertfordshire to address a multi-agency seminar held to explore the possibility of establishing a similar scheme on Wearside. This meeting was very well attended and was characterised by great enthusiasm for the idea. A steering group was established, as a result of which a panel was established with a co-ordinator specifically appointed by the Probation Service to undertake this task. It was set up on a pilot basis terminating on the 30th June 1992 and the experiment is currently being evaluated. However, preliminary results indicate the following:

The plan to develop a true multi-agency partnership in the assessment and diversion of mentally disordered offenders (where appropriate) from the Criminal Justice System, suffered three important set backs:

i   Social Services were unable to commit any resources to the proposed scheme
ii The part time CPN post was lost in the Health Authority's round of budget cuts
iii No agreement could be reached with the local psychiatrists - around seven to eight in Sunderland - for one of their number to commit themselves to the work of the Panel for the duration of the Pilot.

Effectively this necessitated a total reevaluation of what the project should direct itself towards. The outcome of consultation with other agencies through the steering group was that the scheme should seek to improve the assessment process and should attempt to develop a model of more effective communication, shared assessments, pre-report planning, production of one joint report to the Court and, finally, post sentence joint work.

The Pilot Project began on 6th January 1992 and is currently in the process of evaluation. To date 40 referrals have been to the Panel Co-ordinator. Of these, 22 have resulted in a Social Inquiry or Panel Report being submitted to the Court. Initial findings have produced a number of important lessons to be considered by the agencies involved.

Community Psychiatric Nurses have been involved in the assessment of all cases in which reports were eventually submitted to the Court. This is a major area of new work for them. None of the local CPNs had prior experience of undertaking assessments for a Court document, nor had they knowledge of the Court system, its processes and the Criminal Justice system in general.

The Scheme operates much more effectively where an agency nominates one member of staff as that agency's representative to the panel. Evidence of this has been in the high degree of co-operation and speed of response from CPNs, psychologist and the hospital based Approved Social Worker. This has not been the case in our experience of work involving psychiatrists, where cases are allocated to psychiatrists on a number of different criteria, often depending largely on the surname and postal address of the client/patient.

The Scheme has highlighted an area of need which is still largely unmet. 'Personality Disorder' is a term with which many are familiar. Whether it is treatable is debatable and depends often on the individual clinician's own interest. In Sunderland, in a department willing to undertake such treatment, there is a current waiting list of six months. We have found ourselves in the uncomfortable position of identifying a need, discussing a treatment plan, but admitting that this cannot be delivered. This is a major frustration to Magistrates who are then left with the difficult decision as to sentence.

Overall, the scheme has succeeded in raising awareness of the needs of this client group. It has succeeded in engaging with those outside of the Criminal Justice system - particularly those in Community Psychiatric Nursing and Social Work - in undertaking joint assessments, consultation and planning. It has lead to increased awareness among Probation Officers of Mental Health as an issue in their client group and that group's pattern of offending behaviour.

We are developing the Scheme now through the award of a £10,000 grant from the Department of Health which will allow us to part fund an Approved Social Worker post which will be used to undertake pre-release assessments on those prisoners in HMP Durham who will return to Sunderland upon release. We would ideally want to extend the scheme in the other direction - i.e. pre-sentence, by undertaking in Court Assessments to increase either the use of cautioning, diversion or Section 35 remands to hospital for assessment. At this time the resources are not available to undertake this.

b) The recently established Mental Health Trust in Newcastle was approached to ascertain their interest in providing a Duty Psychiatrist Scheme to Newcastle Magistrates Court, the largest Magistrates Court in the region. As a result of an affirmative response a steering group consisting of representatives from the Probation Service, the Crown Prosecution Service, Police, Magistrates, Clerks to the Justices and Social Services Department as well as the Trust was established. It was decided to try and ascertain the scale of the problem by undertaking a survey of all those detained overnight to appear before the Court the following morning over a period of three months. Those in this category were all interviewed by means of a structured questionnaire by a member of the nursing staff from the Trust. What the service showed was that out of a total number of 663 interviewed, 12 i.e. 1 per week, was suffering from mental illness and 70, i.e. about 5 per week, had mental health problems. Those categorised as mentally ill had either recently received hospital in-patient treatment for an identified mental illness or, in the opinion of the researcher, should be receiving treatment on an in-patient basis. In general, those in this category had a major mental illness i.e. schizophrenia or a bi-polar affective disorder. Those with mental health problems suffered from a wide range of such matters either receiving treatment on an out-patient basis or could/should be referred to local outpatient services. They were not considered to have a major mental illness. In passing, one should mention that the Trust in Newcastle is currently intending jointly with another provider in the region to establish a psychiatric service to local prison department establishments. The problem that persists is that although all the agencies are committed to move forward on establishing a scheme there is no decision on funding. Finance was allocated to the Home Office by the Treasury in the Chancellor's last Autumn Statement but because of administrative problems this money has not been spent and no advice given on the basis for bids. Although the administrative problem has now been resolved, because of the present economic climate further discussions are going on with the Treasury about whether or not the money is to be released.

c) Prompted by some initial encouragement from the Home Office and more recently the Reed Committee on support for specialist bail hostels, a multi-agency group consisting of representatives of three Probation Services within the region, Health Authority, and voluntary sector providers was set up to explore the feasibility of establishing such a project in the North East. The two major issues to surface have been whether or not it would be right to establish a separate facility for mentally disordered offenders with the result of pre-stigmatisation and secondly the resource issue, whether the Home Office might make funding available and if so on what basis. Discussions are continuing and it may be that there are other options to developing separate facilities by means, for instance, of providing specialist staff in existing facilities.

I do hope that I have given you at least a flavour of how one probation area has responded to the challenge presented by Home Office Circular 66/90 and what progress, faltering though it might have been, we have made. There is only so much that a service like ours can achieve in isolation. There is a real need to work together for the good of this disadvantaged group but in the long term much depends on whether or not there is the political will to translate the good intentions of the Reed Committee into reality. If not, especially in today's contract culture, nothing much, I am afraid, will change, with all the attendant consequences.

48 Promoting the mental health of those who offer psychological help and support to individuals following a major disaster

M. Wonham

Abstract

This paper examines evidence that mental health workers, both lay and professional, who offer support to those affected by disasters may suffer an enormous affective impact. It identifies issues relating to the selection, preparation and support of individuals to undertake this work. It describes an on-going multi-agency project in Mid Staffordshire to set up and sustain an effective service for the provision of such help after a major disaster. A priority in this work is to maintain and promote the mental health of those who help others following a disaster.

Beginnings

In July 1989, Dr Chris Cooper, Medical Director of the Mental Health Foundation of Mid Staffordshire NHS Trust called a meeting to discuss providing a volunteer counselling service in Mid Staffordshire to help those involved in major accidents. The multidisciplinary group included Police, Fire and Rescue and Ambulance from the emergency services; Social Services and CEPU (the County Emergency Planning Unit) from the County Council; Staff from the Mental Health Foundation of Mid Staffordshire NHS Trust, and the Shropshire and Staffordshire College of Nursing and Midwifery and one of the Chaplains at the District General Hospital from the Health Service; British Red Cross, Salvation Army, Relate, Stafford and District Bereavement and Loss and WRVS from the voluntary sector.

We decided that a counselling service is desirable and necessary and that we would like to continue to work within a multi-disciplinary framework. We identified two necessary tasks: the development of an operational policy for this service and the recruitment and training of suitable counsellors. As many here will know from personal experience, it is extremely difficult and time consuming to get these initiatives working with so many different agencies; there are different values, expectations, management frameworks and structures and different methods of working. It was also difficult for us because the same brief was taken up by two very different groups: our group and a group based on the District Psychology Service. The two groups had different values, service principles and objectives and different models for the way forward. We tended to be very pragmatic with a rather rough and ready approach whereas the psychology group decided to work out the theoretical framework first. It was not possible to combine the two groups and so when Social Services took over the leading role and responsibility in February 1990, it was decided that clients who attended the District General Hospital would be the responsibility of District Psychology and we would provide a service to the rest of the community.

For many months we wrestled with the task of identifying issues as well as trying to resolve practical considerations and by November we felt as though we were in a log-jam. At this point I presented a paper to the group relating to the operational policy and training issues and this enabled us to move forward. Subcommittees for training and operational systems were set up and these reported to the main group in March 1991. We were fortunate in that Social Services were able to fund a number of delegates to attend two courses run by Michael Stewart from the Centre for Crisis Psychology, Four Arches, Broughton Hall, Skipton, North Yorkshire. In May and June 1991, we trained our first cohort of counsellors and included in the group several people who had attended the Michael Stewart course. We hoped they would provide us with suitable tutors and facilitators for our on-going training and preparation. We were beginning to realise that the 'helper stress' was the major issue for us to face.

Helper stress

Many individuals are affected by disasters indirectly and those who seek to help others do so at great personal cost. Popular stereotypes of helpers see them as strong and resourceful, compared with the 'victims' who are viewed as helpless and resourceless. (Short, 1979) Helpers do not expect to be at risk, they put the needs of the victims before their own needs and frequently use denial as a coping strategy. (Shepherd, and Hodgkinson, 1990). It is now clear, however, that short-term psychological aftereffects include emotional, cognitive, behavioural effects, somatic components, motivational changes and effects on relationships. Debate continues over the existence of longer-term effects. (Raphael, 1986; Berah et al., 1964; Duckworth, 1986, 1988; Taylor and Frazer, 1982; Raphael et al., 1980, 1984; Miles et al., 1984)

There is a real danger that unprepared or poorly briefed professional helpers may inadvertently add themselves to the list of casualties (Stewart, 1989). Michael Stewart, who has been actively involved in this work as a trainer and consultant as well as actually working with those who have been involved in major disasters, comments:

> *'...anyone who gets involved in the work of supporting survivors during a period of unthinkable loss and powerful psychic pain is bound to experience distressing reactions of his or her own'.*

Staff frequently experience what Stewart calls a 'mirroring reaction', mourning the potential loss of their own families and becoming suddenly aware of fragile vulnerability in their own lives. They reported being bewildered by sensations of 'waves of grief', similar to the feelings of those they were endeavouring to help. They were also distressed and surprised by the emergence of jealously and resentment among their colleagues and by acrimony between helping agencies.

Raphael (1986) suggests three sources of extreme stress:
* The close encounter with death, reminding helpers of their own vulnerability
* Sharing anguish of victims, and the close empathetic identification that often results
* Role-related difficulties.

Bartone et al., (1989) identified four major areas of stress:
* Distress of the bereaved
* Initial period of confusion associated with lack of information and poor communication
* Delay over body identification producing feelings of helplessness
* Difficulties resulting from 'identification' with the deceased and strong association with the deceased's families.

Preparation and training

Clearly it is no light matter to offer oneself for preparation to help should a major disaster occur. For this reason we ask that potential helpers should be trained and experienced counsellors (or, in some cases, individuals not formally trained but with extensive experience in counselling) who are able to reflect on their own feelings, strengths and weaknesses as well as the needs of future clients. They must be willing and able to attend additional training and preparation which will need regular updating and to receive counselling supervision. Individuals need to come to terms with the fact that they are being asked to invest considerable personal energy preparing for an eventuality which we hope will never happen.

Proper training and emotional preparation are essential; our first course was of 12 hours, spread over seven weeks. Key features were:
* experiential learning with theoretical input as required
* peer-group input which included building up a support group for later
* personal growth, 'coming to terms with the chaos within' and the external chaos inherent in disaster situations
* flexibility to address issues specific to individuals

At times the sessions were painful and tense. We were expecting anger, frustration and other negative feelings to emerge because individuals were becoming open to how they may be affected in a personal way by a major disaster, coping with what Stewart (1989) terms their 'fears, fantasies and terrors as well as their wishes and hopes about the work'. Pain, introspection and talking are the usual means by which we come to terms with and cope with terrible events. Stewart (1989) further comments,

'There can be no absolute certainty that talking about it and facing up to trauma always helps, but it is this belief which underpins the whole of counselling, and psychotherapy, allowing for some exceptions. Helpers have to look to their own survival'.

We would agree with this last remark to some degree but also feel that we as facilitators, trainers and initiators of this service have a degree of responsibility to help volunteers to consider whether they are willing and able to do this work to provide an effective framework for support with on-going quarterly meetings, facilitating peer-group support and counselling supervision. We need to ensure that the spiritual needs of counsellors are met and they receive sensitive, non-directive and affirming pastoral care. (Not everyone will wish to receive this from the Clergy and so we also make parallel arrangements with a lay-person able and willing to work with people of different faiths and none.)

The present situation

We have been asked to extend our work to cover the whole of Staffordshire and this, coupled with reorganisation of the County Council's Social Services Department, will involve further development of the operational policy. New people will be involved and we will need to take time to come to a new shared understanding of our task, our service principles, values and objectives. We already need to change and develop for there are still important unresolved issues.

Who are our clients?
- those directly injured,
- those who witness the disaster,
- those whose work involves them - the emergency services, the press, health workers, social workers and others,
- relatives and friends of all these people,
- our volunteers and other helpers,
- ourselves.

What are the needs?
- counselling those with post-traumatic stress several weeks after the event
- 'being with' relatives waiting for news ..... waiting to identify bodies
- offering support and comfort at inquests and enquiries (months and years later)

What will it be like?
- will our plans be effective when we are preparing for the totally unexpected, unprecedented event?

Can we cope with this?
- do I want to?
- can I be effective in helping others to prepare?
- can anyone?
- perhaps our efforts are better than nothing.

What if it never happens?
- is this all a colossal waste of time, distress and energy?
- how do we maintain skills, interest, commitment and emotional preparedness in a sufficient number of volunteers over perhaps years of waiting?

These are the issues we continue to wrestle with. We do it because we know it *may* happen and if it does we want to be in as good a position as possible to help people in deep trauma and distress. We know that it will be personally costly, perhaps sacrificially so, for our volunteers, and we want to protect and promote their mental health as far as we can.

Acknowledgements

I would like to acknowledge, with thanks, the help and support of Dr. Chris Cooper, Medical Director of the Mental Health Foundation of Mid Staffordshire NHS Trust.

References

Bartone, P., Ursano, R., Wright, K. & Ingraham, L. (1989). Impact of a military air disaster. *J. Nerv. Ment. Dis.*

Berah, E., Jones, H. & Valent, P. (1984). The experience of a mental health team involved in the early phase of a disaster. *Aust. NZ J. Psychiat.* 18, 352-358.

Duckworth, D. (1986). Psychological problems arising from disaster work. *Stress Med.* 2, 315-323.

Duckworth, D. (1988). Disaster work and psychological trauma. *Disaster Man.* 1, 25-29.

Miles, M., Demi, A & Mostyn-Aker, P. (1984). Rescue workers' reactions following the Hyatt Hotel disaster. *Death Educ.* 8, 315-331.

Raphael, B., Singh, B. & Bradbury, L. (1980). The helper's perspective. *Med. J. Aust.*, 2, 445-447.

Raphael, B., Singh, B., Bradbury, B. & Lambert, F. (1984). Who helps the helpers? *Omega* 14, 9-20.

Raphael, B., (1986). *When disaster strikes*, London: Hutchinson.

Shepherd, M., & Hodgkinson, P.E. (1990). The hidden victims of disaster: Helper stress. *Stress Med.* 6, 29-35.

Short, P. (1979). Victims and helpers. In R. Heathcote & B. Tong, (Eds.), *Natural hazards in Australia*. Canberra: Australian Academy of Science.

Stewart, M. (1989 February 2). Mirrors of pain. *Community Care.*

Taylor, A. & Frazer, A. (1982). The stress of post-disaster body handling and victim identification work. *J. Hum. Stress.* 8, 4-12.

49 Evaluating the Wirral Healthy Mind project: Looking at information uptake and participants' responses

R. Woodward

Abstract

This paper describes a two part evaluation of the Wirral Healthy Mind project. In part one an observational study of the uptake of information is presented. In part two the results of a retrospective questionnaire of the workers involved in the project is described. The results give data on the success of the project in terms of information uptake, and also highlight the importance of underlying differences and problems in continuing mental health promotion ventures beyond this initial stage.

Introduction

Primary prevention in mental health has several aims (Edwards, 1989):
* to foster the development of a competent community
* to design and implement early intervention for 'at-risk' groups
* to educate the public about mental health and maximise the coping skills of the community.

Wirral Healthy Mind Week was a project which focused on the latter aim. For three days mental health workers from a variety of settings, together with voluntary groups and users of services, staffed displays and stalls in a large local shopping precinct. Information on a wide range of mental health topics was available to the public, together with free 'Healthy Mind' balloons and hats. In general, little seems to have been done previously to evaluate this type of venture. This paper describes a two part evaluation of the Healthy Mind project, measuring information uptake by the public and attitudes of the workers involved.

Method

The structure of the project

Planning for the project started approximately one year before the event. A multi-agency steering committee was formed and four task groups were set up to coordinate the displays and information to be given out on a variety of mental health topics. Each task group consisted of up to ten members from various organisations and voluntary groups. The steering committee dealt with the many administrative tasks relating to the project as a whole e.g. venue, publicity, practical planning, finance, etc. Some resources to back the project were made available from Health and Social Services Departments. Attempts were also made to get resources from sponsors in the community, mostly with little success. In the month prior to the actual week, an open general meeting was held to explain the project and draw in people to staff the stands. Wirral Healthy Mind Week took place on 4-6 September 1991, in a large shopping precinct in Birkenhead on the Wirral.

Evaluation

A two part evaluation of the Healthy Mind project was attempted. The first part was an observational study of the days themselves. The second stage of the evaluation looked at the effect of the project on the network of workers involved, retrospectively.

Observational study

In this study three types of data were recorded:
* total number and type of mental health leaflets taken by the public,
* contact with the displays by members of the public,
* engagement or enquiries on mental health issues by members of the public.

Each of the four stand areas nominated an observer who recorded contact and engagement. A *contact* was defined as anyone who approached the stand, took a leaflet, balloon or hat, or read information but did not speak to a volunteer. An *engagement* was defined as someone who spoke to a volunteer about a topic. Different people acted as observers for each morning/afternoon period for each of the four stands over the three days. The data was recorded according to age, sex and enquiry topic.

Retrospective study

An important part of the Healthy Mind project seemed to be the breaking down of the traditional work boundaries and roles of the mental health professionals and users on the Wirral. To attempt to measure this, a retrospective questionnaire study was made of the people involved in the project. A questionnaire which looked at four main areas was sent to everyone involved.

* level of practical involvement
* satisfaction with involvement
* attitudes towards mental health
* the effect on likely future interaction

Results

Observational study

In total, over the three day period, nearly 13000 different leaflets on various mental health topics were given out to the public. The type of leaflet available and the numbers of each taken are listed in Table 1.

Table 1
Number and type of mental health leaflet taken

Topic	Number taken
General mental health leaflet	5600
Anxiety	1200
Depression	1100
Women and anxiety	850
Caring for Women	550
Well-woman leaflet	950
Men and stress	1200
Positive old age	500
Mental illness	200
Elderly fears	125
Local organisations description	410
`Mind' leaflet	85
Wirral Rehabilitation	45
Other local organisations	90
Total	12905

In total 3392 people made contact with stands, the ratio of men to women being approximately 2:5. Table 2 presents these contacts analysed according to estimated age and sex. The male and female contacts are given separately, but both expressed as percentages of the full total.

Table 2
Contacts recorded by age and sex

Age	Male	Female	Total contact
under 20	5%	11%	16%
20-40	8%	29%	37%
40-60	7%	20%	27%
over 60	7%	13%	20%
	27%	73%	100%

In total 2078 people made enquiries or 'engaged' volunteers staffing stands on a mental health topic. This data was recorded by sex and enquiry topic. A ratio of approximately 1:4 male to female enquiries were made. An analysis of the topics of interest are presented in Table 3. Enquiries are expressed as percentages of the totals for men and women separately.

Table 3
Enquiry topics recorded by sex

Topic	Men (% of total for men)	Women (% of total for women)
Anxiety / stress	25	25
Depression	12	11
Man's problem	13	3
Woman's problem	4	14
Family problem	2	1
Older person's query	4	6
Mental illness	5	3
Personal difficulty	7	1
Organisation (local)	5	5
Social Services / Health Dept query	6	11
Other e.g. smoking, physical health	17	20

Retrospective study

Of the 100 people involved in the project 40% returned the retrospective questionnaire. In general the highest percentage of replies came from the smallest organisations: voluntary and user groups (57% replied), health community unit (67% replied). The smallest percentage of replies came from the largest organisations: Social Services (28% replies), Health Trust (37% replied). Further analysis of the results are presented in three categories comparing Health, Social Services, voluntary and user responses. Table 4 presents some of the practical data on range and average time spent per person on the project and estimated cost. Based on these figures and the project 'cost' 233 working days in total and £23000 in personnel staffing costs, excluding the cost of all materials, displays, etc.

The data on satisfaction with involvement is presented in Table 5. In all groups, between 64% and 73% of people reported making new contacts

Table 4
Time spent and "cost" per person

	Average time spent	Cost per person
Health	22.6 hours (range 2 - 114 hours)	£273
Social Services	19.6 hours (range 2 - 96 hours)	No figure available
Voluntary / Users	9.6 hours (range 2 - 32 hours)	£190

Table 5
Satisfaction with involvement and contact

	Not at all satisfied	Fairly satisfied	Very satisfied	
Health	0	77	23	Satisfaction
Social Services	23	38.5	38.5	with own
Voluntary/Users	0	63	37	involvement
Health	18	45	36	Satisfaction
Social Services	10	70	20	with
Voluntary/Users	20	60	20	contact

in different agencies through the project and 80% to 100% of people wished to maintain these contacts. However, 100% of respondents did not report a change of attitude to mental health problems. Neither had attitudes to other professionals or users been altered in most cases. Thus only 29% of Voluntary / Users felt that their view of other mental health professions was better. Similarly, 23% of Social Services staff and a slightly higher percentage of Health Department staff (42%) reported a changed view in a positive direction.

In the future direction part of the questionnaire, 100% of respondents felt the project should continue in some form. However, assessment of the actual achievement of the project varied. 56% of voluntary workers and users felt the project achieved its goal, compared with 95% of Social Services replies and 100% of Health Department replies.

Discussion

One of the aims of Healthy Mind Week was to attempt to educate the public about mental health. The results of the observational study suggest that this aim was achieved, at least in part. Many thousands of leaflets on key mental health topics were given to interested members of the public, with anxiety, depression, women's health and men and stress being particularly popular. The more traditionally stigmatised areas of mental illness such as schizophrenia and the elderly, attracted less interest. Between six and seven hundred leaflets on different sorts of local self help organisations and user groups were also given out. How this information affected the attitude or coping skills of those who read it, was not assessed.

The project did attempt to attract the interest of younger people. Balloons, cartoons, youth theatre, disco and an opening by a local television personality were all part of the event. Despite this, only 16% of contact was by the under 20 age groups. The 20 to 40 and 40 to 60 age groups were all more willing to approach the stands and take information. This may reflect several factors e.g. timing of the project during the day in school terms, sex and age of workers, unwillingness of young people to involve themselves in discussions about mental health. Similarly, men were far less willing to approach or engage than women. However, the percentages of men and women who were interested in anxiety, depression, physical health, etc., were the same. Men were most willing to engage about mental health topics, if focused on something they related to directly e.g. physical health, men's problems etc. These results might suggest that following up this general blanket approach with some more focused contact aimed at specific groups and topics might be appropriate, particularly for young people and men. Specific talks or contact with work places, youth and community centres would be worth considering, to increase the involvement of young people, men and ethnic minorities in a dialogue about mental health.

The retrospective study gave some interesting, if limited results. All groups were potentially equally involved in the setting up and running of the project. However, differences emerged between these groups in the amount of time spent, satisfaction and attitudes expressed. Paid mental health workers on average spent more time on the project, using both work and personal time. Volunteers and users of services spent about half the average amount of time and reported feeling less satisfied with the project as a whole. This might reflect a number of factors, including possibly, a feeling reported by some users of services, that their involvement in the project was 'cosmetic' rather than essential. Volunteers and users of services also commented that they were working purely in their 'own time', not as paid working time. Other possibilities include difficulties with the organisational set up of the project. Task groups were based on informal committees. Volunteers and users again reported feeling less familiar or at ease with this format and so tended to remain a little outside the structure, feeling less able to contribute. There were also indications that members of large organisations did not always feel completely satisfied either. For example, 23% of Social Services staff involved, reported not being particularly satisfied with their involvement. It may also be of note that this group had the lowest return rate of questionnaires anyway, in comparison with users of services and the smaller community health unit, where reply rates were higher.

Replies relating to future prospects were unanimously positive, with 100% of respondents feeling that the project should continue in some form. Despite this, nearly a year on from the Healthy Mind Week, no further plans have been made by the group as a whole. There are many possible reasons for this, including the possible 'burn-out' of the small numbers of workers on the steering committee who masterminded the project. They contributed extremely high levels of work time and personal time, which would be very hard to maintain. Clearly, continuing the project requires sustained leadership from one of the existing team, or someone else, which without specific resources, is difficult to achieve. After the project people tended to return to their original well defined professional or voluntary camps, without the force of a high profile, focused 'fun' project to overcome such barriers. Perhaps, paradoxically, the lack of resources initially, allowed traditional arguments and differences to be dropped temporarily and the project to develop at all. However, to continue, resources are needed and long established differences and problems of multi-agency cooperation again become of significance.

Conclusions

Wirral Healthy Mind Week was a very successful multi-agency initiative which promoted interaction with the local community on mental health issues. The evaluation has shown the success of the project, but also highlighted the gaps in attempting a broad spectrum project. Some groups, such as young people, men and ethnic minorities tended to be less willing to engage in this type of approach. Ideally, specifically focused initiatives with these groups in the community would enhance the broad spectrum of a general mental health week.

The retrospective study gives some indication of the effect on workers. In general, paid workers from medium-sized organisations gave most time and felt most involved and satisfied. Members of larger organisations, although equally involved, reported less satisfaction. Perhaps, interestingly, users of services and voluntary groups seemed very committed in terms of response rate, but also reported slightly more cautious negative results. They felt able to contribute less time, felt less satisfied and less optimistic about the true success of the project.

The lack of continued work on the Healthy Mind project, to date, might suggest that some of these underlying differences, although bridged temporarily, need real solutions before positive mental health initiatives can become an integral part of the community as they should be.

Acknowledgements

This paper would not exist without the help of the other steering committee members of the Wirral Healthy Mind project, particularly Irene Findlay, Derek Farrell, Linda Jones, Mary O'Malley, Bev Dingle and Neil Grice. Thanks are also extended to everyone who completed questionnaires and participated in the project as a whole.

References

Edwards, G. (1989). Finding the Broad Street pump: Primary prevention in mental health. *Changes*, **7** (2), 61-64.

50 Promoting mental health

A. Wylie

Introduction

The promotion of physical health is dependent on a number of factors, but one significant factor is the individual's ability to manage and accept change. (Personal, social, occupational, environmental, etc.), and to be sufficiently motivated and skilled to make behavioural changes when appropriate.

The promotion of mental health is possibly linked to the acquisition of skills necessary to anticipate and manage change. The experience of change and the consequences of change will be both varied and unique for each individual.

Promoting mental health, therefore, lies not in the problem solving case study scenario, although that has a place, but in the development of skills, by the individual, others involved and organisations.

It could be argued that promoting mental health will play a part in preventing mental illness and reducing the effects of mental illness.

However, I would suggest that promoting mental health should be done for its own sake, and not solely for the expected benefits in reducing mental and physical illness.

While people are experiencing change in transition, they may be seen as more vulnerable in terms of mental illness, but it may be that change was merely the catalyst for an illness that was sooner or later going to manifest itself.

In preparing the courses for the promotion of mental health, I moved away from medical models and developed Educational Life Skill models.

The skills incorporated into the courses, to various degrees, were:

* Relationship skills
* Inter-personal skills
* Acceptance of loss
* Communication skills
* Time and stress management
* Conflict management
* Assertiveness
* Listening skills

Defining mental health

Few people have attempted a definition of mental health, but with definitions of health, one can find some references to mental health. Dufos (1990) suggests that health in total, is related to the ability of the individual to function in a manner acceptable to himself, and to the group of which he is a part.

What is acceptable is a variable. The Human Trait makes medicine a philosophy that goes beyond exact science. Mankind is made up of independent individuals with free will. New urges will develop and result in new problems requiring new solutions. Human life implies adventure - adventure brings struggle, risk, danger and excitement. Also the dignity of mankind is such that according to Dufos (1990), we will value certain ideals above comfort, and above life itself at times.

Reaching a state of mental well-being

Most people, who are not deemed mentally ill, will experience periods in their life when they feel anything but mentally well. Brown (1990) suggests that depression (non-clinical) is essentially a social phenomenon, as some societies experience this more than others. Those societies where depression is experienced, have many factors contributing to this phenomenon, such as:

1) Deprivation and Social Class
2) Lack of intimate relationship
3) Loss of mother (death or other loss) before the age of 11 years
4) Three dependants under the age of 15 years

Brown (1990) suggests that these factors plus contributory life-events, may play a causal role in depressive disorders, i.e. they are factors influencing vulnerability, but not on their own the cause. There is a cumulative effect, and essentially they affect the level of self-esteem.

It is, therefore, an essential component of any Mental Health Promotion programme to address issues affecting/influencing self-esteem of the individual, the family, the community and organisations.

What are we doing to promote mental health?

The work of a Health Educator is varied, and a significant amount of the work relates to the promotion of Mental Well-being.

In our department we have produced booklets and leaflets, we have purchased and developed resources and we have run eight training courses that relate to the promotion of mental health. The courses have been available free of charge, (that will change) and equivalent to a one day course, to wide variety of professionals, voluntary workers, and some to the specific groups. This allows a shift in Health training from the medical approach to the multisectorial approach (Kickbush 1991). None of the courses have attempted to address mental illness, the therapy, the treatment and the management of mental illness.

The courses we provided in 1991-1992, and which we intend to continue, have the following aims. To help individuals, families, communities and organisations to achieve or maintain mental health and to offer appropriate guidance to those working with, living with, or caring for the mentally ill. All courses are based on research.

Defining mental health is a difficult task. The medical professionals have focused on the task of defining mental ill-health. Even in this area, diagnosis is difficult, treatment is variable, and families suffer from ignorance. However, the psychologists and the social scientists suggest that we are all in a state of perpetual change and transition. Some of us may be more vulnerable to mental illness during these transitions or major life changes, than others.

Our course considered whether we can improve our ability to manage change and therefore not only reduce our vulnerability to mental ill-health, but also to develop a state of emotional, spiritual, and mental well-being, develop an acceptable level of self-esteem, self-worth, confidence and assertiveness, developing client-centred approaches to mental health (Tones 1990).

    * An ability to respond and adapt to challenge

    * An ability to make and manage relationships (Nelson-Jones 1986)

The course titles were:

1) Ante-natal Education - a study day based on the findings of local research

2) Parenting courses for professionals and volunteers, jointly presented with Parent Network

3) Stress Management for professionals working with clients in stressful situations

4) Stress Management for individuals in statutory, commercial and voluntary workplace

5) Confronting Difficult Issues - Part 1 - Taboo and Fear::
   This course was offered to professionals and volunteers aiming to help participants focus on 'what is **their** problem, what is their managers/clients problem' and what can they control and what is beyond their control?

6) Confronting Difficult Issues - Part 2 - Dealing with Death and Bereavement.:
   The course aimed to help participants become more comfortable with the life event of death, and consider their role, if any, in support of their client's bereavement.

7) Preparation for Marriage. The course was primarily for couples preparing for a Christian Marriage, although the focus was on the development of effective communication as an essential foundation for the commitment of a long term relationship.

8) Drinking Patterns and Health. This course explored the development of drinking patterns and what intervention may be useful when clients' drinking is a cause for concern.

All the courses were over subscribed. A comfortable number for the courses was sixteen, with the exception of the Preparation for Marriage course. This course had four couples. Some of the courses had in excess of sixteen, with an absolute maximum of twenty-four. Subsequent courses will have a maximum of sixteen. There are physical and practical reasons for limiting the numbers as well as professional reasons.

The courses

Ante-natal education - a study day based on local research

The findings of my research on Consumers' Assessment of Ante-natal Education, demonstrated a need for more exploration on the emotions and feelings surrounding pregnancy, labour, childbirth and breast feeding. Whilst the educators impart facts with confidence, parents felt a need for more emotional preparation. Fathers were frequently excluded both physically and by implication. Issues around sexuality, the new relationships and self-esteem were not addressed. The findings of my research were similar to the findings of an HEA research project. The course presented the participants with some new ideas and resources based on the recommendations of my report, followed by group work looking at three different scenarios.

  a) The challenging and enquiring group of expectant mothers and fathers in an affluent area, - an evening session.
  b) A group of Asian women, in the final stages of pregnancy, and full of fears regarding procedures, presence of men, and other fears not easily expressed - a morning class.
  c) A group of young single mothers, in temporary accommodation, - an afternoon session.

The tasks were to plan an hour's session, to define needs, aims and objectives, and methods of evaluation.

For many health professionals and others working as ante-natal educators, this was an innovative approach, but ante-natal education is controlled by the Director of Midwifery. She feels that midwives are 'doing a good job' and only two midwives attended the study day. The other participants were health visitors, a GP (we had PGEA approval), obstetric physiotherapists and NCT tutors.

The birth of a child is a major change, both emotionally and physically, it is a unique event. To help parents to meet the challenges of this event, educators must consider their needs, rather than the physical and physiological nature of the event if they offer 'Ante-natal Education'.

Participants found the study day:

Practical	70%
Well structured and organised	90%
Recommended to colleagues	100%

Comments from participants:

Those who felt it offered them personal development	40%
Those who felt they gained practical and professional skills	60%

A number of participants experienced personal development and felt they gained practical skills.

My comments on this day:-

Health Professionals have been trained to be didactic, to impart information to give advice. To expect them to change dramatically is unrealistic. They, as individuals need training days to develop skills in dealing with emotional issues which may threaten them, make them feel vulnerable and conflict with their own personal values.

Parenting course - a study day for professionals and volunteers jointly with Parent Network

My colleagues are very involved in the issues around Parenting Skills, how and what professionals advise, how and what problems parents present to professionals and others. The relationship of parent and child is one that is in a constant state of transition, where the health professional input has been about physical needs. Parents' ability to deal with difficulties, everyday demands and their responsibilities, is varied and influenced by many factors, but particularly by their own experiences. If their own experiences were inappropriate, they need to learn skills to deal with the issues. Parents also have needs, and their needs have to be acknowledged, although they may not always be met.

The study day explored the above statements and asked, what is a family? The conventional family is alive and well, but within our society there are many different models of family life. Parenting skills need to be developed within the context of the particular model of family life for that parent, without being judgemental about the structure of that particular family.

My particular interests are in the final stages of parenting - the management of change from parent - child relationship to parent - young adult son or daughter relationship. In this area of parenting, the skills needed are listening, acceptance, trust and flexibility. The final part of the day was a communication task. The participants discovered how difficult this was, and how easily misunderstandings occur. Some key points were made surrounding the 'ownership of feelings'.

The course was attended by Health Visitors, teachers, social workers, and volunteers with Parentlink and Homestart.

Participants found the day:-

Practical	72%
Well structured and organised	90%
Recommended to colleagues	100%

As all the participants were parents they all felt the course offered them some personal development.

The majority felt they gained practical and professional skills.

However, 2 participants felt that the day was exploratory and thought provoking, but they had wanted a more practical approach.

- A problem solving approach.

My comments on this day are as follows:-

We don't like being challenged on our own ability as a parent. Those present could see where their clients could improve their skills as parents, but felt vulnerable when they examined their own skills and experiences

594

of parenting. This helped participants develop empathy. If we start well, then we can develop our parenting skills. If things have gone wrong, 'repairing relationships' is very challenging and the question is 'can the relationship be repaired, or is it necessary to build a new one?'

What arose out of this day, was a reminder that a good parent-child relationship was likely to promote the mental well-being of parent and child, a poor relationship based on power, dominance, and control would expose the child and the parent to mental distress both short-term and long term.

Stress management for professionals working with clients in stressful situations

This course was considerably oversubscribed, so it was repeated within a few weeks. The majority of professional and voluntary care workers have clients in stressful situations. The professional has the skill to deal with the physical needs of the client, but may frequently find the client's stress and the family's stress are a cause for concern.

The course aimed to help the professional define stress, help the client explore the causes, and consider relevant methods of coping. The possibility of preventing some of the stress and communicating more effectively is also explored. The day takes the form of a stress management day for the participants in order to develop empathy with their clients, and then case studies, based on participants' experiences, are worked on. Can the principles of stress management be applied?

The focus was educational and skills based. No attempt was made to provide skills for therapy, but participants were encouraged to be familiar with local services if referrals were appropriate, to offer accurate and constructive advice as required, e.g. benefits. It was vital that if participants don't know the answers, they say so, and either do no more, or endeavour to find some information for the client.

These courses were attended by Health Visitors, Practice Nurses, District Nurses, School Nurses, Teachers, other professionals, including Occupational Nurses, those working with mentally ill clients and their families, those working with clients who have learning difficulties and voluntary workers working with the homeless and those who offer counselling to HIV positive people.

Participants found the study day:-

Practical	80%
Well structured and organised	95%
Recommended to colleagues	100%

Comments from participants:

    Those who felt the course offered personal development   95%

    Those who felt they gained practical skills   90%

My comments:

Stress management is a popular term used in clinical and non-clinical settings. By defining the course clearly to potential participants, the course met their expectations. It was developed, based on ideas and studies reported by Professor Anthony Clare, Professor Cooper, HEA stress material, and my reading on the subject during my masters course.

The course helped participants feel more confident in dealing with and accepting their own stress, which many felt was the key to being more helpful to their clients. However many felt one day was insufficient, and much more extensive study was needed. This is extremely difficult for a number of reasons and unlikely to happen in the near future.

However, I have produced a small in-house booklet on Stress Management resources and services.

Stress management for individuals

The course was offered on a commercial basis to statutory, commercial and voluntary workplaces.

None of the 10 courses run were promoted, they were all in response to general requests. Before offering the course, I discussed with management their reasons for wanting the course, and if there were any organisational issues to be addressed.

The courses were simplistic in approach, non-threatening and based on developing listening skills. The six themes were:-

    What is stress?

    Am I stressed?

    Can I cope?

    Preventing stress

    Responsibilities to others

    Where do I go from here?

I was aware that most participants in the first instance were just enjoying 'an away day' with the support of management. This in itself is part of a positive approach to stress management in the workplace.

Participants found the days:

            Practical   96%

            Well structured and organised   94%

            Recommended to colleagues   100%

Comments from participants.

These were varied and predominantly reflected satisfaction with the day especially the free refreshments made available via management.

My comments.

These courses could be run by a number of people, such as personnel officers, occupational health nurses, and training officers. The recession is not an ideal time for the development of these courses, although the need may be increased. It is necessary that the tutor manages the group effectively, to avoid any unnecessary questioning. such basic skills as listening can diffuse or avoid conflicts in the workplace.

Confronting difficult issues - part 1 - taboo and fear

This course aimed to explore some of the taboos and fears that professionals and volunteers have when working in difficult situations. A pre-course, anonymous questionnaire was sent to all course participants, and based on the returns, we considered how we would plan the day. What was most interesting from these questionnaires, was the fact that many professionals were dealing with difficult situations frequently in their work. It was an integral part of their workload, however, there was a denial of this. Somehow these difficulties were intrusions, and differed from their expectations of what their workload should be.

Professionals and voluntary workers on this course had been ill-prepared in their training, and frequently felt at a loss.

The day examined:
1) The ownership of feelings
2) The acknowledgement of difficult situations as part of their work.
3) Defining their professional role and limitations
4) Management and organisational problems - separating these from the field work responsibilities.
5) What are the problems and who owns the problems?
6) What is within my control, and what is beyond my control?
7) Verbalising exercises -
   - Opening statements when faced with situations:
   - Why am I here?
   - What are the difficulties?
   - What do I propose?
   e.g. I've come to discuss Jim's truancy, but I find it difficult to talk with the television on, and with your visitor present. Can we go into another room?

This day could have been no more than a talking shop - that would have been therapeutic, but it was a constructive and productive day.

Participants found the study day:

Practical	80%
Well structured and organised	89%
Recommended to colleagues	100%

Comments from participants.

Felt the course offered Personal development	96%
Those who felt they gained practical skills	90%

My comments.

This was, for us, a very innovative day, and I was assisted in presenting this day by a male colleague. We had felt that two tutors would be of mutual benefit to each other, as well as being able to offer any one-to one support with participants if the need arose. In the event, there were no problems and the day was very stimulating for all concerned. One comment: 'felt so much better at the end of the day, felt able to disclose problems and share issues with other disciplines'.

All participants want a follow-up day (or half day) to assess progress and they want to encourage colleagues to come on this kind of study day.

Reports from managers about all our courses have been favourable, but this one in particular, was seen by managers as 'extremely useful'.

Confronting difficult issues - part 2 - dealing with death and bereavement

This course aimed to help participants become more comfortable with the life-event of death and bereavement, and consider what role they may have with their clients. A pre-course anonymous questionnaire was sent to participants in order to design the day to help meet their needs.

The first part of the day considered the changing face of death over the last 100 years, and how our experiences of death have dramatically changed. The local Registrar gave a short presentation on the legal requirements of registration, and some examples of how procedures can be delayed.

Having dealt with death, the day proceeded with a study on bereavement. The previous evening, Dr. Colin Murry-Parkes had given a lecture in Reading and I was comforted in the fact that I was thinking in a similar way to him. Much of my reading and research made reference to his studies.

We consider the concept of 'spiritual ambiguity', the deceased, the bereaved and the course participants, and how this may influence the nature of the bereavement.

We consider the nature of the death and how that influences bereavement.

Support for the bereaved needs careful consideration, using examples from 'Good Grief', and my list of organisations, participants were encouraged to consider:

Does the client need referral? (Am I delegating, or abdicating?)

Which agency would I refer the client to, and why?

How will I know if it was useful?

We then had a speaker from CRUSE, talking about the service they provide and the training programme for their counsellors. We summarised the day, and provided all participants with:

a list of referral agencies

a folder with information on benefits

a pamphlet of helpful contacts, produced by the local Forum for Mental Health.

As a member of the Forum, I was instrumental in having this pamphlet produced.

This study day was considerably oversubscribed and very successful. Participants found the study day:

Practical	89%
Well Structured and organised	91%
Recommended to colleagues	100%

Comments from participants:

Felt the course offered personal development	94%
Those who felt they gained practical skills	80%

My comments.

The success of this course (or the need) has encouraged me to produce packs with information on issues such as Coroner's Court, benefits, and helpful contacts. We have also arranged to put this course on all subsequent training programmes, and in one part of the district, I have modified the course for 'Churches Together', in order to develop the skills of lay people in the community.

Drinking patterns and health

This course was quite different in style from the previous courses, and I did not participate in the actual day. The aims of the day were to explore the development of drinking patterns and how professionals can help clients whose drinking patterns may cause concern.

The participants were professionals from health, Probation and Social Services. The first part reviewed current understanding of what influences our attitudes to alcohol and how we develop our drinking patterns. When does use turn to misuse, and who defines misuse, was explored.

Following an alcohol free bar and lunch, participants looked at methods and styles of self-monitoring alcohol consumption, assessment of risky/

vulnerable situations and experiences of craving.
Participants found the day:

Practical	90%
Well-structured and organised	94%
Recommended to colleagues	100%

Comments from Participants:

Felt the course offered personal development	10%
Those who felt they gained practical skills	90%

My comments.

These comments are based on the presenters remarks and personal evaluation. The day was innovative, light-hearted and enjoyable - an unusual and very different approach for professionals in the Community Alcohol Services, who are normally working with people who have major problems with alcohol misuse. It helped the participants realise they may have a preventative role with the minimum of intervention and they could advise in a constructive way.

Since the course, we have produced diary cards and other support material for people who need to self-monitor their alcohol consumption.

Preparation for marriage

This course was for four couples preparing for marriage and equivalent to a one day course, but given over a period of six weeks with four evening sessions.

The course aimed to develop communication skills between couples and was broadly based on the marriage promises - what do they mean, what is the commitment?

The first session was:-

To Love, Honour and Cherish, for Better and for Worse.

Each person had a worksheet asking them about their partner, (very superficial, light questions), they then discussed together, and with the group.

The next worksheet was asking:-

What does 'for Better' mean? What does 'for Worse' mean?

They again did this individually, then compared their findings and shared some issues with the group.

The format followed each of the sessions, and the second session looked at sexuality, contraception and related issues.

Fidelity was considered at the third session, relating in the main to the breaking away from family and friends, rather than being unfaithful, although this was discussed.

Managing changing relationships with family can cause major difficulties for young couples.

The final session, was about the wedding, the rituals, the celebrations, the costs, etc. At each session, a poem was given to participants (my selection), these poems tried to reflect the theme of the session and hopefully helped couples to own and explore their feelings, rather than deny or suppress them.

Churches have increasingly been involved in planning courses for marriage, none has been presented in this way - with active participation. It is also difficult to know how useful the different types of courses are.

Participants found the course:

Practical	90%
Well-structured and organised	100%
Recommended to friends	100%

Comments from participants were all complimentary, but some added that it wasn't what they expected,

- they enjoyed coming
- 80% liked the poetry
- 20% didn't see the point of poetry (male comment)

My comment.

This course, together with a number of other Preparation for Marriage Courses are going to be discussed at Diocesan level.

There are possible ways forward in this area, but couples who experience marital problems suggested that they can't talk to each other and have never really talked.

Hence the course I did was based on developing communications skills, examining expectations, and accepting differences.

As the wedding approaches, it becomes more difficult for couples to focus on the long-term commitment of marriage, their thoughts are with wedding plans. Therefore courses need to be available some time before the wedding if potential areas of conflict are developing and need to be addressed.

The White Paper 'The Health of the Nation'

A need to concentrate on Health Promotion as much as health care.

Promoting mental health and well-being may play a significant role in facilitating the five key areas for Action and National targets, adding years to life and life to years.

1) Mental health and coronary heart disease and stroke

If, as most experts suggest, Coronary Heart Disease and Stroke are influenced by life-style and health related behaviour, then individuals needing to make changes or maintain a healthy life-style, need to have a high level of motivation to reduce Coronary Heart Disease and Stroke risks. Those suffering from these illnesses, and their carers, are likely to cope better if they are mentally well.

2) Mental health and cancers

Some cancers are associated with life-style and health related behaviour, and could be prevented. Some cancers may have a better prognosis if detected early and some cancers will remain with us, causing unpleasant side-effects during treatment, fears about ability to cope, and dealing with premature death.

The individual's and the professional's mental state will probably influence life-style change, attitudes to screening services, and the ability to deal with any diagnosis.

Knowledge alone will not bring solutions, but those who are mentally well, will be more likely to manage any life-style, change, and the death of a family member or friend.

3) Mental health and mental illness

Many patients who suffer from mental illness experience further stress as they can feel (and indeed are, in some cases) rejected. This is a problem for them and their carers.

Again the promotion of mental health may facilitate an improved understanding of the needs of people with mental illness, and acceptance of mental illness and an improved situation for carers and a respectful recognition of their burden of responsibility.

The suicide targets are directly linked to a person's mental health. A rational person who is not mentally ill, may be suicidal if they feel they are in a hopeless situation, e.g. low self-esteem, problematic relationship. How such people can be directly helped is difficult to say, but surely any programme facilitating mental well-being may potentially be useful.

4) Mental health and sexual behaviour

This area of people's personal lives is charged with emotion. Knowledge alone will not change people's ability to develop safer sexual practices. Confidence and self-esteem are also essential and these can be particularly vulnerable.

The consequences of sexual activity can have long term effects on mental health and well-being, from being extremely beneficial and satisfying, to harmful and demoralising.

Any work in this area must address mental health.

602

5) Mental health and accidents

Accidents probably bring about a change in mental health for those involved, but the state of the individual's mental health before the accident may also have been poor and may have been a factor in the events leading up to the accident, e.g. inability to concentrate, carelessness.

Conclusion

In the field of Health Promotion, medical facts and disease prevention have a part to play, however motivating people, facilitating behavioural change, and enabling people to make informed choices about how they manage life events and transitions, is arguably dependent on their mental health and well-being and there is, therefore, a need to try to promote mental health and well-being and develop ways of doing so.

It is difficult to define how useful the courses have been in the pursuit of mental health and well-being, but judging by the evaluations, they have been acceptable to the participants, and give me the confidence to continue to develop them on Education Life Skill models, modifying as necessary.

References

Bellack, A. S., & Herson, M. (1990). *Handbook of comparative treatments for adult disorders*. New York : John Wiley and Sons.

Brown, G. (1990). Depression; a sociological view. In N. Black, D. Boswell, A. Gray, S. Murphy, & J. Popay (Eds.), *Health and disease*, Scotland: Open University.

Dutos, R. (1990). Mirage of health. In N. Black, D. Boswell, A. Gray, S. Murphy, & J. Popay, (Eds.), *Health and disease*, Scotland: Open University.

Kickbush, I. (1991). Foreward. In L. Barié, (Ed.) *Health promotion and health education Module 1. Problems and solutions*, England: Barns Publications.

Nelson-Jones, R. (1986). *Human relationship skills training and self-help*. East Sussex: Cassell Education Ltd.

The Health of the Nation. (1992). Government White Paper H.M.S.O. London.

Tones, K., Tilford, S., & Robinson, Y. (1990). *Health education effectiveness and efficiency*. Chapman & Hall: London.

Section Three
PLENARY AND WORKSHOP

51 Mental health promotion in older adults

R. Barry

The session began by examining the changing definition of 'old' in society and accepted that since, for service provision, the definition is taken as 65 plus, we would have to work within that, whilst acknowledging that this definition is, in itself, ageist.

However, since much of the focus of the session was on promoting good mental health throughout the life cycle with the ultimate aim of achieving good mental health in old age, any definitions of old became irrelevant.

We looked at negative stereotypes of older people and how these become self-fulfilling prophecies, so that older people often deny themselves enjoyable experiences because they believe the stereotypes, or they are concerned that others will. For example 'You do not ride a bike at my age' 'You do not flirt at my age'. Also traits which may be viewed positively in younger people e.g. determination, strength of mind, become negative in old age. For example 'he is stubborn', 'will not listen to advice'.

Ageism, defined as 'prejudicial attitudes, discriminatory practices and institutional policies and practices' (Butler 1980) was examined in terms of how it is perpetuated in society. This is through the use of patronising terminology, negative media images of old people, negative expectations of society and the use of segregated groups and segregated housing which force older people to live unnatural existences, in isolation from different age groups (and the high levels of depression amongst old people living in A.P.H's was noted). This also denied younger people opportunities to know and mix with older people thereby dispelling the negative stereotypes. Also forced retirement, low pensions and age barriers to jobs,

605

adoption, community care schemes etc.

Factors which contribute to poor mental health in older people clearly include loneliness and isolation (Murphy 1984), bereavement and all that entails (Samaritans 1989) as well as lack of a role, negative expectations and attitudes as well as poor physical health.

Strategies to promote good mental health

These could be split roughly into four groups:
1. Political or policy
2 Life development
3. Roles
4. Services for older people

Political or policy

It was felt that a certain level of income is necessary to maintain a basic level of health, both physical and psychological and that the basic pension in this country is below that level. While money cannot buy happiness, lack of it certainly contributes to poor health and unhappiness in terms of increasing isolation and access to activities as well as basic lifestyle. So higher state pensions were considered important, but perhaps within a framework of more flexible working and retirement practices e.g. job sharing older and younger people, flexible retirement age and part time working.

It was felt that older people should have more voice in the services offered through, for example, surveys of needs/wants, which should be given higher profile, both by having older people representing themselves on planning committees, and through the use of younger professionals as advocates to lobby on their behalf. As in other areas of discriminatory practice, the ideas of positive discrimination and targeting of older people in the fields of education (both as providers and users), voluntary work, community services etc. was suggested.

Life development

To improve mental health in the long term it is important to begin early. A programme beginning in schools which would familiarise children with older people via discussion groups actually led by older people would (a) provide positive images (b) dispel negative stereotypes (c) help to integrate different ages (d) help young people to begin to think about how to live well into old age. Added to this might be discussion groups about life and death issues so that taboo subjects come out into the open thereby beginning the preparation to deal with them.

These could be followed by regular life review interviews offered perhaps by health centres to individuals or groups of certain ages e.g. ten yearly at ages 18, 28, 38, 48 etc. in which could be discussed individual needs, activities, opportunities relevant to that age group with the intention of identifying early potential sources of distress and planning against them. These might include encouraging people to take up physical and social activities which can be continued into old age, identifying skills deficits in advance and encouraging people to fill them before a crisis, such as death of a spouse, leaves them feeling incapable and vulnerable.

Health centres or educational establishments could also run sessions on how to cope with life crises, teaching people what to expect, how to cope and normalising, rather than medicalising, the experiences so that the first thought is not of medical help.

Roles

One of the sources of distress in older people is the loss of a role. In days gone by (and indeed in other cultures) older people were valued for their experience and continued to have a role in society both as workers and advisors. Increasing division of skills and family mobility has removed the opportunities for this. The grand-parent role, for example, which was once so important is denied to many due simply to lack of proximity. Various schemes were suggested which aimed to address this loss of roles.

(a) Involvement in schools, as suggested above.
(b) Mixed drop-in centres maximising the skills of older people e.g. to teach housekeeping skills to young mums instead of professionals doing it.
(c) Adopt a granny.
(d) Fostering of children by people aged over 65.
(e) Increased involvement in community services generally by targeting older people.
(f) Flexible working practices with older people maintaining some level of involvement if they want.

Services to older people

Good health in old age will be facilitated by an approach which starts in the cradle and spans the life cycle. However, for people who are already old, services are needed now to help them to live well. The over-riding theme here was that of choice. To give older people choice involves making the environment safe. For example, good street lighting, physical access to buildings, good, safe, reliable and regular public transport and community transport. Many older people are frightened to go out after

607

dark and simply cannot walk long distances so need these services if they are to have access to the social support networks which are such important mediators on the road to depression and suicide. They should have the choice of mixed housing where they can live a more natural life alongside different age groups (but also fulfilling their special needs) instead of always being grouped together in aged persons sheltered housing schemes etc. Also mixed groups both community and health, for example, assertion groups, anxiety management groups, loss groups for all ages.

Community based groups for older people are an essential means to provide support and companionship. These could be instigated by professionals but then left to be run by the people in their own homes, rather than health bases. The voluntary agencies such as Cruse and Age Concern already play an important role here but are left to do it with very little in the way of funds or professional help. Since these organisations often contain older voluntary members they are often the best sources of ideas as to what is needed but they need financial and professional help. (They also fulfil the dual purpose of providing a role for older people plus helping less able older people).

Schemes like the widow-to-widow scheme in the U.S.A. are not available here. In this, newly bereaved are contacted (i.e. it is proactive) by widows who have been through the worst of their grief, and offered support and counselling.

More practical support should be available to carers, who are often older, to ease the physical burden of care thus mitigating against the physical and psychological impact of exhaustion upon the death of the cared for.

Finally, greater training of health professionals, and particularly G.P's, who are often the first point of contact in recognising the early signs of distress and providing a point of contact and access to appropriate services.

Conclusion

To facilitate healthy ageing a programme is needed which spans the life-cycle. Starting with education in schools aiming at integration of older people back into a useful role in society and to dispel current negative stereotypes which often become a self-fulfilling prophecy. This needs to be continued throughout the life-cycle and finally supported in old age by the provision of accessible, community based services aiming mainly at promoting integration, preventing isolation and loneliness, educating all ages and normalising rather than medicalising the ageing process so that people look to other sources than their G.P. to help them deal with the distressful experiences. Whatever you may think when you are young the chances are getting better by the day that one day you will be part of it.

52 Mental health issues in relation to HIV/AIDS

S. Benn

Exploring issues around the alternative and complementary therapies in relation to quality of life when facing life threatening illness.

Terminology always features strongly in any HIV/AIDS discussion and this was a starting point, not so much in relation to specific HIV/AIDS issues but certainly defining 'alternative' and 'complementary'. Both terms were felt appropriate but the most important aspect is to accentuate the real issue which is one of CHOICE and not imposition. Allied to this must be respect for an individual's right to choose but also respect for the individual's right to choose not to choose. It was agreed that this was not an arena for complementary versus orthodox approaches to the treatment of ill health.

Looking at ill health and the needs of an individual in a holistic way was agreed to be the preferred route. The association between the effects of HIV infection on the body's immune system and the well documented research on the effects of stress on the same system was addressed.

This formed the basis of the session and agreement held that whatever choices could be offered to individuals in their quest for quality of life, **whether** immune **compromised or not**, should not only be offered but also made more accessible. This is an issue to be addressed by planners and policy-makers alike.

Finding BALANCE between an individual's needs in relation to illness and the orthodox medical interventions is both difficult and important. The facilitation to enable an individual to reach the balance appropriate to his/her needs is an issue carers need to address.

Complementary therapies have an important role in increasing confidence, giving people a sense of control, alleviating stress and improving quality of life. Debating the orthodox/complementary issue does a great injustice to both: only by being sympathetic and critical to both can we help an individual address the balance of therapy for his/her needs.

53 The Magic Shop: Applying the personal store of images in the assessment of health needs

H. Graham

This paper elaborates on material presented by the writer at the first conference on the Promotion of Mental Health 1991 which, while emphasising the importance of personal needs to both physical and mental health, challenged assumptions about the nature of such needs and the ways in which they are assessed, arguing for an imaginative approach which utilises imagery as a means of accessing, exploring and articulating unconscious needs. What follows here is an example of the way imagery can be used to facilitate awareness of personal needs and flexibility of mental functioning - two key factors in the promotion of health - illustrated with examples drawn from the writer's therapeutic practice.

Countless people world-wide have seen the film **Shirley Valentine**, based on a stage-play of the same name by Willy Russell, which has been a huge critical and commercial success. The eponymous heroine is a Liverpudlian housewife, married to a hard-working man, and with a son and daughter who have grown up and left home. Shirley spends much of her time alone, shopping, cooking and cleaning, and a good deal of it talking to her kitchen wall. It is by way of these monologues that she reveals the circumstances of her life, and many of her conflicts and concerns.

As a girl Shirley was bright, lively and intelligent but her potentials were not recognised, encouraged or developed. She rebelled, dropping out of school, and into marriage and motherhood, where she has remained. Many of her dreams and ambitions have not been realised. She has, for example, always wanted to travel, but has never been out of the country.

Nevertheless, Shirley is not unhappy with her lot, simply unfulfilled, and somewhat perplexed; as is revealed by her question: 'Why do we have so much life, when we live so little of it?'

It is clear from the reaction of audiences - from their laughter and tears - that both men and women find much to resonate with in Shirley's life, which appears to portray some universal truth. This is because it exemplifies what the psychologist Abraham Maslow (1966) described as the 'psychopathology of the average' - the ordinary state of disease - which results from unmet needs.

Needs, health and illness

Maslow viewed health in its etymological sense as synonymous with wholeness, which he conceived as being the fulfilment of all a person's needs - physical, psychological and spiritual; - and illness as an indication that important needs are being denied. In a society where illness is viewed primarily in physical terms most people recognise that if a person's physical needs are unmet they will not thrive and are likely to succumb to illness. However, the importance of psychological and spiritual needs tends to be overlooked. Nevertheless, failure to meet these needs can result in illness which manifests at the physical level as psychosomatic disorder, or at the psychological level as neuroses or psychoses. Moreover, illness is not merely a **consequence** of unmet needs but a **way** - for some people, perhaps the only way - of fulfilling them.

Illness may enable a person to say 'no' to unwanted responsibilities, avoid unpleasant and stressful activities or situations; or permit them to do what they want to , such as paint or write. It may be a way of asking for love, care and attention; or it may serve as an excuse for failure. Illness thus often provides that which a person is otherwise not gaining from life; and therefore serves as a signal for change. However, the benefits of illness may not be consciously recognised by the sufferer so its inherent meaning or message is often overlooked. Indeed studies (LeShan 1966, Soloman 1969, Abse et. al. 1974, Achterberg et. al. 1977) suggest that people who succumb to serious physical or mental illness characteristically lack awareness of their needs, are rigid in their thinking, attitudes, beliefs and behaviours, and resist change.

By comparison survivors, whether long-term hostages or prisoners of war; those who considerably outlive medical prognoses for serious illnesses such as cancers or AIDS; or reverse their HIV status from positive to negative, **unlike most people**, characteristically function in a wholesome or healthy manner, pursuing all their needs simultaneously, albeit with an implicit hierarchy of what is important in a given situation. In so doing they demonstrate both **awareness** of the situation and their needs within it, and **flexibility** in responding so as to meet those needs (Siegel 1990, Newton 1980, Achterberg 1975).

Arguably if the qualities of awareness and flexibility intrinsic to health and survival could be more widely encouraged and personal needs met in ways other than illness, much pain, discomfort and distress might be avoided. Certainly illnesses often remit or go away, sometimes quite dramatically, when important needs are met in other ways, as is illustrated in the following real-life examples. A woman's breast cancer began to regress and eventually disappeared once she 'got off her chest' the intense dislike she felt towards her daughter, which she had previously failed to either acknowledge or express. Another woman who had been profoundly deaf for many years found that her hearing was restored three weeks after the death of her husband, when she realised that the only way she had endured forty-five years of a very unhappy marriage was by 'turning a deaf ear' to his demands (Graham 1992a).

Both these women were denying their own needs and, being unaware of them, were unable to meet them. In so doing they were acting quite normally inasmuch that from early childhood onwards people are encouraged to be aware of and meet the demands of others rather than identify and act upon their own needs. Everyone is thus conditioned to believe that he or she needs what others want him or her to; and these wants are imposed through life. Most of these demands relate to gender roles, which are the bedrock of social identity.

Social roles and illness

Irrespective of nationality, race, religion or creed, - which all impose their own demands, - and so-called equality of opportunity, different patterns of life tend to be prescribed for males and females. Marriage is still the primary universal standard by which women are evaluated, and work or career the standard for men. Males are told from childhood onwards that they need to work in order to be fulfilled, and females that they need marriage and a family. Accordingly, males are expected to be 'breadwinners' and to strive and achieve in the world outside the home. They are encouraged in the belief that in order to do so they need to be competitive and assertive, to suppress emotionality, vulnerability and all signs of weakness. These traits are encouraged in early infancy and reinforced throughout subsequent development, so boys quickly learn to be self-reliant and controlled. Their aptitudes and interests are channelled into scientific and technological endeavours, into 'hard' and logical manly activities and away from artistic and aesthetic pursuits.

By comparison, females are still expected not to achieve outside the home but to confine themselves to the domestic sphere and depend on, or care for others. As babies and children their interpersonal sensitivity and emotional expression are encouraged more than physical activity, exploratory behaviour and curiosity. They are not expected to display intellect, initiative, independence, drive and ambition; and schooling generally reinforces these expectations by encouraging girls in domestic 'science', 'home economics', the creative arts and languages.

The implications of these gender assumptions for health and illness are now widely recognised. There is a marked tendency for males to succumb to certain types of physical illness (Friedman & Rosenman 1971, 1974, 1986: Kissen & Eysenck 1962, 1963, 1964, 1967, 1969). Moreover, the cultural expectation that men are self-reliant, independent and strong often results in those who are most at risk dismissing the possibility and failing to seek help (Hughes & Molloy 1990). Not uncommonly men find relief in alcohol, which is one of the few socially acceptable ways in which they can express emotions such as sadness, guilt and fear. Frequently, however, drinking leads to aggression and violence, thus reinforcing socially accepted patterns of male or 'macho' behaviour, and to both physical and psychological illness.

Women are encouraged to express emotions and weakness, to be helpless, and dependent on others, and these traits are frequently reflected in the illnesses to which they succumb (Greer & Morris 1975; Derogatis 1979; Mears 1977; Simonton 1975; Moos 1965; Moos & Solomon 1965a; 1965b). Their use of drugs is also consistent with this pattern, tranquillisers usually inducing further passivity and helplessness (Hewitt 1986). However, as women increasingly enter the same professional areas as men and are subjected to similar stressors they more frequently succumb to the same diseases and resort to the same 'remedies'.

Traditionally mental health has been seen as largely dependent on the successful adoption of the personality traits and behaviours considered appropriate to the individual's gender. This view still prevails within the health professions, with the inevitable consequence that standards of mental health differ for men and women. Whereas it is healthy for a man to adopt the characteristics or traits associated with his sex, an inverse relationship holds for women, because the 'normal' feminine traits of dependence, passivity and irrationality are not positive correlates of mental health (Broverman et. al. 1970). High levels of femininity have been found to correlate positively with anxiety and negatively with such indices of health as adjustment, autonomy and assertiveness. Not surprisingly therefore women are twice as likely to seek help or treatment for mental disorder than men and exceed the latter in psychiatric out-patient clinics and hospital wards by a ratio of 2:1. Moreover the conditions they suffer show consistent sex differences. Men tend towards conditions characterised by destructive hostility or self-indulgence, to be assaultative, impulsive and more inclined to acts of violence, whereas women show higher levels of nervousness, nightmare, confusion and depression.

From the foregoing it is easy to presume that the roles men and women play in society predispose them towards certain types of illness or disturbance. Certainly there is some evidence to suggest that conformity and compliance are characteristic of those persons who succumb to serious physical and psychological illnesses (Greer & Watson 1985; Shekelle et al. 1981, Schmale & Iker 1971; Brown et al. 1978; Gove & Tudor 1972; Llewelyn 1981). Arguably, however, there is nothing inherent in these roles that necessarily predisposes a person to illness of any kind. It is more likely to be that which is **left out** that gives rise to difficulty inasmuch that needs perceived as inappropriate to these roles are re-pressed and are therefore not expressed or satisfied. (That this is the case is certainly borne out by research on carers conducted by the Health Education Council and reported in Graham 1992b). Thus in attempting to conform to their central social roles people tend to suppress or disown features of themselves, and in so doing effectively deny much of their own nature. Having done so they are unable to articulate or act upon their needs because they don't know what they are. Moreover, the profession-als charged with assessing the needs of these people are in no better position to do so as they invariably make assumptions based on what they and society want for them rather than what is appropriate (Graham 1992b).

Rigidity in the interpretation of social roles thus tends to lead to lack of self-awareness and to problems, many of which can be avoided through greater flexibility. People who achieve this therefore tend to be healthier, more adaptable and better adjusted than those whose behaviour is stereotypically determined (Bem 1975,6;). Accordingly the cultivation of self-awareness and flexibility should be fundamental to the promotion of health.

Promoting flexibility and self-awareness through imagery

Shirley Valentine was provided with the opportunity to travel when a friend won a Greek island holiday and offered her a ticket. For Shirley, however, the much longed for trip abroad became an even more needed journey of self-discovery in the course of which she discovered and began to meet important needs that had previously been denied. In so doing she was transformed from a rather dull and dowdy housewife into a healthy and vital individual.

Unlike Shirley, most people are not given a ticket for self-discovery. Even when such a journey is free for the taking they do not know how to embark; how to begin to discover who and what they are; and what they need to become and remain wholesome and healthy. However, throughout history traditional healers have guided people on this journey through the landscapes of the self using the vehicle of the imagination which they recognised as giving expression to unconscious processes and important clues to features of the self which are normally hidden. By exploring the products of imagination, -imagery-, they were able to facilitate awareness of the insight into unconscious and unexpressed aspects of a person. In more recent times these imaginative methods have been utilised within the field of psychological medicine, most notably by Sigmund Freud and Carl Jung; and psychologists have investigated imagery as it has become clear that most leading scientists and creative thinkers of modern times have attributed their insights to this source. As a result there is now better understanding of the psychological functions of imagery. Cognitively it affords a way of representing issues non-verbally, as opposed to verbally, which is the predominant representational mode. As such it provides, quite literally, a new perspective on or way of looking at issues, and in so doing increases the range of flexibility of mental functioning, providing a new tool which greatly benefits problem solving, decision making and creative thinking. It is particularly suited to addressing issues which are by nature non-verbal - health, illness, physical processes, emotions,; - the whole complex of the self. In addressing emotions it gives rise to feelings which might otherwise not gain expression. It also promotes mental absorbtion, a key feature of relaxation, and in so doing promotes flexibility of mental and physical functioning and increased awareness - the two key characteristics of healthy functioning and survival.

While most therapists prefer to work with the imagery spontaneously produced by the individual it is widely recognised that in many instances a person's representational style may be too limited and inflexible to enable coping in a given area. In order to provide a person with a means of representation which has previously been lacking or inadequate, and which challenges his existing representational mode guided imagery is often utilised to good effect. It can be thought of as a situation where a 'storyboard' is provided for a 'movie' in the mind, which the individual casts, enacts, produces and directs himself. It can be likened to a waking dream, a process whereby a person, guided by another, creates in the imagination a new experience for himself, and in so doing can confront the contents of his personal unconscious and relate them directly and often dramatically to his problems. By exploring his own symbolism and transforming or translating it, it is possible to establish contact with the generally unrecognised aspects of himself and thus effect a healing, or integration. As guided imagery tends to be highly absorbing, it generally promotes relaxation and so preliminary relaxation procedures are usually unnecessary.

Identifying personal needs through guided imagery

For the reasons outlined above many people have inadequate inner dialogue and therefore take insufficient notice of messages concerning physical, psychological and emotional needs. The exercise which follows is directed towards the recognition of needs. It is particularly powerful and versatile, often yielding dramatic insights, resolution of problems, and personal transformation, and for this reason gives its name to the book from which it is extracted, **The Magic Shop** (Graham 1992a). This presents a series of specially focussed imaginative exercises directed to promoting awareness of aspects of the self relevant to health and illness. As in the book, the commentary which follows is drawn from the contributions of those people who have undertaken the exercise in a therapeutic context.

The Magic Shop: an exercise in guided imagery

Take a few moments to make yourself comfortable and to withdraw your attention from your surroundings and bring it to your inner self, closing your eyes as you do so. Imagine it is the late afternoon of a day towards the end of the year and you are shopping in a familiar street. It is already dark and the shop windows are brightly lit and full of vivid and colourful displays.

As you are walking along the street looking in various windows, it suddenly begins to rain very heavily, and looking about for shelter you see an opening which you may or may not have been aware of previously. You step into this opening and, having done so, glance back into the street from which you have come, briefly observing the scene there.

Then you glance down at yourself, noting your appearance, clothing, sex, age and how you feel. When you have done so, you begin to explore your surroundings, your feelings and reactions to them. Looking ahead, your attention is drawn to what appears to be a shop window. You approach it and peer in, noting what, if anything, you expect to see there, what you do see, what, if anything, you are particularly attracted to, and how you feel about it.

As you are looking in the window you become aware of a door to one side, and as you turn to look at it the door opens and a figure appears in the doorway and beckons to you. Responding to this gesture you approach the figure, noting every detail of its appearance as you do so, and how you feel towards it.

You follow it over the threshold, and the door closes behind you. The figure then communicates to you in some way that you are in a magic shop which contains the entire universe. You may have whatever you want and take it away with you on condition that you leave something in its place. The figure then withdraws, leaving you to browse around the shop. Take time to look around the shop, noting what you see or experience there, and what you don't see or experience that you might have hoped or expected to. Take note also of whatever you are drawn to, and why, and what considerations influence your choice.

After a while you again become aware of the figure urging you to make your choice, if you have not already done so, and reminding you that you must leave something in its place.

Having made this transaction, you become aware that you are being propelled towards the open shop door. You find yourself outside the shop, and the door closes behind you and disappears from view.

Take note of how you feel, and looking down at yourself observe your appearance.

When you have done so, walk back towards the street from which you first came, and then back into your present surroundings, opening your eyes when you have done so.

Commentary on the 'Magic Shop' exercise

Apart from the basic 'storyline' provided, every feature of the exercise is the individual's own creation, and as such is potentially very meaningful. The significance of some features will be immediately obvious but others may need considerable work for their latent meaning to be discovered. This is accomplished by the person relating their experience, noting the key features and their feelings about them. The listener(s), whether a therapist or other group members, may assist in uncovering the meaning of the experience by amplifying its content in various ways, such as indicating 'missing' elements of the story, or those which are only sketchily described; asking about the feelings associated with each feature; inviting associations - of words, thoughts, memories or other images - and offering their own associations and suggestions (but **not** interpretations); and encouraging the person to draw, paint, model or enact features of the imagery. Each of the key features of the fantasy is examined in this way.

The 'opening' scene

The street in which the person is shopping is usually known to the person, whereas the opening in which they seek shelter may not be. The latter may be a side-road, alleyway, doorway, subway or shopping mall, but irrespective of whether or not it is open to the sky the person invariably reports that it is not raining there, in contrast to the street where it is still raining, and that it is daylight. This is some indication that 'conscious' control of the process has been relinquished, because, were this not the case, one might expect the conditions in the street and in an area open to the sky to be much the same.

Some people immediately feel anxious on leaving the street, suggesting a fear of the novel, unexpected or unknown, and a few experience anxiety reactions such as sweating, trembling, dry mouth or goose-flesh, which indicates the effect of imagery on physiological processes. Many rationalise this reaction in a number of ways, for example as a fear of being mugged, raped or assaulted. This is in itself significant because they have produced this scenario as opposed to non-threatening alternatives, and, to the extent that they are unable to change it or its inherent possibilities, suggests a rigidity of expectation or attitude which is essentially negative. The fear may be quite unspecific, and indicative of unconscious factors that may limit ordinary behaviour just as they constrain fantasy activity. Many of those who experience anxiety will overcome or endure it, while others will be unable to do so and go no further. Were they to do so, they might well find that other features of the experience would highlight their fears, anxieties and concerns. One man was obliged to do so because a portcullis descended behind him, barring the entrance to the alleyway and preventing his return to the street.

The latter may be of interest in itself, providing insights into a person's way of life, and features of it which they may need to change. When viewed from the perspective afforded by the alley or entry these may be striking. One woman saw that her street was a blur of frenetic activity, and another described the stressful hustle and bustle of London's Oxford Street crowded with Christmas shoppers. In another instance, hindsight revealed a familiar street as it might have appeared in a bygone era, with horse drawn vehicles clattering over cobblestones.

People are often startled by the discovery that their appearance has altered. They may find that they are wearing strange or unfamiliar clothes or costumes, from earlier stages of their life or periods in history; or different cultures; items of dress they do not possess or have never owned. Their sex, age, skin colour, race or ethnic character may also have undergone change, as might their height or weight. These features are symbolic and need to be explored if their meaning is to be discerned. Notwithstanding their personal significance, they also indicate that conscious control has been relinquished. In some cases this awareness prompts an immediate reaction, often panic or fear, and an attempt to restore conscious control by censoring or directing the ensuing imagery. Again this suggests a certain rigidity in the person's mental operations or representational mode, and a dis-ease with the less rational features of the self.

It is not unusual for people to find themselves minus items of clothing or even body parts. Some, when looking down at themselves, can see no body at all. This often reflects a poor body image or sense of self; or a tendency to be excessively cerebral. It may indicate that they have a tendency to be overwhelmed by situations, and to lose themselves as a result. Missing feet and legs may indicate lack of security or 'groundedness', or their 'poor standing' in the world. These individuals may have difficulty in adjusting to new situations or change, and in establishing their personal boundaries or self in relation to the environment.

Other aspects of the setting may also be significant, especially if they promote strong personal reactions, and should be examined more closely.

The shop front

For most people the shop and its window are the most salient features of their surroundings. Shops of every conceivable kind emerge in varying degrees of illumination and clarity. Their windows may be well-stocked, or empty, featuring only a single item, or a few, some or only one of which attract attention. The contents may be clear or vague, difficult or easy to see or sense, and may give rise to various feelings, thoughts, memories, associations or past experiences. When examined in more detail it is frequently the case that the window and its contents reflect the person's wants, albeit represented in symbolic form. These may correspond to the contents of the shop and to what they eventually take from it, but usually they are totally different, reflecting the fact that what a person wants is not necessarily related to what they need. For example, a young woman who saw a window full of compact record discs, entered the shop eagerly, expecting it to be a lively, noisy disco, only to find nothing except calmness, which she gladly took away with her.

The 'shopkeeper'

The figure in the doorway is a key feature of the fantasy, standing as it does at the threshold of the shop and thus symbolically at the threshold of the person's inner self. It may be a friend, foe or family member (alive or dead), or an unknown person; a fictional, fairytale or mythological character, creature or animal; a film, television, comic or cartoon figure; an inanimate object, or one, such as a skeleton, strangely animated.

There may be no figure as such, only a feeling or vague sensation: a light, colour or indistinct form. The clarity of the figure is greatly variable. Some are perceived in vivid detail, whereas others may be hooded or concealed in some way; headless, or without discernible features of any kind. In other instances, the figure spontaneously changes identity or form, or may be a kaleidoscope or collage of different images or impressions. Irrespective of its appearance, people are usually emotionally moved by it in some way. Reactions vary enormously from delight and great happiness to sadness and fear. Frequently people experience spontaneous outbursts or emotion, and can be perceived crying, smiling, frowning or laughing.

Usually the figure relates to a person's needs - often unmet needs, especially in respect of unfinished business and past relationships. Hence dead or distanced relatives, friends, lovers, teachers, business and social acquaintances or pet animals commonly appear. Many people are astonished to encounter a person or animal they haven't consciously thought of, much less seen, for many years, and they cannot understand why they should do so. Similarly people may be perplexed to find themselves in the company of Donald Duck or Mary Poppins, and it is important to remind them that it is not necessarily the character **per se** that is important but what it symbolises or represents. Thus, while for one person the figure of his mother may represent some matter directly relating to her, for another the mother figure may signify an aspect of his childhood or later experiences; past or present aspects of his life; particular issues, problems, feelings, situations or conflicts; or it may symbolise motherhood, caring, nurturance, submissiveness, repression or hardship. Sometimes the significance of the figure may be discerned only after a lot of hard work. A specific feature of the figure may be particularly puzzling. An example from my own experience illustrates this. In one of my 'journeys' to the magic shop I was quite baffled to find my doorkeeper attired in a long white apron. I realised I would not have produced this were it not in some way significant, but its meaning continued to elude me despite my attempts to understand it. Much later, after producing various word and image associations, I realised that it was a cobbler's apron, which initially did little to clarify the issue, until I asked myself what a cobbler does, and came up with the answer that 'he mends soles'. The pun was not lost on me, as I recognised immediately that my doorkeeper was in fact concerned with the **mending souls** - psychotherapy in its literal sense - a highly significant issue for me at that time, as I was planning to write a book on the subject. However, a former student provided an alternative suggestion, which is that my imagery was simply 'cobblers'!

The shop interior

The inside of the shop may be consistent with its outside appearance or totally different; vast and full of items, as in a chain store or mail order catalogue warehouse, or apparently empty. Once in the shop many people find themselves drawn immediately to particular objects, such as cars, compact disc players, dishwashers. This materialism is very evident in some people, especially the young. However, objects may not always be what they seem. A woman who took a diamond subsequently realised that what she needed was some 'sparkle' in her life; and a woman who chose a lamp realised she needed to 'brighten up'. Others are drawn to more abstract qualities such as love, peace, tolerance, health; or to objects which they recognise as symbolising these. Some take an object, often against their inclinations, only to discover later that it represents a more abstract issue of which they were unaware at the time. This proved to be the case for the man who took the only available object, a bell, only to find that when rung it emitted colour. He took this as indicating his need to 'sound out' his 'true colours' - an appropriately mixed metaphor for this apparent synaesthesia.

Some people enter the shop with a very clear idea of what they are looking for, and may be disappointed if they don't find it. In some cases they fail to see anything else, which indicates how desires can often limit one's vision and prospects for fulfilment or satisfaction. One woman went into the shop looking for the only thing she wanted, the elixir of permanent youth. All she could find was an ornate Greek vase, which she refused to take, continuing her search until she found the elixir. However, she was disappointed to find that on coming out of the shop with it she neither looked nor felt any different, which might not have been the case had she taken the vase which was presented. Others, having seen what they want in the window, are then surprised to find something in the shop which they need or value more. A man who wanted some gift-wrapped marzipan was rather surprised to leave the shop with a spiral working-model of the universe.

Some people find there is nothing they want. The experience enables them to realise that they are not really concerned with material possessions, and that many of their everyday wants are not needed. One young woman exchanged all the clothes and ornaments she had been collecting since her teens for a feeling of profound calmness. Others recognise that even their non-material wants may not be what they need.

Some people find what they need, but then fail to strike a bargain because they feel they should make an equivalent exchange and can find nothing of equal value to leave in its place, as in the case of the woman who left the shop empty-handed because she had not had time to assess the value of the item she had chosen, or the woman who did likewise because the item she wanted had no marked price, and so she did not know the value of the item she should leave in exchange. Such people can justifiably be regarded as knowing the price of everything and the value of nothing. Others fail to recognise the opportunity offered them, and, assuming that they are required to 'buy' something, don't - thereby betraying the tendency of 'looking a gift-horse in the mouth'. This trait was epitomised by the woman who refused the tiny gold coach drawn by tiny live horses she wanted, and later acknowledged her tendency to turn down golden opportunities.

Failed transactions may also reveal the way in which codes of conduct or morality lead to self-denial, or how other self-imposed 'shoulds' and 'should nots' limit their chances of fulfilment. A graphic example of this was provided by a young woman who realised she needed space, which was symbolised for her by a large house. However, religiously-inspired self-denial led her to reject this and to leave the shop, apparently with nothing. Back on the street she was horrified to find that she had become an old, lonely, and 'dried-up' monk with a begging bowl, and she immediately recognised the 'poverty' of her moral principles and the possible consequences of her self-denial. Less dramatically, but no less significantly, a man who saw several things he wanted, took none of them because it seemed wrong to him to take something priceless in exchange for something cheap. Similarly another man took nothing because he believed that real exchanges have to be equal. In some cases a failed transaction can highlight a person's uncompromising attitudes, or tendency towards extremes, as in the case of the man who did not take the woman he loved because he would have to give up art for her. That such tendencies can be highly self-destructive is suggested in the case of the man who gave both of his legs in exchange for the resolution of past relationships; and the woman who exchanged health for a semi-precious stone, and emerged from the shop weak and disabled.

Some people make exchanges because they feel they have to. They believe they must do as they are told, follow instructions and abide by rules. These people are so governed by what others want or expect of them that, in the absence of precise guidelines they cannot act; as in the case of the man who could make no exchange because he didn't know the precise terms of the transaction; or that of the woman who went into the shop as a child wearing school uniform, and found herself so indecisive and uncertain that she left empty-handed. She subsequently acknowledged that her childish attitude and approach had resulted in many missed opportunities.

Others may take something they don't particularly want or need because they feel they have to. One young woman, finding few material items in her shop, felt cheated to 'have' to leave with a bottle of shampoo, which was the best thing on offer. She didn't want to consider any possible significance it might have such as her needing to 'wash something out of her hair', or 'to come clean', or other suggestions made to her. She said simply that she found the shop boring and merely did as she was told. When asked if she normally did this she replied that she didn't know and the questioner would have to ask her husband, clearly implying that he knew her mind, and presumably her wants and needs more than she did.

It may be hard to accept that the offer of anything in the universe could possibly be boring. However, the universe of some people is unbelievably restricted, confined to the known, certain and habitual, and lacking all novelty, challenge, excitement and interest. Such was the case for this woman who admitted that she had expected her shop to be dull, and it was, providing a clear example of self-fulfilling, albeit in this instance self-denying, prophecy.

One young man was annoyed to discover only one item in the shop, and therefore only one choice - take it or leave it. He took the item, feeling resentful as he did so, only to realise later that it was something he needed badly but might not have recognised or taken away if given more choice. Similarly, a student was given an object and told she would need to give years of her life for it. Thinking that this meant she had to 'give up' or lose some years off her life, she made the exchange somewhat reluctantly, only to recognise it as her 'calling' in life once out of the shop.

The tendency not to seize the opportunities presented or to make the best of them, to be inhibited by doubts, indecision, negativity, scepticism, and guilt may be highlighted in this exercise, and help individuals to understand the consequences of self-denial. Frequently those who don't complete a transaction feel depressed, disappointed, upset, angry, regretful, resentful, or older, darker, heavier afterwards; and these traits may characterise them and their reactions to everyday life. A man who wanted to leave his parents in exchange for a house did not do so because he felt guilty, and came out of the shop wearing old, dull clothes and feeling depressed. He recognised in this his need to gain independence from his parents, whose old-fashioned out-moded ways he resented.

While some people fail to make an exchange because they have nothing of value to leave behind, there are others who are reluctant or refuse to give up what they have. Often this betrays a general difficulty in letting go, even of pain, problems, negativity, unhealthy attitudes and behaviours. This in itself may prove highly revealing when examined in detail. One woman, whose long-term uncertainty about whether or not to seek a divorce from her husband had led to physical and emotional difficulties, found on entering the shop that she wanted her husband as he had been when she was first married to him, but not enough to give up anything. Initially she reported that she had nothing to exchange for him, although when questioned she admitted that she had thought of leaving her inexpensive handbag but had decided against it. This shocked her because it suggested that she didn't regard her husband as being of much worth, which she knew was not the case. However, when asked about the importance of her handbag she declared that it meant 'everything' to her and that 'she would be lost' without it because it contained her Filofax full of business and social engagements - precisely the things she would have to give up if she remained in the marriage. She recognised that her uncertainty about the marriage arose because she was holding on to an outmoded and idealistic idea of her husband, just as he was holding on to an unrealistic view of her as a housewife and mother who should be content to stay at home. She realised that in holding on to her handbag she was in effect holding on to herself, and she decided to continue to do so, and thus 'save' herself rather than her marriage.

By comparison, some people conduct their transactions easily and strike very positive deals, exchanging items or features of themselves or their lives that they don't want or need for ones that they do. Examples of these include the man who acquired a magic wand for 2p; and the one who took love in exchange for self-pity; the woman who exchanged her lack of confidence for the 'parts of herself she knew were missing'; the man who left stress and took calmness; the woman who took maturity in exchange for the pain associated with her childhood; and the woman who took a prescription pad she could fill out for herself in exchange for someone else's vision, in the form of their spectacles. These individuals invariably gain a great deal from the exercise, often finding solutions to problems. This was certainly the case for the young woman who exchanged her engagement ring for the bloom of youth, symbolised by a crocus, and emerged wearing men's clothes. Initially alarmed by what she saw as the loss of femininity resulting from her refusal of marriage, she subsequently realised that the masculine attire represented her career and independence, which her future husband insisted she give up after marriage in favour of motherhood, his view being that the man 'should wear the trousers' in marriage. She recognised that this imagery gave expression to deep-seated reservations she had about her imminent wedding, which she called off shortly afterwards.

This example highlights another feature of the exercise which is that the transaction is not always what it seems and the person often gets rather more than they bargained for. A woman who entered a jeweller's shop, dressed completely in black and wanting jewels, found only wonderfully coloured lights which she wanted to take away, but did not, taking instead a jar labelled 'discipline' because she thought she should. However, once outside the shop again she found everything brightly illuminated and all her clothes vividly coloured. She then realised that what she needed was not discipline but to lighten up and get some colour into her life. Similarly, a man who exchanged his dark coat and hat for a bicycle realised that these had been hiding his true colours, which were very bright indeed, and that he needed to show these rather than conceal them.

Many people leave the magic shop feeling rejuvenated, lighter, brighter, better, healthier and happier. This is illustrated by the very obese woman who was embarrassed to reveal that her shop contained sexy, slinky dresses, such as the red one she had been drawn to in the window, which she could not possibly fit into. Once inside the shop, however, she found to her astonishment that she could do so, being very much smaller and slimmer; and she exchanged her mother for this image of herself. On leaving the shop she felt lighter, in every sense, and described herself as looking and feeling 'terrific'. Such people are generally positive in attitude and outlook, and make the best of the opportunities they create or that are presented to them. They tend to enjoy new experiences and self-discovery, and to act on the insights derived thereby. For many the insights are profound, as in the case of the man who left behind his illusions, having recognised them for the first time. Typically these people appreciate the power of the exercise in shedding light on significant aspects of themselves and their lives, and its potential for transformation. Indeed few people who undertake the exercise fail to recognise its power in accessing formerly unconscious aspects of the self, and enhancing self-awareness. This potential should not be underestimated. Transformation resulting from the exercise may be dramatic, not only life-changing, but in the case of the sick, life-giving.

When Shirley Valentine identified her needs and began to act on them, her husband, family and friend refused to listen to her. They were so wedded to their own wants that they were unprepared to acknowledge or allow her needs. Those using imagery in the assessment of personal needs must therefore possess the very qualities they seek to facilitate in others, namely awareness and flexibility of response. Accordingly they should be suitably trained in listening skills and sensitive to the subtleties of symbolism, never imposing their own or culturally prescribed meanings on to the symbols inherent in a person's imagery, but rather facilitating a process whereby a person uncovers their own meaning through translating the message conveyed by their unique use of symbols. They must also recognise that anything which has the power to heal can also hurt, and be capable of supporting a person through the often painful process of self-discovery and growth.

References

Abse, D. W., van der Castle, R. L., Buxton, R. L., Demars, W. D., Brown, J. P., & Kirschner, L. G. (1974). Personality and behavioural characteristics of lung cancer patients. *Journal of Psychosomatic Research*, 18, 101-113.

Achterberg, J. (1985). *Imagery in healing: Shamanism and modern medicine.* Boston and London: New Science Library, Shambhala.

Achterberg, J., Simonton, S. M., & Simonton, O. C. (1977). Psychology of the exceptional cancer patient: A description of patients who outlive predicted life expectancies. *Psychotherapy: Theory, Research & Practice*, 14, 4. Winter 416-22.

Bem, S. L. (1975). Sex role adaptability: One consequence of psychological androgyny. *Journal of Personality and Social Psychology*, 31, 634-43.

Bem, S. L. (1976). Probing the promise of androgyny. In A. G. Kaplan & J. P. Bean, (Eds.) *Beyond sex role stereotypes: Readings towards a psychology of androgyny.* Boston: Little, Brown.

Broverman, J. K., Broverman, D.M., Clarkson, F. E., Rosenkrantz, P S., & Vogel, S. R. (1970). Sex role stereotypes and clinical judgements of mental health. *Journal of Consulting and Clinical Psychology*, 34, 1-7.

Brown, G. W., & Harris, T. (1978). *Social origins of depression: a study of psychiatric disorder in women.* London: Tavistock Publications.

Derogatis, L., Abeloff, M., & Melisarotos, N. (1979). Psychological coping mechanisms and survival time in metastatic breast cancer. *Journal of the American Medical Association*, 242, 1504-8.

Friedman, M., & Rosenman, R. H. (1974). *Type A behaviour and your heart.* New York: Alfred A. Knopf.

Friedman, M. & Rosenman, R. H. (1986). Type A behaviour: its association with coronary heart disease. *Annals of Clinical Research*, **3**, 300-312.

Graham, H. (1992a). *The magic shop: An imaginative guide to self-healing*. London: Rider.

Graham, H. (1972b). Imaginative assessment of personal health needs. In D. Trent, (Ed.) *Promotion of Mental Health* Vol. I Avebury.

Greer, S. & Morris, T. (1975). Psychological attributes of women who develop breast cancer: A controlled study. *Journal of Psychosomatic Research*, **19**, 147-153.

Gove, W. K. & Tudor, J. (1972). The relationship between sex roles, marital status and mental illness. *Social Forces*, **51**, 34.

Hewitt, L. (1986). Women and Drugs. Paper presented at the annual Standing Conference on Drug Abuse. York University.

Hughes, H., & Molloy, F. (1990). Type A behaviour and attitude towards coping strategy when faced with stress. Unpublished dissertation submitted in fulfilment of the requirements for B.A. Hons. Keele University.

Kissen, D. M., & Eysenck, H. J. (1962). Personality in male lung cancer patients. *British Journal of Medical Psychology*, **36**, 123-7.

Kissen, D. M., & Eysenck, H. J. (1963). Personal characteristics in males conducive to lung cancer. *British Journal of Medical Psychology*, **36**, 27-36.

Kissen, D. M., & Eysenck, H. J. (1964). Relationship between lung cancer, cigarette smoking, inhalation and personality. *British Journal of Medical Psychology*, **37**, 203-16.

Kissen, D. M., & Eysenck, H. J., (1967). Psychosocial factors, personality and lung cancer in men aged 55-64. *British Journal of Medical Psychology*, **40**, 26-43.

Llewelyn, S. (1981). Psychology and women: An examination of mental health problems. *Bulletin of the British Psychological Society*, **34**, 60-63.

Maslow, A. (1966). *Towards a psychology of being*. New York: Van Nostrand Reinhold.

Meares, A. (1977). Atavistic regression as a factor in the remission of cancer. *Medical Journal of Australia*. **2**, 132-3.

Newton, B. W. (1980). The use of hypnosis in the treatment of cancer patients: A five year report. Presented at the Annual Science Programme of the American Society of Clinical Hypnosis, Minneapolis.

Schmale, R. B., & Iker, S. H. (1971). Hopelessness as a predictor of cervical cancer. *Social Science and Medicine*, 5, 95-100.

Shekelle, R. B., Raynor, W. J., Ostfield, M. D., Garron, D. C., Bielianskas, L. A., Lin, S. C., Maliza, C., & Paul, O. (1981). Psychological depression and 17 year risk of death from cancer. *Psychosomatic Medicine*, 43, 117-25.

Siegal, B. S. (1990). *Peace, Love and Healing*. London: Rider.

Simonton, O. C., & Matthews-Simonton, S. (1975). Belief systems and management of the emotional aspects of malignancy. *Journal of Transpersonal Psychology*, 8, 29-47.

Solomon, G. F. (1969). An emotional life-history pattern associated with neoplastic disease. *Annals of the New York Academy of Science*, 335-342.

54 What does assertiveness have to do with women's sexual health

P. McKenzie

We started with 3 different aspects on Women's Sexual Health:-

1. Sexual health cannot be separated from wider political, cultural and social contexts. Women's position in society has far ranging implications for the way we feel about ourselves, our self-esteem and self confidence. In order to address assertiveness and sexual health we have to be aware of the context in which we are living, e.g. the influence of history, religion and male dominated institutions including the media.

2. The second area to consider is the relationships women have with professionals in relation to their sexual health. The way women interact and communicate with professionals and vice-versa is often not given consideration, and women often come away with many unanswered questions. Women are also physically at a disadvantage in some situations: It is difficult to feel assertive lying flat on your back with your legs in stirrups!

3. The third area is sexual relationships. These can be fraught with difficulties for women in communicating their needs and desires and in taking responsibility for their sexual well-being, emotionally and physically. The advent of H.I.V. has brought along another guilt trip for women - 'I should have made him use a condom....'

Sexual health is not just about our reproductive systems, it is part of the core of our existence, about emotions and intellect as well as physical health.

In the session the group of 11 women split into 3 groups each looking at one of the three areas highlighted. each group was asked to answer the questions:-

'How can women be assertive in this area'?
'How might being assertive/non-assertive affect your sexual health'?

Responses from the Groups

Group 1. Considered the media portrayal of women as sexual/sensual. Conclusions were that 'Woman' is a cultural construction. We aspire to the culturally constructed image of what and who we are. This aspiration causes pain when physically we cannot ever attain that image. The lowering of confidence and self-esteem affects how we feel about ourselves as sexual beings.

Women can be more assertive in this area through;

Educating and empowering other women to believe in themselves as being O.K.

Contradicting assumptions about women's images wherever possible and particularly working to promote positive images of older women.

Lobbying to ban 'image' advertising to sell everything from cars to tampax.

Form women's co-operative groups to lobby the Government.

Group 2. The group considered the medicalisation of women's sexual health to be a form of rape - women's wisdom converted to men's power, with the speculum as a symbol of torture (heavy stuff!)

Women can be more assertive by:-

Educating health professionals about things they are unhappy with. Challenging and confronting assumptions of professionals that women are reproductive objects. Complaining about poor treatment.

Being non-assertive in this area, devalues, debilitates, derides and degrades women. 'I' can be more assertive and 'we all' can be more assertive to enhance, value and improve women's sexual health.

Group 3 There is conflict in sexual relationships between wanting to be sexually desirable and still maintaining yourself as an individual. Assertiveness in the area of relationships relies heavily on negotiation with a partner. Women can be active in educating men that sex does not necessarily rely on the penis!

There is anxiety around expressing sexual needs to partners for fear of their anger/resentment/frustration. Women can be assertive in demanding **time** for discussion around sexual needs in relationships.

Conclusion

Assertiveness is the basis of improving women's sexual health in all aspects. Women can be assertive by expressing needs and wants, by joining together, by educating others; by negotiating, but first by assertively being themselves.

55 Mental health promotion: A political issue

A. Norman and S. Hunter

Workshop attenders came mainly from the statutory (Health Service) sector.

Aims

The aim of the workshop was to address the political issues of ACCESS, STIGMA, RESOURCES AND POLICY by adopting the principles of Health For All.

* promoting community participation
* addressing inequalities in health
* encouraging multi-sectoral collaboration

The method we were encouraging was a community development approach, starting from people's needs as they themselves define them, encouraging collective action and self-activity and moving onto affecting policy more generally.

We aimed to furnish participants thereby with the tools to develop local events which could promote mental health. Our underlying philosophy is that the models and principles we provided are more appropriate to promoting mental health than simply targeting people with services without their involvement. It also assumes that it is important to reach disadvantaged sectors of the population, and that it is both efficient, effective and mentally healthy to encourage agencies to work together.

We started from the WHO definition of health, namely
'not just the absence of disease, but a state of complete mental, physical and emotional well-being'
We conceived of mental health as a continuum as illustrated below:

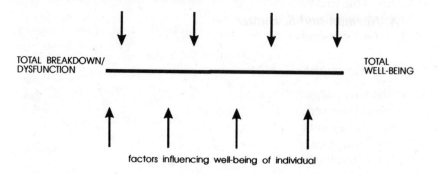

TOTAL BREAKDOWN/
DYSFUNCTION

TOTAL
WELL-BEING

factors influencing well-being of individual

Outline

The workshop attenders were given some guidelines in order to consider the topic:
MENTAL HEALTH PROMOTION: A POLITICAL ISSUE
These were the 3 main principles of the World Health Organisation's Health For All BY the Year 2000, a continuum model of mental Health and the World Health Organisation's Definition of Health. (see above)

The workshop took the following form:
    Introductions to facilitators, group members
    A brief introduction to the topic
    A group brainstorm of words associated with mental health
    Dividing into 2 groups, to each choose and plan an event to promote mental health in a city/ town/ neighbourhood. (To do this each group would refer to the Health For All Principles and the political issues identified by the facilitators of ACCESS, RESOURCES, STIGMA, POLICY)
    Each group then presented the outline of their event to the other group

Discussion of events

Summing up and feedback about the workshop

Group brainstorm of factors enabling mental health

    * A sense of belonging to a community

638

* feeling good about yourself
* personal ownership of one's feelings
* being able to give/receive love
* feeling in control
* being able to develop coping strategies
* feeling you have access to choices
* having a sense of value

Planning the event

A checklist was suggested for planning the event
    * what is the event you want to plan?
    * aims of the event
    * target audience/s
    * who is involved?
    * resources needed
    * how are aims to be achieved? i.e. methods
    * anticipated outcomes/benefits
    * how will event be evaluated?

Questions arising from workshop

- do you plan within resources available or try to do something with wider impact which involves fund-raising?
- multidisciplinary working has advantages but also difficulties in terms of whether there are shared values.
- it is important to acknowledge the extent to which you have to work with the process and the different agendas brought by different sectors, which can be useful as well as problematic.
- is work with users of services more difficult to plan and envisage?
- are awareness-raising and training events easier to envisage and plan?
- Perhaps awareness-raising is necessary before strategic work?
- it might be best initially to focus in on something specific rather than attempt an ambitious event.
- it is valid to concentrate on a group you feel comfortable working with, whilst recognising the wider aims of community participation, addressing inequalities and multi-sectoral collaboration.

56 The stigma of 'the dependant'

C. Ormston and J. Thornton

This plenary session explored the stigmatising labels attributed to, and often accepted by, people with a drug or alcohol problem. The presenters examined ways in which groupwork as a therapeutic technique can be a useful vehicle for the promotion of Mental Health and presented the Intervention Course - a specific programme for people with a drug or alcohol problem.

The presenters highlighted the ways in which negative and restrictive labels dictate the roles, and possibilities open to individuals - e.g. 'once an alcoholic, always an alcoholic' - the continuation of the problem seems almost inevitable. It was felt, however, that although outwardly unhelpful, people can receive subtle benefits from accepting these labels; e.g. 'Don't expect much of me, I'm an addict'. If people are viewed as deviant, hedonistic or mentally ill, then they will be the passive recipients of punishment, external restraint or treatment.

A tentative definition of mental health was made which emphasised the need for a balanced outlook, and personal resilience to enjoy the 'ups' of life, and cope with the 'downs'. It was felt that 'mental health' constituted the recognition of one's own power and possibilities, and the ability to access and utilise them.

The group considered the notion of power and whether clients need empowering by their therapist. This seemed somewhat arrogant on the part of the latter, since the group believed that clients already hold their own power and therefore do not need it given.

It was agreed that, in groupwork, the powerbase lies firmly with the group members and, as such, has much value in the promotion of mental health. Inherent group processes emphasise the responsibility of its members, their value as individuals, and to each other. The session explored Yallom's (Yallom I.D., 1975) factors for group effectiveness in promoting mental health.

The 'Intervention Course for Problematic Drinkers and Drug Users' was introduced. The course acts as a catalyst for change, capitalises on clients' strengths, and can provide a detailed assessment. The Intervention Course runs over two weeks as a closed group and is deliberately eclectic in its content. It was felt important that a wide variety of approaches was available which would therefore not dictate how the clients problem was viewed and determine the treatment pursued.

Preliminary research has indicated that the intervention course benefits approximately 66% of its participants; however, empirical evidence of the longer term results of the course, is difficult to establish. It was felt that research methodology which somehow indicates an intervention's 'success', in its widest sense, perhaps based on clients' own perceptions and subjective evidence of change, would be of value.

The presenters highlighted how the intervention course attracted a higher ratio of female to male participants than the ratio of referred clients to the Northern Regional Drug & Alcohol Service as a whole. The delegates explored some possible explanations which included - were women more attracted to groupwork than men? or perhaps more men referred to the unit were in paid employment compared with women and therefore unable to attend? Again, it was thought that further research into this would be useful.

The balance of power within therapy was examined and it was acknowledged that the therapist can take power from clients and expect them to be grateful when it is given back! The delegates felt strongly that any therapist should be clear about their own agenda within therapy, being clear sighted regarding which issues belong to the client - and those which are their own.

In general this plenary session recognised the personal power and possibilities each person possesses, and the ways in which interventions can enhance, or detract from this. In promoting mental health for drinkers and drug users, or for anyone, we can use the empowering elements of groupwork in combatting passivity and helplessness, allowing the individual to utilise the power which is theirs.

References

Yallom,I.D. (1975). *The theory and practice of group psychotherapy*. Basic Books: New York

Errata: In *Promotion of Mental Health, Volume 1, 1991*

In 'Between psyche and society: The role of the community mental health promotion officer'.

   p.145 Fig.2 This is drawn from Caplan R. 1986
   p 147 Fig.4 Should read as follows:

The Sociology of Radical Change

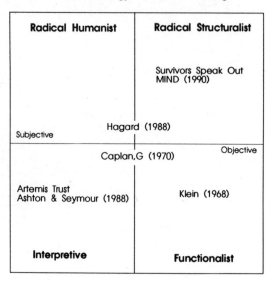

The Sociology of Regulation

Figure 4 Four paradigms for the analysis of social theory(Burrell and Morgan, 1979, p.22). Locating theories of community mental health promotion

With regard to the two appendices referred to in this chapter, but omitted, further information can be obtained from the author.

Acknowledgements

To L. J., thank you for being there.

D. R. T.

'It makes far better sense to rely on a fence
Than an ambulance down in the valley.'

Anonymous